GRANT APPLICATION WRITER'S HANDBOOK

Fourth Edition

Liane Reif-Lehrer, PhD

Tech-Write Consultants/Erimon Associates

JONES AND BARTLETT PUBLISHERS

Sudbury, Massachusetts

BOSTON   TORONTO   LONDON   SINGAPORE

World Headquarters
Jones and Bartlett Publishers
40 Tall Pine Drive
Sudbury, MA 01776
978-443-5000
info@jbpub.com
www.jbpub.com

Jones and Bartlett Publishers Canada
2406 Nikanna Road
Mississauga, ON L5C 2W6
CANADA

Jones and Bartlett Publishers International
Barb House, Barb Mews
London W6 7PA
UK

The cover of this book was designed by Anne Spencer of Jones and Bartlett Publishers and incorporates *Over the Tiger's Den,* a painting by Damon Lehrer, the author's son. The painting was reproduced with permission of the artist.

Library of Congress Cataloging-in-Publication Data
Reif-Lehrer, Liane, 1934–
   Grant application writer's handbook / Liane Reif-Lehrer.
     p.   cm.
   Includes index.
   ISBN 0-7637-1642-1
   1. Proposal writing in medicine.   2. Medicine—Research grants.   3. Proposal writing for grants.
   I. Title.
   R853.P75R439 2005
   808'.06661—dc22

                                      2004018267

Production Credits
Acquisitions Editor: Kevin Sullivan
Production Manager: Amy Rose
Associate Production Editor: Renée Sekerak
Editorial Assistant: Amy Sibley
Marketing Manager: Ed McKenna
Associate Marketing Manager: Emily Ekle
Manufacturing Buyer: Therese Bräuer
Composition: Auburn Associates, Inc.
Text and Cover Design: Anne Spencer
Printing and Binding: Malloy, Inc.
Cover Printing: Malloy, Inc.

Printed in the United States of America
08 07 06 05 04   10 9 8 7 6 5 4 3 2 1

Dedication

To my husband, Dr. Sherwin (Sam) Lehrer, and our children, Damon and Erica, for all I have learned from them and for always "being there for me";

To my father, Dr. Gerson Reif, who, because of the terrible events that took place in Vienna at the start of World War II, died in 1938, before I was old enough to get to know and remember him;

To my mother, Clara Reif, who, at great sacrifice to herself, made it possible for me to have the luxury of a lengthy education;

To my brother, Dr. Fred Reif, for all that he taught me and for taking it for granted that I would have a career;

To all those who taught me, and encouraged me;

To Cho Cho San, Kitty, and Pete, now all gone, for sharing their lives with us;

And, as always, to "The Little Prince" (A. de St. Exupéry).

Contents

RESOURCE APPENDIX, available at the online catalog page for this title on the Jones and Bartlett Web site, www.jbpub.com.

INTRODUCTION

This fourth edition of *Grant Application Writer's Handbook* is my last book on proposal writing. As I would like it to be useful for some time to come, I am omitting many of the details that are likely to change and cause the book to fall into oblivion in too short a time. Thus, I have focused primarily on the general concepts that will help the reader write good proposals, Grant Applications, research papers, and other types of documents that require good expository writing. Since the publication of my previous book, *Grant Application Writer's Handbook* (Jones and Bartlett Publishers, 1995), a large amount of information has become available online via the Internet. This has made available to anyone with access to a computer and modem a wealth of information about many subjects related to the Grant Application process, including funding sources. The digitization of information has also made it possible to rapidly update changes in rules and regulations about forms, Application procedures, and the like in a timeframe that was not readily possible with printed information about these matters. As a result this book discusses primarily conceptual issues; it is left to the reader to get additional necessary details from the appropriate websites. You can visit the *Resource Appendix* at the online catalog page for this title at www.jbpub.com.

Please use the material conveyed in this book as a guide rather than as a set of rules. Every Study Section is different, every granting agency is different, every Reviewer is different, and every Principal Investigator is different! You are responsible for your proposal. When you mail your Application, YOU must feel comfortable with what you submit.

Please do not use this book in place of reading the instructions provided by the National Institutes of Health (NIH) or other granting agencies to which you plan to apply for funding. Much of this information is now available on the Web. This book is intended as an aid. It is your responsibility to read the instructions of the granting agency **carefully** and to follow them **meticulously**. You will be in a good position to compete for funding if you

—have a good project idea that interests the funding agency to which you plan to apply.

—respond to the needs and instructions of the granting agency to which you are applying.

—practice the principles of good proposal writing set forth in this book.

Although the principles of good proposal writing presented in this book are unlikely to change for some time, the specifics *may* change periodically. With changes toward electronic grant administration, the rate of change at the NIH, at the National Science Foundation (NSF), and at other government agencies is likely to accelerate in the next few years. It will be worth your while always to check with your potential granting agency about changes in policy and procedures—and to determine whether the agency is interested in your proposal objectives—**before** investing time to prepare an Application.

It would be unwise for a Grant Applicant to permit redundancies to creep into her/his proposal and thereby squander precious space in a document with stringent page limits.

However, this book has no page limits. Therefore, I have intentionally introduced redundancies on occasion for reasons of emphasis or convenience to readers, especially those who use this book as a reference rather than reading it from cover to cover. I hope readers will find these repetitions helpful rather than annoying.

A MATTER OF CORRECT USAGE

Although grant-seekers often make statements such as "my grant is due," or "I have to write a grant," they are actually referring to the Application. The grant is the award they get if their Application is successful. Also, be aware that the NIH and some other agencies have very specific definitions of words such as "agency," "institution," "Applicant," "investigator," and "grantee." "Agency" technically refers to the funding agency; that is, the organization that awards the funding. The "institution" generally refers to the organization that applies for the funding. The word "applicant" refers to the institution of the Principal Investigator (PI); "grantee" refers to this institution after it has been awarded funding. These terms are often used more casually in the scientific community, and I have also taken this liberty, referring sometimes, for example, to a PI who has received an award as a "grantee," and to her/his institution as the "grantee's institution." Likewise, strictly speaking, at the NIH, an Application that is funded results in a grant for the PI, whereas a proposal that is funded results in a contract for the PI. Also, in common usage, the "proposal" often refers primarily to the Research Plan, whereas the "Application" tends to refer to the completed packet of information submitted to the funding agency. However, as is common in the scientific community, I have used the terms "Application" and "proposal" more or less interchangeably.

In some parts of this book I have included direct quotes from government documents without specific attribution. Thus, when I have wanted to convey information from the NIH instructions (PHS-398 or PHS-2590) that was clear as stated in the NIH instructions, and for which I did not think I could improve on the clarity by rewording the text, I have inserted in my book, verbatim, the text in the instructions (or other NIH publications) without quotation marks. I have used quotation marks only when I specifically wanted to emphasize that the wording was unchanged from that of NIH. Because government documents are not copyrighted, because my major goal is to inform the reader, and because this book is not an exercise in creative writing, I trust that no one will be offended by my taking this liberty.

Throughout this book I have included a variety of resources that might be helpful to researchers and proposal writers. Many of the listings came to my attention in the course of my work. Some of the items listed are resources that I have found particularly useful. Others are items that have been recommended by colleagues, or about which I have only read. They may not necessarily be the only or best in their category. I am not endorsing or (with a few exceptions) recommending these items. I am only trying to make the reader aware of some of the resources that are available to

    —help you work faster and more efficiently,

    —relieve you of certain tedious chores that can be done by computers, service agencies, and the like,

    —leave you the greatest possible amount of time to do your creative work,

    —and visit the additional "Resources Appendix" found on the catalog page for this book at the Jones and Bartlett web site, www.jbpub.com.

Please use these items and this information as a guide to find additional resources. Before investing time and money in a book, a software program, or a service, you should
—ask colleagues what else is available in a particular category,

—get recommendations from people whose opinions you trust, and keep in mind that technology is advancing very rapidly.

Books and software programs are revised and upgraded frequently, and superb resources of today often succumb to newer and better technologies within a relatively short time. In the computer industry especially (but not uniquely), products often appear and disappear within a few years. You may on occasion, with very short notice, find yourself without further support for a product and without appropriate upgrades as computer system requirements change.

The demise of a product is not necessarily a reflection of its quality. Some very useful products have disappeared after only a brief existence, presumably for "market" reasons. It is in your interest to check into the history and stability of a vendor prior to making an expensive purchase. Thus, before using the services of any vendor, investing money to purchase any product, or committing time to learning to use the product, it is important to
—read reviews of the vendor and the product,

—get advice from colleagues who may be familiar with the product, and/or the vendor.

PREFACE

The first edition of *Writing a Successful Grant Application* was originally written as a monograph, in response to a request by an administrator at the Eye Research Institute of Retina Foundation [now the Schepens Eye Research Institute (SERI)] that I put together a document to help my colleagues improve their proposal-writing skills. The guidelines in the first book were based largely on my experience serving on an NIH Vision Study Section, Vis. A (Visual Sciences A) (later called, Vis. Sciences A ad hoc) from 1976 to 1978. Additional information was obtained from various publications written by the U.S. Department of Health and Human Services, and from seminars presented by NIH administrators.

In 1984, I began to give workshops on grant proposal writing throughout the United States. The second edition of the book incorporated material from a handout that I developed for my workshops. The third edition was based on my workshop experiences after the publication of the second edition. Since the mid-1990s, I have conducted seminars and workshops at universities and professional meetings, including several in the former Soviet Union, sponsored by the American Association for the Advancement of Science, and a week-long workshop in Beijing, China, sponsored by the China Medical Board. As I presented these seminars I continued to learn more about the needs of the people who attended. NIH Study Section members, Scientific Review Administrators, other grant administrators, and well-funded senior faculty members have occasionally attended my workshops, and it has been gratifying that they almost always concurred with what I said, and I have been grateful to receive additional useful information from them. Officers in charge of the grants offices at the various universities where I have lectured have also been generous in sharing information—and in some cases cartoons—with me. I also learned much from researching responses to questions that have come up in the course of the workshops, from grant applications I have critiqued for clients, and from discussions with scientists at universities and at the NIH and NSF who have been involved, more recently than I, in the grant process as grantees, reviewers, or administrators.

I have tried to stay current about changes and events at NIH and NSF via the agencies' Web sites and publications, by keeping in touch with scientists who serve on Study Sections/Review Boards, and by maintaining contact with people at the funding agencies. Thus I was able to incorporate updated information to this edition about changes to forms and procedures at NIH and NSF that have been instituted since the last edition. I trust that the basic advice in this book will be valid for many years. Agencies do, however, periodically change procedures, forms, and so on, and as a result it is not possible for all the specifics in my book to remain current. Thus I must leave it to you, the reader, to keep abreast of changes at the agencies of interest to you. Please note that another change new to this edition is that the "Resource Appendix" is not printed in the current edition but is, instead, on the Jones and Bartlett Publishers Web site, www.jbpub.com, by clicking on the catalog page for this book, where it will be accessible to those who purchase this book and where it is scheduled to be periodically updated.

The basic principles in this book are useful for writing many types of grant applications/proposals to both government agencies and private foundations, as well as research papers, business plans, and other similar documents. However, a National Institutes of Health (NIH) investigator-initiated research grant application (R01) is used as the primary example for discussion throughout this book. One Appendix, written and subsequently revised by scientists with experience with applying for NSF grants, addresses some of the similarities and differences in grant application and review at the National Science Foundation (NSF). There is also an Appendix with information about applying to private foundations. Although the review process may be different at the various funding agencies, the kinds of information that reviewers look for in a grant application are not very different. Therefore, the information given in this book can easily be extrapolated for use with applications to many other agencies. As in the second edition, some of the information in this book is intentionally presented in outline form, and in some cases in both narrative and outline form. I have also retained the excellent suggestion of Dr. Janet Rasey (made for the second edition) to include a "Recap" section at the end of each part of the book. I hope this will satisfy the variety of readers who may require or prefer more or less information about specific topics. Above all, I must emphasize the importance that the reader always remains aware of what is happening in the funding arena. Establish a good relationship with your institutional Grants Office, use the Web, and share information with astute colleagues.

Acknowledgments

My sincere thanks go to many colleagues, associates, and friends who have been involved in reviewing or administering proposals at NIH, NSF, and other funding agencies and who took the time to help me make this a better book. Although there are too many people to name, they all helped to improve this and/or earlier editions of this book and I greatly appreciate their help and wisdom.

- Anthony M. Coelho, Jr., PhD, Donna J. Dean, PhD, Sam Joseloff, PhD, Sonny Kreitman, William E. McGarvey, PhD, Robert Moore, Clifford Scharke, DMD, MPH, George Stone, PhD, all now or previously at NIH.
- Stephen H. Vessey, PhD, Amanda Voight, MS, and a former NSF Program Director who did not wish his name listed, for helpful comments about the Appendix about NSF.
- Jane F. Koretz, PhD, Director, Center for Biophysics, Professor, Department of Biology, Science Center, Rensselaer Polytechnic Institute, Troy, NY, and a former member of the NIH Visual Science–A Study Section.
- Erin B. Lindsay, Administrative Technology Center, California Institute of Technology.
- Julie T. Norris, Director, Office of Sponsored Programs, Massachusetts Institute of Technology.
- Richard Pharo, PhD, Vice President for Administration, Forsyth Dental Center.
- Janet S. Rasey, PhD, Director of the Research Funding Service and former Professor of Radiation Oncology, University of Washington Medical Center, Seattle, WA and a 2-term member of an NIH Study Section.
- Bruce Trumbo, PhD, who wrote the original Appendix about NSF for earlier editions of this book, and Hartmut Wohlrab, PhD, Senior Staff Scientist, Boston Biomedical Research Institute and a former member of an NSF Review Panel, and an NSF Program Director who wished to remain anonymous for updating this Appendix.
- C.L. Albert Wang, PhD Deputy Director and Senior Scientist, Boston Biomedical Research Institute, Watertown, MA and current member of the Biophysical Chemistry (BBCB) Study Section at NIH.
- Pamela A. Webb, Senior Director, Sponsored Research, Office of Research Administration, Stanford University.

Thanks also go to:
- Philip R. Conley, former Director of Library Services, Associated Grantmakers of Massachusetts, Inc., who graciously helped me find information about foundation grants over the years.

- Sherwin (Sam) Lehrer, PhD, Senior Scientist, Boston Biomedical Research Institute, my husband, for his help and support and for graciously accepting the premise that "the book comes first."
- To our children, Damon and Erica, for their support and advice during the process of writing this book, and to Damon for again allowing me to use some of his artwork for the chapter openers and the image of one of his paintings for the cover of the book.
- The Principal Investigators who graciously gave permission to publish, anonymously, their Summary Statements and, in some cases, parts of their grant applications.
- The many investigators and grant administrators with whom I have had helpful discussions over the years about grants and the peer review process. I am especially indebted to the institutional grants officers who have recommended my workshops and other services to their colleagues and to those who have sent me interesting materials to use in subsequent workshops.
- The many people who have attended my workshops, especially those who have taken time to give me thoughtful, constructive feedback about how to improve the workshops and, hence, also the book.
- The many people not specifically mentioned above at NIH, NSF, other granting agencies, book publishing and software companies, and various libraries who were helpful in my efforts to gather up-to-date information for the book—especially for the Resource Appendix.
- Don Jones, Sr., Clayton Jones, Kevin Sullivan, Renée Sekerak, Amy Sibley, and the many other people at Jones and Bartlett Publishers who have supported my efforts in the preparation of the current and the three earlier editions of this book.
- Anne Spencer of Jones and Bartlett Publishers for a beautiful cover design based on a painting by my son, Damon Lehrer.

ABOUT THE AUTHOR

Dr. Liane Reif-Lehrer was born in Vienna, Austria in 1934. After the death of her father in September 1938 and the frightening events of "Krystallnacht" on November 10, 1938, she left Europe on May 13, 1939 with her brother and mother on the infamous ship, the *St. Louis*. The ship, bound for Cuba, was denied entry into Cuba and the United States. After almost 6 weeks at sea, the *St. Louis* was ordered to return to Europe.* The Reif family was assigned to go to Loudun, France, but after less than a year there, the Germans invaded the town and the Reif family escaped to Limoges, in southern France, where Dr. Reif-Lehrer had her first year of schooling.

After two and a half years in France, Dr. Reif-Lehrer was finally able to come to New York with her mother and brother in November 1941 under the sponsorship of Dr. Reif-Lehrer's father's sister, Lena Klinghoffer, and Lena's children in New York. It is notable that one of these children, Leon Klinghoffer, was killed in 1985 when the Achille Lauro, the cruise ship that he was on with his terminally ill wife, was highjacked and Mr. Klinghoffer, who was in a wheelchair because he had suffered a stroke, was thrown overboard. Abu Abbas, the person who masterminded the highjacking, died in jail of a heart attack in March 2004, while Dr. Reif-Lehrer was working on this book. Dr. Reif-Lehrer has submitted a book manuscript about her life story to the Holocaust Memoir Project sponsored by Random House Publishers.

Dr. Reif-Lehrer graduated from Erasmus Hall High School in Brooklyn, New York, in 1952, received a B.A. degree in chemistry from Barnard College, Columbia University, in 1956, and a PhD in physical organic chemistry from the University of California at Berkeley (UCB) in 1960 under the tutelage of Professor Andrew Streitwieser.

Following two years of research at AVCO Corp., Dr. Reif-Lehrer and her husband, Dr. Sherwin (Sam) Lehrer, whom she had met as a fellow graduate student at UCB, took a year off and traveled around the world for nine months.

From 1963 to 1966, Dr. Reif-Lehrer was a postdoctoral fellow with Dr. Harold Amos in what was then called the Department of Microbiology and Immunology at Harvard Medical School (HMS), where she became interested in control mechanisms in animal cells, especially in the retina. In 1966, she was invited by Dr. Jin Kinoshita to become an instructor at the Howe Laboratory of Ophthalmology of Harvard Medical School, headed by Dr. David Cogan, and located at the Massachusetts Eye and Ear Infirmary. She was later promoted to assistant professor. In 1972, while retaining her HMS appointment, she moved her laboratory to Boston Biomedical Research Institute and in 1975 to the Eye Research Institute of Retina Foundation (now called the Schepens Eye Research Institute), where she held an appointment as Senior Scientist. In 1977 she attained the rank of associate professor at Harvard Medical School. From 1964 until 1985, Dr. Reif-Lehrer supported her research almost entirely with grant funds, obtained primarily from the National Institutes of Health.

*(The voyage of the *St. Louis* has been documented in many books, e.g., *Voyage of the Damned* by Gordon Thomas and Max Morgan-Witts, 1974, 1994; ISBN # 0-87938-909-5.)

From 1976 to 1978, Dr. Reif-Lehrer was a member of a National Institutes of Health Initial Review Group ("Study Section"). From 1978 to 1979, she was a Senior Visiting Fellow in the laboratory of Dr. Mary Voaden, at the Institute of Ophthalmology, University of London, England.

It was her experience as a member of the NIH Study Section as well as a request from the administration at the Eye Research Institute that she write a monograph to help her fellow faculty members prepare better grant proposals that prompted Dr. Reif-Lehrer to write the first, abbreviated (82 pages), edition of *Writing a Successful Grant Application,* published in 1982. The book was published as a 282-page second edition in 1989.

In October 1985, Dr. Reif-Lehrer left the Eye Research Institute and Harvard Medical School to start Tech-Write Consultants/Erimon Associates (TWC/EA), a consulting firm to help people write better grant applications, research papers, etc. and also give workshops about how to write a good grant application.

In 1995, Dr. Reif-Lehrer wrote a new book on the subject of proposal writing: *Grant Application Writer's Handbook* (Jones and Bartlett Publishers, 1995; 472 pages). Shortly thereafter, Jones and Bartlett Publishers also published a companion video of Dr. Reif-Lehrer's workshop, *Getting Funded: It Takes More Than Just a Good Idea.*

Dr. Reif-Lehrer has given workshops and seminars and provided private consulting in a number of areas, including proposal writing, business writing, giving good oral presentations, and good time management. Her workshops and seminars about proposal writing have been well received at many universities and professional meetings throughout the United States, in several countries of the former Soviet Union, and in Beijing, China.

A veteran lecturer and writer of grant proposals, and the author of some 40 publications in the scientific literature, Dr. Reif-Lehrer has also published articles in *The Scientist, Journal of Science Education and Technology, Journal of the National Grantseekers Institute, SciTech Journal, Science's Next Wave, Trends in Cell Biology, HMS Beagle, Boston Magazine,* the *Boston Globe,* and the *Christian Science Monitor.*

◾ PART I ◾

GETTING STARTED

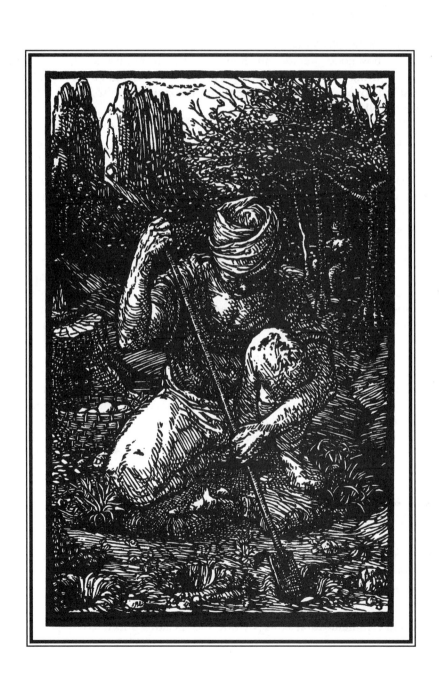

INTRODUCTION

Success in obtaining grant funding depends on many factors; the major ones are

- a good—preferably innovative—research idea (project)
- a good match between the proposed project and the mandate (mission) of the funding agency to which you plan to apply
- a carefully thought-out approach to the project
- a focused, well-written proposal

The Mission of the funding agency

No matter how good your idea and how well-written your proposal, if the agency to which you are applying is not interested in your project, you will not be funded! Thus, you should understand, for example, that the **scientific mission** of the United States National Institutes of Health (NIH) is

> "To improve the health of the people of the United States by increasing our understanding of the process underlying human health and by acquiring new knowledge to help prevent, detect, diagnose, and treat disease."

That is, **the mission of NIH is NOT to fund good research—but rather to improve the health of the people in the United States.** This understanding should have a great impact on how you present your project and may, other things being equal, enhance your chances of success.

Granting agencies change their funding priorities—and even their missions—from time to time, as problems get resolved, more pressing problems arise, or the administrators and/or trustees of the agency change. Sometimes the changes are major—sometimes they are subtle. Thus, you should understand that an idea rejected one year might have a high priority at a later time! Likewise, an agency may, over time, lose interest in projects it had previously given high priority. The cost of a long distance phone call is a small price to pay to avoid spending time "barking up the wrong tree." Before you spend any time on a grant application, call the program officer(s) at the agency to which you intend to submit the proposal, and be sure the agency is interested in your research idea. Also try to find out what aspects of the project are of greatest interest to the agency so that you can optimize the match between your research plans and the agency's funding priorities. **Please note that there is NO insinuation here that you be dishonest.** It is just important that you emphasize those aspects of your project that are of greatest interest to the funding agency. It is also important to explain to the potential funding agency how—and to what extent—your work is likely to result in a return on their investment in you.

SOME TRAITS OF A SUCCESSFUL GRANT-GETTER

Successful grant-getters need

1. Good research skills
2. Salesmanship skills
   - to convince the granting agency that your idea is worth funding
3. Good communication skills (writing and speaking effectively)

- **Good writing skills** are necessary to:
  —write a good grant proposal
  —write high quality publications that will build your reputation
- **Good speaking skills** are necessary to:
  —give good talks that will help bring your work to the attention of the scientific community
  —make a convincing presentation during a site visit
  —successfully negotiate the interactive process that may be involved in foundation grant Applications

4 Ingenuity and flexibility
- to take advantage of current program relevance and funding priorities. Determine what aspects of your project best match the mandates of the funding agency and make those sufficiently prominent to capture the attention of the Reader/Reviewer.

5 Administrative skills (from leadership to accounting)
- Keep informed

  Although grants policy interpretation and oversight is the principal role of the grantee organization's Office of Sponsored Research (or equivalent office/officer), it is important that the Principal Investigator (PI) is aware of the scope of policy responsibilities, and makes it her/his responsibility to comply with post-award reporting deadlines and other NIH (or other funding agency) regulations. The NIH Grants Policy Statement is online at

  http://grants.nih.gov/grants/policy/nihgps_2001/

- Leadership
  —You must be able to gather and maintain a cohesive, productive workgroup that is motivated to help you fulfill your research goals. You must be able to convince a potential funding agency that you have this capability.
  —Know where, how, and when to get information about available funding. If in doubt about any aspect of the grants process, don't guess, call the program officer or other grants personnel at the potential funding agency(ies).
  —Periodically evaluate your progress.
- Accounting

  Keep close tabs on your grant budget once you are funded. Although there may be a support service at your institution that keeps track of your expenditures, you (the Principal Investigator) are responsible for working within your budget.

6 Good human relations
- It is important to have the ability to motivate and gain the cooperation and confidence of
  —your immediate staff
  —people in your department
  —people in other departments
  —people in your institution whose help you may need
  —colleagues at other institutions
  —granting agency officials

Scientists often have not been trained in good human relations skills. If you tend to be brusque—or fail to consider the sensitivities of the people around you—these people will tend to shy away from you and you may, thus, be cheating yourself out of some superb resources. If, on the other hand, you have good "people skills" and tend to help people, others will often be pleased to help you and relieve you of certain tasks that allow you to spend more time on your important work, i.e., the things that only you can do. In other words, **people who are adept at social skills and know how to motivate others can often enhance their own productivity via help from others.**

7. Persistence, dedication, patience, and the ability to work hard
   - Don't give up. Keep revising wisely and applying for grant funds until you get funded, but also know when it is time to change to a different project.

8. Political awareness and action
   - Be aware of funding sources and funding levels.
   - Scientists can help themselves and their peers by lobbying for their own cause. Write and/or call your congressional representatives when your professional associations request that you do so.
   - Make your voice heard: Vote for officials who support research.

9. Integrity
   - Guard against
     —possible questions concerning your integrity
     —poor judgment that may impair/blemish your reputation

KNOW WHAT YOU PLAN TO DO BEFORE YOU APPLY FOR FUNDING

Some questions that SUCCESSFUL grant-getters should be able to answer before starting to write a Grant Application:

NOTE: I have maintained the list of questions shown below for a long time and have modified the list as my views about writing proposals have evolved. Somehow, the reference for the list became separated from the list many years ago and I do not recollect where the original list came from. Thus, I profusely apologize to the originator of the list, as I would like to acknowledge the originating entity.

1. **What do YOU plan to do?**
   - What is the hypothesis to be tested or the question to be answered?
   - How easy—or difficult—will it be to collect new data and to repeat experiments in the system you plan to use?
   - What is the rationale for your proposed project?
   - What is novel/unique/useful about your idea/concept?

2. **Why is the work worth doing? (Significance)**
   - Is it original?
   - If it is not original, why is it worth doing again?

3. **What is the broad, long-term objective**/long range goal (the "carrot" at the end of your stick)?

4. **What are the specific aims**/objectives/goals that you are likely to accomplish in one or two project periods?

5. Is the **methodology** "state of the art"?
   - If you propose a new method, why is it better than the methods currently in use?

6. **Who will do the work?**
   - How good is the **reputation** of the grantee (PI) and her/his team? How can you document this?
   - What are the **qualifications** of the grantee (PI) and her/his team? How can you document this?

7. **Why should "they" let YOU do the project?**
   - What are your **unique qualifications** and background to carry out this project?
   - What is the extent of your **experience** in relation to your ability to carry out this project?

8. **How long will the work take?**
   - Have you formulated a realistic timetable for the project?

9. **How much will the project cost (Budget) and why (Budget justification)?**
   - If you can't justify something in the context of the project, don't ask for it.

10. **What other funds are—or might be—available to support the project?**
    - Many funding agencies appreciate cost sharing.

11. **How will the project be supported in the future?**
    - That is, after the funding you are requesting is used up.
    - Where will the work be carried out?
    - Are there **colleagues** for you to talk to about your work?
    - Is the **environment** conducive to good information exchange and other support?

12. **What facilities will the work require?**
    - Do you have adequate access to such facilities?

13. **How will the results of the project benefit the granting agency?**
    - How will the results of the project benefit the **advancement of science** and the work of other scientists?
      - —NIH has developed formal guidelines for sharing unique research resources ("Research Tools"). See

      http://ott.od.nih.gov/NewPages/RTguide_final.html

      - —NIH requires PIs to include a plan for sharing of research data, or to state why data-sharing is not possible. Sharing of research data will apply to extramural scientists seeking grants, cooperative agreements, and contracts, as well as to intramural investigators. See

      http://grants.nih.gov/grants/guide/notice-files/NOT-OD-02-035.html

      This Document ("NIH ANNOUNCES DRAFT STATEMENT ON SHARING RESEARCH DATA") is reproduced on page 23.

14. **How will the results of the project benefit society?**
    - For example, what is the **Health Relatedness** of the project?
    - For corporation grants also discuss:
      —How will the project increase the stature of the corporation?
      —How will the project increase the financial gain of the corporation?
15. **What are the expected results?**
    - What are your contingency plans if you encounter a problem?
16. **Are you and your team aware of what has been done in this and related fields? (Background)**
17. **Does the agency require a pre-application or letter of intent/inquiry?**

WHAT DOES IT TAKE TO BE A SUCCESSFUL GRANT-GETTER?

Successful grant-getters understand
1. The essentials of grantsmanship (psychology)
2. The **mission** of the potential funding agency
   - keep in touch with the agency
   - stay informed about the funding situation at the agency
   - keep up to date about changes in the mandate and/or the budget of the potential funding agency

> **NOTE:** It is not sufficient to simply take the written or stated mission/missions at face value. Talk to an officer at the potential funding agency and try to ascertain which aspects of the overall mission the agency is currently most interested in pursuing. Also determine whether your proposed project fulfills some aspect of the agency's mandate.

3. The nature of the **review process** (psychology)
   - How does the process function at NIH? At other agencies, especially the one to which you plan to apply for funding?
   - What are Reviewers looking for?
   - What are the factors that influence the grades the Reviewers assign?
4. The concept (psychology) of writing for
   - the reader (the Reviewer)
   - the wider audience (the potential funding agency administrators)
5. The "art" of responding to a set of instructions
   - **Understand how to read and follow the instructions.**
   - Keep in mind that the people who write the instructions may NOT know the "art" of writing a good set of instructions.
   - It is YOUR job to
     —understand the basic principles of good expository writing
     —respond to the challenge of responding to less-than-ideal instructions by "artful" responses which are clear and concise
     —follow the instructions in a complete and logical stepwise manner

6 The basic elements of **good expository writing**
  - Note that the word "expository" is based on the root word **"to expose."**
  - A grant proposal should never sound like a novel or mystery story.
  - The Reviewer wants to get the **maximum information in the minimum number of words.**
  - The Reviewer wants **accuracy and clarity.**
  - The Reviewer should never have to guess what you mean.
    - —Your proposal should always maintain **good logical flow** so that the reader (Reviewer)—who may not be in your specific field—can easily perceive how you got from point A to point B.
    - —What may seem obvious to you and your close colleagues may not be at all obvious to a reader not intimately knowledgeable about your specific field of research.
    - —Keep in mind that many bright scientists may have had no formal training in expository writing—or even in any kind of writing!
    - —Keep in mind that many very bright native English speakers may not have a very extensive English vocabulary. Test a few of your colleagues with some words such as impecunious, parsimonious, and perspicacity, words which most graduates of good colleges would have known in the 1950s. The results of this little exercise may convince you to **use relatively simple vocabulary** in science-related grant proposals!
    - —Keep in mind that **many scientists** now working in the U.S. (some of whom may be Reviewers) **are not native English speakers!**

7 Successful grant-getters should be aware of the sequence of steps that can help optimize their chances of success in obtaining funding:
  - Research the topic meticulously
  - Formulate the ideas/hypotheses/questions for your proposal
  - Plan the project in detail
  - Do sufficient **preliminary studies** to convince yourself and the Reviewers that what you propose to do is feasible and stands a good chance of yielding results that will advance your field of study
  - **Make an outline** for your proposal
  - Revise the outline until all necessary information is included and everything is in good logical order. (Do NOT weigh the outline down with prose until you are 99.9999999% satisfied with your outline.)
  - Convert your outline to an easy-to-understand prose document that conforms to agency page limits
  - **Proofread** your proposal and **revise** as necessary
  - **Send your proposal to 3 readers** for evaluation of
    - —content (accuracy)
    - —clarity
    - —consistency
    - —brevity
    - —style (emphasis, tone, and presentation)
  - During the time the Readers have your proposal, **allow yourself time to distance yourself** from the proposal; this will help you to view the proposal with a fresh viewpoint when it is returned to you with your Readers' comments.

- **Incorporate appropriate suggestions** from Readers
  - —Do not allow your emotional responses to your Readers' comments to cloud your reactions to the comments.
  - —Remember that you are not obliged to use all of your Readers' comments. The grant application is, after all, yours. However, in return for the work your Readers have done for you, you are obliged to **seriously consider the Readers' comments** in a dispassionate manner. You must assume that the Readers you chose have your interest at heart and are trying to help you. If you cannot do this, you have probably chosen the wrong Readers!
  - —If you feel hurt or angry in response to some/any of your Readers' comments, put the proposal away for a day and then look at the comments again when you feel calm. Use only those comments that **you** consider appropriate!
- Do a final revision and proofread, and then finalize the proposal and the rest of the application.

SOME GENERAL INFORMATION FOR BEGINNING GRANT APPLICATION WRITERS

What is a grant?
A grant is a form of sponsorship for a project, the ideas for which generally originate with and are designed and carried out by the Applicant. Grants can be classified according to:

- Type of activity or activities supported (research, training, service, etc.)
- Degree of discretion allowed the awarding office (mandatory or discretionary)
- Method of determining amounts of awards (negotiated or formula)

The project may be
- education
- research
- a performance
- creation of a work of art
- construction of a housing development
- a plan for other community improvement
- organizing a conference
- travel with a purpose
- acquisition of equipment

NOTE: Although the examples used in this book focus on grants awarded in response to Applications or proposals for biomedical research projects, the general principles put forth in the book are applicable to many fields of endeavor.

The grant may provide funds for
- part or all of the expenses associated with the project
- only direct operating costs and indirect (overhead) costs
- only direct operating costs

Direct costs

Costs readily identified as necessary for carrying out the project, such as

- salaries
- fringe benefits
- equipment
- supplies
- project-related travel
- publication costs

Direct costs are requested by the grantee and are subject to approval by the grantor.

Indirect costs (overhead)

Costs incurred by the grantee institution to provide support services that are generally shared by other projects. These costs include, for example, administrative expenses and plant operation and maintenance such as

- library
- restrooms
- cafeteria
- electricity
- other utilities
- security
- institutional store
- parking facilities

Indirect costs are generally negotiated between the grantee institution and the grantor. The "negotiated indirect cost rate" is generally a percent of salaries and wages or a percent of total direct costs.

> **NOTE:** Grants from agencies that do not provide overhead may be considered unacceptable by some grantee institutions. But it is sometimes possible to charge certain items, normally considered overhead, as direct costs (for example, administrative costs). This must first be cleared with the grantee institution and must be consistent with its normal accounting practices.

Be aware that many granting agencies will award a grant only to an institution, i.e., the agency will NOT award funds to an individual who is not affiliated with an appropriate institution. For example, when you apply for funding to NIH, strictly speaking, it is not you but your institution that is applying for the award. If the award is granted, it is granted not to you but to your institution. Your institution sets up an account for you upon which you draw for funds to carry out your project. A few agencies do give funds to unaffiliated individuals. The National Science Foundation (NSF) is one example.

Categories of awards

- **Fellowships**

  Support continuing or advanced education of researchers or other scholars.

- **Grants, Cooperative Agreements, and Contracts**

  Provide recipients with the means to carry on their work in the sense that the grantee has a commitment to perform work that fulfills the expectation of the grantor.

—Grants and Cooperative Agreements come out of assistance programs.
—Contracts result from acquisition programs.

The characteristics of these 3 types of awards are as follows:

Grant

- An agreement to support research.
- Ideas originate with and are defined by the Applicant.
- Generally for basic research.
- Allows the recipient a reasonable amount of freedom. No programmatic involvement by the sponsoring agency, but the grantee is expected to make substantive scientific progress and to contribute to the general body of knowledge of the field of the research.

Cooperative Agreement

- Identical to a grant except that there is substantial programmatic involvement by the sponsoring agency.
- According to the Federal Grant and Cooperative Agreement Act, Public Law 95-224 (Feb. 3, 1978), the only difference between a "Grant" and a "Cooperative Agreement" is the amount of programmatic involvement by the sponsoring agency.
- At NIH, grant Applications are reviewed by Study Sections within the Center for Scientific Research (CSR), whereas Cooperative Agreements are generally reviewed by Study Sections assembled and administered by staff at an NIH Institute or Center (Institute Review Groups).

Contract

- An instrument to procure research.
- Generally for applied research.
- The work required is spelled out by the funding agency.
- Usually has defined deliverables: either in the form of products or services.
- The funding agency exercises more control over the recipient than in the case of a grant.
- Involves stricter financial accountability than a grant.

Types of granting agencies

Government

- Most abundant source.
- Lots of materials and information available.
- Trendy (e.g., may change with the federal administration), but must be responsive to voters and the democratic process, so response to external changes is slow.
- Information about review procedures is public information and is readily available.

Private Foundations

- Funding depends on matching specific interests.

- Some materials and information are available.
- The mandate may remain the same over a long period or may change frequently. For example, following the advent of the polio vaccine, the focus of the March of Dimes Foundation changed from polio to birth defects.
- Can respond quickly to new ideas/unique needs.
- Information about review procedures may be considered proprietary information and may not be readily available.

Business and Industry

- The least abundant source of funding for academic institutions.
- There is no good readily available central source of information.
- Identifying a corporation that will sponsor an activity or a research project may be difficult.
- Finding a funding source takes time, initiative, energy, imagination, and persistence.
- Information about review procedures may not be readily available.

    Building relationships with the appropriate staff members—before there is any mention of money—is an important aspect of getting funding from the business community. See *Get Funded! A Practical Guide for Scholars Seeking Research Support from Business*, by Dorin Schumacher, Ph.D., Sage Publications, 1992.

About NIH

Special awards for beginning grant seekers

Some government agencies, such as NIH, offer special awards for certain categories of grant-seekers such as young investigators (first-time Applicants), investigators whose projects are high risk but have the potential for high "pay off," etc. These special categories tend to change more often than the more standard categories such as "Investigator-initiated research grants." It is important for potential Applicants to remain aware of new funding vehicles and new sources of funding. If you are a young investigator, contact NIH and other appropriate agencies and ask about special programs for first-time Applicants and other special programs that may suit/match your particular situation. Watch especially for new "Requests for Application" (RFA) and "Requests for Proposal" (RFP). A good place to get a current list of special programs is the "NIH Guide for Grants and Contracts," which is published weekly. The NIH Guide—including a searchable index—may be accessed at

http://grants.nih.gov/grants/guide/index.html

Comprehensive Archives of Published NIH Guide Articles can be accessed via

http://grants.nih.gov/grants/guide/index.html#desc

Near the beginning of the above Web site, **you can request that the Index for each issue of the NIH Guide be e-mailed to you** each time an issue is posted (see details below).

Where to get information about available grants

- Internet (e.g., Agency Web sites/electronic mail)

grantsinfo@nih.gov
http://www.nih.gov
http://grants.nih.gov/grants/index.cfm

- Toll-free numbers are available for certain NIH Institute contacts:

Arthritis and Musculoskeletal and Skin Diseases	877-226-4267
Child Health and Human Development	800-370-2943
Complementary and Alternative Medicine	888-644-6226
Deafness and Other Communication Disorders	800-241-1044
Heart, Lung, and Blood	800-575-9355
Kidney and Urologic Diseases	800-891-5390
National Library of Medicine	888-346-3656
Network of Libraries of Medicine	800-338-7657
Neurological Disorders and Stroke (Brain Resources and Information Network)	800-352-9424

- Direct line to NIH: 301-435-0714 (8:30 AM to 5 PM workdays); press 5 to speak with someone.

- **NIH Guide for Grants and Contracts**
  To receive the *NIH Guide* Table of Contents each week, send an e-mail to **listserv@list.nih.gov**
  In the **first line of the email message** (not in the "Subject" line), type:
  subscribe NIHTOC-L your name
  (where "your name" is the name you wish to use).

- **National Science Foundation (NSF)**
  http://www.nsf.gov
  http://www.nsf.gov/home/grants.htm
  https://www.fastlane.nsf.gov

Information about agencies other than NIH and NSF

- **GrantsNet**: Research Funding Database

  http://www.grantsnet.org
  A resource to find funds for training in the sciences and undergraduate science education. The service is free. It is supported by the Howard Hughes Medical Institute (HHMI) and the American Association for the Advancement of Science (AAAS). From the **GrantsNet** site, you can also access an International Grants and Fellowship index.

- **FirstGov**

  http://www.firstgov.gov
  The first-ever U.S. Government Web site that provides easy, one-stop access to all federal government online information and services

- **GrantStation**

  http://www.grantstation.com
  Weekly news about new funding programs, upcoming deadlines, conferences, seminars, and more! There is a substantial membership fee.

■ GrantSelect

http://www.grantselect.com

A list of over 10,000 funding opportunities, including funding from state and federal governments, corporations, foundations, and associations. The list is updated daily. An e-mail Alert Service delivers funding information directly to your e-mail inbox. Flexible pricing.

You can subscribe to one or more of 7 customized segments of the research grants database:

—Arts and Humanities

—Biomedical and Health Care

—Children and Youth

—Community Development

—K–12 and Adult Basic Education

—International Programs

—Operating Grants

■ **Resource centers and libraries**

There are several resource centers and libraries dedicated entirely to information about funding sources. Some examples are:

—**Associated Grant Makers**

55 Court St., Suite 520

Boston, MA 02108

Telephone: 617-426-2606

E-mail: agm@agmconnect.org

http://www.agmconnect.org

Kenneth Liss, Director of the Resource Center

Associated Grant Makers is a resource center for philanthropy; the research library has a reference collection of publications and other information on foundation and corporate grant making and nonprofit management including Massachusetts grant makers, national foundations, corporate giving, IRS 990-PF forms, journals, newsletters, fund raising manuals, and proposal-writing guides. Associated Grant Makers has orientation sessions twice a month for first-time users. Call or e-mail to get the schedule.

—**Donors Forum Library**

208 South LaSalle Street, Suite 735

Chicago, IL 60604

Telephone: 312-578-0175

Fax: 312-578-0158

TDD: 312-578-0159

http://www.donorsforum.org

The Donors Forum of Chicago is an association of Chicago-area grant makers. Its mission is to advance philanthropy by serving its members and by promoting an effective and informed nonprofit sector. Through education programs, workshops, publications, research projects, and a Library, they provide resources for grant makers, nonprofit organizations, the media, researchers, and anyone seeking information on the nonprofit and philanthropic sector. The Donors Forum has more than 180 grant making members and 1,000 nonprofit Forum Partners, and is committed to promoting and encouraging active relationships between grant makers, nonprofits, and the community at large.

—The Foundation Center
79 Fifth Avenue/16th Street
New York, NY 10003-3076
Telephone: 800-424-9836; 212-620-4230
Fax: 212-807-3677
http://fdncenter.org
http://fdncenter.org/funders/
http://fdncenter.org/about/contact.html

Founded in 1956, the Foundation Center is dedicated to serving grant seekers, grant makers, researchers, policymakers, the media, and the general public. The Center's mission is to support and improve philanthropy by promoting public understanding of the field and helping grant seekers succeed.

The Foundation Center:

Collects, organizes, and communicates information on U.S. philanthropy

Conducts and facilitates research on trends in the field

Provides education and training for the grantseeking process

Ensures public access to information and services through their
—World Wide Web site
—print and electronic publications
—5 library/learning centers
—national network of Cooperating Collections

The Foundation Center online orientation to the grant-seeking process can be accessed at

http://www.fdncenter.org/for_individuals/

Some other Foundation Center tools available to help grant seekers succeed are:

Foundation Finder – allows you to search by name for basic financial and contact information for more than 70,000 private and community foundations in the U.S.

Grantmaker Web Sites – 4 distinct directories of annotated links to grant maker Web sites organized by grant maker type allows you to search or browse summaries of the collected sites.

Sector Search – a specialty search engine that indexes every page of the most useful non-profit sites on the Internet.

990-PF Search – a searchable database of the 990-PF tax returns filed with the Internal Revenue Service by all domestic private foundations.

The Foundation Directory Online – a monthly or annual subscription service that allows you to search the Foundation Center's database of over 76,000 grant makers and more than 350,000 grants.

Online librarian – The Foundation Center has an Online librarian at
http://fdncenter.org/learn/librarian/
—The Grantsmanship Center (TGCI)
1125 W Sixth Street, 5th Floor
PO Box 17220
Los Angeles, CA 90017
Telephone: 800-421-9512; 213-482-9860
Fax: 213-482-9863
http://www.tgci.com

The Grantsmanship Center is primarily a training organization. The Center sponsors workshops on writing grant proposals; publishes a funding newsletter, *The Grantsmanship Center Magazine*, available free to qualified agencies; and sells reprints of articles related to proposal writing and fund raising. The Center deals primarily with government agencies and non-profit agencies and concentrates on grant-seeking organizations rather than on individual grant seekers.

- **General libraries**

General libraries usually also have listings of grants and sources of grant money, such as:

The Foundation Directory

The Foundation Grant Index

Much of this information is now also available on the Internet.

- **Databases of available funding**, such as

—**InfoEd International, Inc.**
1873 Western Avenue, Suite #201
Albany, NY 12203
Telephone: 1-800-727-6427; 518-464-0691
Fax: 518-464-0695
E-mail: office@infoed.org

SPINPlus, including **SPIN** (Sponsored Programs Information Network), **SMARTS,** and **GENIUS** systems

SPINPlus, an Internet-based database, helps faculty and administrators locate federal, nonfederal, and corporate funding sources for research, education, and development, in science/medicine/technology.

GENIUS is a searchable expertise profile system that contains faculty Curriculum Vitae (CVs) and can generate the NIH 398 Biosketch Form. Free searches are available to sponsors, industry, and subscribers to SPINPlus.

SMARTS matches **GENIUS** profiles with the **SPIN** funding opportunities and automatically delivers daily updates via e-mail to keep investigators informed of new funding opportunities, deadlines, and sponsor updates. If your grants office subscribes, then you can search the database at no cost.

—**The Community of Science (COS)**
1629 Thames Street, Suite 200
Baltimore, MD 21231
Telephone: 800-237-8621; 410-563-2378
Fax: 410-563-5389
E-mail: prodinfo@cos.com
http://www.cos.com

Community of Science, Inc. (COS) is a spin-off company of Johns Hopkins University. COS has a network of more than 480,000 research professionals worldwide. Individual researchers in all disciplines are encouraged to join COS free of charge. But some COS services are available **only** if your institution has a **paid membership**. Researchers can use the COS network to:

- find funding
- promote their research
- track current research activities
- collaborate with peers from around the world

- get research expertise management and alerting systems for:
  - —universities
  - —societies
  - —corporations
  - —governments

COS services include:

COS Expertise®

A database of detailed, first person profiles of scientists and scholars

http://expertise.cos.com

COS Funding Opportunities™

A large inventory of currently available research grant information for all disciplines

http://fundingopps.cos.com

COS Funding Alert™

A customized e-mail service that keeps researchers informed about new funding opportunities in their disciplines

http://www.cos.com/services

(click on "COS funding alert")

COS Abstract Management System™

An online publishing solution for universities and professional societies

http://ams.cos.com

Provides customized access to a range of professional reference databases such as

http://medline.cos.com
http://patents.cos.com
http://georef.cos.com
http://fr.cos.com
http://cbd.cos.com
http://agricola.cos.com

- Other resources:

Institutional grant offices

—Office of Grants and Contracts
—Office for Sponsored Research

Direct communication with agencies that have a specific interest in the area of the proposed application

Research Grants-eNewsletter

Produced by Science Info

Scienceinfo@earthlink.net

to keep scientists informed of the latest information regarding grant and award opportunities in life sciences.

http://www.escienceinfo.com/01-12-04enews.html

Offers subscribers one time FREE listing of Postdoctoral/Research associate positions.

Science Info

Virginia Biotech Research Park
800 E Leigh Street G-25
Richmond, VA 23219

Newsletters from:

—granting agencies

—professional organizations
—private foundations
Commercial newsletters such as:
—Corporate Philanthropy Report
—Education Grants Alert
—Federal Grants and Contracts Weekly
—Foundation and Corporate Grants Alert
—Health Grants & Contracts Weekly
The 5 newsletters listed above are published by
LRP Publications
747 Dresher Road, Suite 500
P.O. Box 980
Horsham, PA 19044
Tel: 800-341-7874; 215-784-0860; Fax: 215-784-9639
LRP Publications also has offices in **Florida and Virginia**
More information about each of the above newsletters (with the exception of "Education Grants Alert") is available at http://www.lrpdartnell.com/cgi-bin/SoftCart.exe/scstore/19_Grants_Nonprofits/cat-Newsletters_Subscriptions.html?L+scstore+USIH749241090013928
Each of the newsletters is also available as an electronic version.
Annual reports of foundations
These reports usually provide a good overview of areas of interest to the foundation and sometimes contain a list of projects they have funded.
Professional and society journals
—Announcements section
—Acknowledgments in journal articles that cite sources of funding for the work described.
News media
Private workshops and seminars
Colleagues (word of mouth)
Requests for proposals (RFPs) and Requests for Applications (RFAs)
RFPs and RFAs are sent to certain institutions, organizations, and publications; e.g., announcements about RFPs and RFAs may be listed in professional organization newsletters. At NIH, RFPs and RFAs are listed in the *NIH Guide for Grants and Contracts*, which is available on the Internet.
—To receive the *NIH Guide* Table of Contents via e-mail each week, send an e-mail to
　　listserv@list.nih.gov
　　In the first line of the email message (not in the "Subject" line), type:
　　　　subscribe NIHTOC-L your name
　　　　(where "your name" is the name you wish to use)

Information to gather before you apply for a grant

From yourself

- Do you have a very clear concept of what your project entails?
- Have you clearly defined what your project is intended to accomplish?
- Have you determined that there are funding agencies that are interested in your project?

- Do you have sufficient preliminary data to convince the Reviewers and the funding agency administrators that your project is likely to succeed and make a valuable contribution to the field?
- Do you know what methods you will use to achieve your goals?
- Do you have a clear understanding of what is necessary to carry out your project?
  —Space
  —Personnel
  —Equipment
  —Supplies
  —Other necessary support services
- Do you have a clear understanding of how long your project will take?
- Do you have a clear understanding of how much it will cost to carry out your project?
  —Have you done some realistic preliminary budget calculations?
- Have you determined what you will need from the funding agency?
  —Some funding agencies want to see a commitment by the Applicant's institution in the form of cost-sharing.
  —Some agencies want to support only part of a project, which may also be supported by other funding agencies.

From your institution

- Is your institution willing to let you apply?
- Will your institution support the project?
- Is your institution willing to cost-share?
- Do you have to file an "intent to apply"?
- Is your institution willing to administer the grant?
- Is your institution willing to put the necessary space and resources at your disposal?
- Have you resolved questions of:
  —Salary?
  —Overhead?
  —Patents?
  —Copyrights?
  —Equipment acquisition, use, and disposal?
  —Relative involvement of the Applicant and her/his institution in the project?
- For government funds, is your institution willing to file assurance of compliance with
  —the Civil Rights Act?
  —affirmative action rulings?
  —the protection of human subjects?
  —the humane treatment of animals?
  —other relevant regulations?

Because of increased emphasis on grants compliance and oversight, it is helpful to specify that the grantee institution has the infrastructure and sufficient resources to comply with all aspects of NIH Grants Policy.

From the prospective funding organization

- Does the agency have printed information/materials to help acquaint you with its
  —Organization?
  —Programs?
  —Research priorities?
  —Grant policies?

For NIH, you can go to

http://www.nih.gov

and type a search word(s) into the relevant space at the upper right of the screen and then click on "**Search**"; this will often lead you to the information you need.

- Does your interest match the purpose of the agency's program (i.e., the current mandate of the agency)?
- Do you qualify to get funding?
  Some agencies have very specific eligibility requirements. Have you checked
  —Eligibility?
  —Restrictions?
  —Special stipulations?
- Have you determined whether the agency is really interested in your project?
- Have you obtained as much information as possible about the agency to which you are considering applying for funds?
- Send for the agency's annual report and/or other printed materials it may provide.
- Find out what projects the agency has funded in the recent past.
  —Ask the agency for a list, or look it up in one of the Foundation directories or indexes.
- Once you have some background information about the agency, speak to a program officer (or other relevant administrator) at the agency before you begin to write.
  —Developing a good proposal is a lot of work.
  —The best-thought-out and best-written proposal will not be funded by an agency that is not interested in the project.
  —Some agencies have written documents describing their funding priorities for the next several (sometimes 3 to 5) years.
- Determine whether your project matches the agency's mandate.
  —Try to get the agency to clarify which aspects of its mandate have priority for possible support, and which aspects are of lesser interest.
  —Some agencies—especially certain private foundations—will help you develop your proposal, a service that is well worth taking advantage of.
  —Try to have the agency clarify which aspects of your project it would be interested in supporting, and which aspects it will NOT support.
  —Try to determine which parts of your project the agency seems most enthused about and emphasize those aspects of your project in your application.
- If you are funded by the agency, do you have any obligations to the agency in the future, e.g., is there a payback clause?

- What amounts of money does the agency grant?
  —Is this amount of funding realistically sufficient to carry out your project? If not, are you confident that you can get the additional funds you will need to complete the project?
- What are the total number of awards and amount of support provided by the agency?
  —What are YOUR chances of getting support?
- Can the agency provide a list of past grantees and their projects?
  —What are the type, length, and amount of support per person?
  —Is this amount enough to complete your project?
- Are the funding agency policies all acceptable to you and your institution:
  —funding level
  —indirect cost policy
  —restrictions

An important caveat: Before you agree to accept funds from an agency—and preferably before you apply for the funds!—it is important that you understand clearly **what your obligations to that agency are in return for the funding**. For example, some private enterprise institutions may offer attractive amounts of funding but may require the Principal Investigator to sign a confidentiality agreement. Signing such an agreement may not be good for your career or your reputation because you may want to:

[1] be free to publish your results, at your discretion, in the general scientific literature, without any restriction from the sponsoring organization

[2] present your latest research results at any scientific conference of your choice without having to get permission from the funding agency

It is wise to get these matters **agreed to—in writing**—before accepting any funds from a private enterprise institution.

It is becoming increasingly common for PIs to request support for a project from both federal and nonfederal sources. Under these circumstances it is important to:

[1] inform both sponsors that you are also requesting funds from another sponsor

[2] communicate to the nonfederal sponsor how use of federal funds will affect the research and its outcome with regard to information sharing, intellectual property licensing, etc.

[3] **Be wary of sponsorship for your research that might involve you in a "conflict of interest"!!!**

Application information

- Is there a formal application kit?
- Does the agency require a pre-application or a letter of inquiry?
- When is the application due? Does the deadline refer to
  —date of postmark?
  —date of arrival at the funding agency?
- Have there been recent changes in requirements or application procedures that differ from the information given in the agency's printed/posted information?
  —At NIH, check with the particular funding component (institute or center) from which you are requesting support about program changes and additional application instructions.

Information about the review process

- Who will review the application?
- Is a site visit required?
- What is the time lag between application and approval?
- What is the time lag between approval and funding?

> **NOTE:** The U.S. Environmental Protection Agency has an interesting tutorial for proposal writers at
> **http://www.epa.gov/seahome/grants/src/msieopen.htm**
> It is worth looking at this site to use as a "practice session."
>
> **NOTE:** You may find it of interest to visit the NIH Image Web site at
> **http://rsb.info.nih.gov/nih-image/**

If you click on "About NIH Image" at the above site, you will find the information below:

About NIH Image

NIH Image is a public domain image processing and analysis program for the Macintosh. It was developed at the Research Services Branch (RSB) of the National Institute of Mental Health (NIMH), part of the National Institutes of Health (NIH).

A free PC version of Image, called Scion Image for Windows, is available from Scion Corporation. There is also Image/J, a Java program inspired by Image that "runs anywhere."

Image requires a color capable Macintosh and at least 4MB of free RAM; 32MB or more of RAM is recommended for working with three dimensional (3D) images, 24-bit color or animation sequences. System 7.0 or later is required. Image directly supports, or is compatible with, large monitors, flatbed scanners, film recorders, graphics tablets, PostScript laser printers, photo typesetters, and color printers.

Image can acquire, display, edit, enhance, analyze, and animate images. It reads and writes TIFF, PICT, PICS and MacPaint files, providing compatibility with many other Applications, including programs for scanning, processing, editing, publishing, and analyzing images. It supports many standard image processing functions, including contrast enhancement, density profiling, smoothing, sharpening, edge detection, median filtering, and spatial convolution with user defined kernels.

Image can be used to measure area, mean, centroid, perimeter, etc. of user-defined regions of interest. It also performs automated particle analysis and provides tools for measuring path lengths and angles. Spatial calibration is supported to provide real world area and length measurements. Density calibration can be done against radiation or optical density standards using user specified units. Results can be printed, exported to text files, or copied to the Clipboard.

A tool palette supports editing of color and gray scale images, including the ability to draw lines, rectangles, and text. It can flip, rotate, invert, and scale selections. It supports multiple windows and 8 levels of magnification. All editing, filtering, and measurement functions operate at any level of magnification and are undoable.

Image directly supports Data Translation and Scion frame grabber cards for capturing images or movie sequences using a TV camera. Acquired images can be shading corrected and frame averaged. Other frame grabbers are supported via plug-in modules.

Image can be customized in three ways: via a built-in Pascal-like macro language, via externally compiled plug-in modules, and on the Pascal source code level. Example macros, plug-ins and complete source code can be downloaded from the Download page.

More information about NIH Image can be found in the Overview section of the manual.

Sharing of research data

The information below, concerning the sharing of Research Data, is reproduced from

http://grants.nih.gov/grants/guide/notice-files/NOT-OD-02-035.html

NIH ANNOUNCES DRAFT STATEMENT ON SHARING RESEARCH DATA

Release Date: March 1, 2002

NOTICE: NOT-OD-02-035 (See NOT-OD-03-032 for Update)

National Institutes of Health

Data sharing promotes many goals of the National Institutes of Health's (NIH) research endeavor. It is particularly important for unique data that cannot be readily replicated. Data sharing allows scientists to expedite the translation of research results into knowledge, products, and procedures to improve human health. THE NIH IS DEVELOPING A STATEMENT ON DATA SHARING THAT EXPECTS AND SUPPORTS THE TIMELY RELEASE AND SHARING OF FINAL RESEARCH DATA FROM NIH-SUPPORTED STUDIES FOR USE BY OTHER RESEARCHERS. INVESTIGATORS SUBMITTING AN NIH APPLICATION WILL BE REQUIRED TO INCLUDE A PLAN FOR DATA SHARING OR TO STATE WHY DATA SHARING IS NOT POSSIBLE. This statement will apply to extramural scientists seeking grants, cooperative agreements, and contracts, as well as to intramural investigators.

Institutions and individuals were invited to comment on the draft policy by June 1, 2002 and expected the policy to become effective as of January 1, 2003.

Background Information

There are many reasons to share data from NIH-supported studies. Sharing data reinforces open scientific inquiry, encourages diversity of analysis and opinion, promotes new research, makes possible the testing of new or alternative hypotheses and methods of analysis, supports studies on data collection methods and measurement, facilitates the education of new researchers, enables the exploration of topics not envisioned by the initial investigators, and permits the creation of new data sets when data from multiple sources are combined. By avoiding the duplication of expensive data collection activities, the NIH is able to support more investigators than it could if similar data had to be collected de novo by each Applicant.

NIH-supported basic research, clinical studies, surveys, and other types of research produce data that may be shared. However, NIH recognizes that sharing data about human research subjects presents special challenges. The rights and privacy of people who participate in NIH-sponsored research must be protected at all times. Thus, data intended for broader use should be free of identifiers that would permit linkages to individual research participants and variables that could lead to deductive disclosure of individual subjects. Similarly, NIH recognizes the need to protect patentable and other proprietary data and the restriction on data sharing that may be imposed by agreements with third parties. It is not the intent of this statement to discourage, impede, or prohibit the development of commercial products from federally funded research.

There are many ways to share data. Sometimes data are included in publications. Investigators may distribute data under their own auspices. Some investigators have placed data sets in public archives while others have put data on a Web site , building in protections for privacy through the software while allowing analysis of the data. Restricted access data centers or data enclaves facilitate analyses of data too sensitive to share through other means. All of these options achieve the goals of data sharing.

However, the NIH also recognizes that in some particular instances sharing data may not be feasible. For example, studies with very small samples or those collecting particularly sensitive data should be shared only if stringent safeguards exist to ensure confidentiality and protect the identity of subjects.

The NIH will expect investigators supported by NIH funding to make their research data available to the scientific community for subsequent analyses. Consequently, the NIH will require that data sharing be addressed in grant Applications (e.g., in sections related to significance, budget, and the end of the research plan) and in the review of Applications. Funds for sharing or archiving data may be requested in the original grant application or as a supplement to an existing grant. Investigators who incorporate data sharing in the initial design of the study can more readily and economically establish adequate procedures for protecting the identities of participants and provide a useful data set with appropriate documentation. Applicants whose research will produce data that are not amenable to sharing should include in the application reasons for not making the data available. NIH encourages investigators to consult with an NIH Program Administrator prior to submitting an application to determine the appropriateness of data sharing and a suitable mechanism to disseminate the data.

This statement on data sharing is an extension of NIH policy regarding sharing research resources, which expects that recipients of NIH support will provide prompt and effective access to research tools. See NIH Grants Policy, Part II Subpart A, Availability of Research Results: Publications, Intellectual Property Rights, and Sharing Biomedical Research Resources

http://grants.nih.gov/grants/policy/nihgps_2001/nihgps_2001.pdf

This statement is also an extension of the PHS policy relating to the distribution of unique research resources produced with PHS funding:

http://grants.nih.gov/grants/guide/notice-files/not96-184.html

Principles and guidelines for sharing biomedical research resources can be found in online NIH reports at

http://www.nih.gov/science/models/sharing.html

and

http://www.nih.gov/news/researchtools/index.htm

Moreover, this statement about data sharing is consistent with the policies of many scientific journals publishing the findings of NIH-supported research.

Department of Health and Human Services (DHHS)
National Institutes of Health (NIH)
9000 Rockville Pike
Bethesda, Maryland 20892

The article below is reproduced with permission of IMV, Ltd, Greenbelt, MD, Publishers SCI/GRANTS News

Perspective

Meeting a Need

Granting agencies exist to meet a need. So do grant Applicants. The grantor is in the business of providing support for projects, programs, individuals and institutions that pursue certain goals. The grantee is in the business of pursuing those goals. Neither can exist without the other.

The concept of grantor and grantee as integral parts of the granting structure is easy to forget during the struggle to obtain grant support. It may also be a bit sophomoric. A failure to understand the concept, however, makes grant Applicants little more than mendicants, and probably even ineffective mendicants.

Effective grants professionals understand that they are giving granting agencies the opportunity to fulfill their mission. They strive to become the perfect client for the right grantor. They aim to meet the needs of the granting institution in order to meet their own needs for support.

You can meet the needs of a potential benefactor by showing that your work goes beyond a simple satisfaction of the guidelines—that it matches the spirit and purpose of the granting agency.

The first step is to find a granting agency with a need that you can meet, to identify a grantor that needs your project or program to make the best use of its funds. Whether you identify an agency through a search service, personal effort and experience, or the advice of a colleague, you must first be sure that there is a reasonable probability that it will at least consider your proposal.

The next step is to identify the grantor's needs as specifically as possible. It is not enough, for example, to know that an agency supports hospital capital campaigns. What types of hospitals? In what types of areas? Serving what types of patients? In short, what type of hospital capital campaign does the grantor *need* to support?

After deciding what a grantor needs, the Applicant must present an opportunity to fulfill that need. The Applicant organization must show that it is the perfect medium for the accomplishment of the grantor's aims. If the grantor needs to serve the needs of the poor, the Applicant must show a commitment to the needs of the poor. Ideally, it should show a record of service to the poor, and an understanding of the poor.

Rarely will the grant Applicant be able to exactly meet the needs of the grantor. Almost always, the match will be close in some respects and looser in others. But wise Applicants will make the most of those areas of grantor needs that they can best serve. They will attempt to show potential benefactors a unity of spirit and purpose.

But they won't lie. If they are smart, they will not counterfeit their aims and philosophies in an effort to persuade a grantor. They will emphasize areas of agreement, minimize areas of disagreement, and present their views honestly, because they know that reviewers are wise in the ways of the world. They know that granting agencies can spot a phony and that phonies don't get grants.

Vol. I, No. 12, December, 1989

RECAP FOR PART I: GETTING STARTED

Success in obtaining grant funding depends on:

- A good match between the proposed project and the mandate (mission) of the funding agency. Consult with the potential funding agency to be sure it is interested in your research idea.
- A good research idea
- A carefully thought-out approach to the project
- A focused, well-written proposal

Successful grant-getters need:

- Integrity
- Research skills
- Ingenuity and flexibility
- Salesmanship skills
- Communication skills
- Good human relations skills
- Administrative skills
- Persistence, dedication, patience, and the ability to work hard
- Political awareness and action

Successful grant-getters should understand:

- The nature of the Review Process
- The concept of writing for the "other" (Readers/Reviewers)
- How to respond to a set of instructions
- The basic elements of good expository writing
- The steps for creating a good Grant Application

Beginning proposal writers should know about:

- Fellowships
- Grants
- Cooperative agreements
- Contracts
- Direct costs
- Indirect costs (overhead)
- Awards specifically targeted for beginning grant seekers
- Types of granting agencies
- Where to get information about available grants
- Information to gather before applying for a grant

PART II

UNDERSTANDING THE NIH REVIEW PROCESS

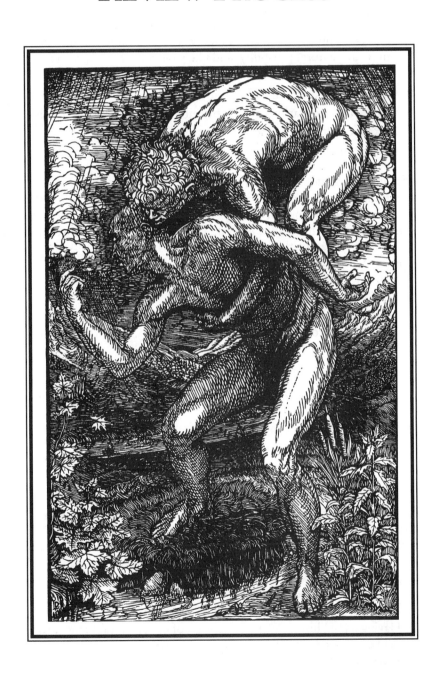

INTRODUCTION

Part II of this book deals predominantly with the review process at NIH. Proposal review at NSF and at private foundations is also briefly discussed in this book. The specifics of proposal review vary from agency to agency. It may be quite codified, formal, and stringent, as at NIH with its dual review system. Or, it may be quite informal, as is the case at some private foundations. Nonetheless, some elements are common to many agencies because, like venture capital firms, banks, and other financial institutions, funding agencies want to be sure that their money is well invested and that they will get the highest possible return on their investment. Thus, virtually all funding agencies want to know about the

- Innovative nature, feasibility, and likely outcome of the project
- Quality and reputation ("track record") of the Applicant
- Quality of the research team
- Quality and reputation of the institution with which s/he is affiliated
- Resources available to the Applicant/project
- Other support available for carrying out the project

A good grant proposal must start with a good idea

A good grant proposal requires a good research idea—a unique, interesting, innovative, important, and well-defined problem for which you can suggest a sound and viable experimental approach that is likely to lead to a tangible solution, for example, a hypothesis that you can test and either prove or disprove.

The good idea must be

- Original/novel/innovative
- Feasible
    —Do-able by you and your staff
    —Do-able at your institution
    —Acceptable to your institution
    —Acceptable to the granting agency and relevant to the mission of the granting agency
    —In conformity with human and animal welfare policies and other funding agency requirements
- Conceptually significant

    The successful resolution of the research idea (solution to the problem) should result in a substantive (nontrivial) finding that will benefit the profession or the public or—in some cases—the funding agency.

The best writing cannot turn a bad idea into a good grant proposal. However, bad writing can turn a good idea into a poor grant proposal. So planning, writing, and revising the proposal are important to the development of a successful Application. These are the aspects of proposal preparation that this book is intended to teach.

Aside from the primary requirement—a good idea—several things will help you prepare a proposal that is likely to receive a good priority score and stands a good chance of getting funded. These are:

- Having a well-focused, well-written research proposal
- Having a long history ("track record") of concentration in a particular research field or problem or—if you are a new investigator—having good training and substantive preliminary results (pilot studies) in the area of the proposed research

- Being prepared to devote a substantial effort to the proposed work

  For new investigators, 75–100% is good, 50% is OK, and below 25% is "iffy" unless you have a very good reason! A smaller percent effort may be acceptable for established investigators. Reviewers also understand that MD researchers with major clinical responsibilities are likely to have limited time for research.

- Maintaining a stable work group
  - —Funding agencies are not happy to have investigators spend agency funds for frequent interviewing and training of new candidates.
  - —A high turnover rate in laboratory personnel often indicates poor judgment in hiring and/or poor interpersonal skills, and may be indicative of poor judgment in other areas.

- Having an ample number of substantial publications, preferably ones on which you are the first author, in well-reviewed, competitive, and (if you are in a non-clinical field) preferably basic science journals
  - —Be aware of the distinction between being the first author and the senior author. The general understanding is that the first author actually did the major part of the work. In contrast, the senior author is often thought to be the director of the research group, who may or may not have done any work on the project, and whose name may have been added as the last author simply as a courtesy.
  - —Understand that a high ratio of abstracts to full-length papers is NOT a good sign.
  - —Be aware that papers in archive-type journals are less meaningful than those in prestigious peer-reviewed journals.
  - —Understand that publications, such as books, chapters in books, or review articles is generally not considered indicative of your ability to do original work. Unless there is a good reason to write one of these types of reviews, it is best to put off such time-consuming projects until you have seniority or tenure.

Understanding the review process will help you write a better grant Application, just as understanding the job description helps you prepare for a job interview. Good expository writing requires that you write for the benefit of the readers. Do not write simply what you want to say. Ask yourself:

- What do the readers, in this case the Reviewers, need or want to know?
- How can I help make the Reviewer's/Reader's job easier?

You should also consider the needs of the wider audience—in this case the potential funding agency—which wants assurance that its money will be well spent.

Thus, you must understand the review process, and the situation of the Reviewers and the potential funding agency within that process, to be able to write a good grant Application.

THE NIH REVIEW SYSTEM

NOTE: In addition to reading the advice in this book, it would be helpful for grant seekers to read some of the resources listed at

http://www.niaid.nih.gov/scripts/search/ncn/query.idq

NIH is perhaps unique in having a dual peer review system, which consists of review by, first, a Study Section (Scientific Review Group) and then by an Advisory Council.

Scientific Review Groups (SRGs)

The first level of review is by a **Scientific Review Group,** constituted by scientific discipline or biomedical subject/topic. The SRG is called an Initial Review Group (IRG) when pertaining to *grant* Applications (as opposed to contracts). The IRGs are composed of sub-committees called Study Sections. In the last decade of the twentieth century, NIH regrouped its Study Sections a number of times in response to government mandates. It is important that those who apply for grant money from NIH keep up to date with the changes that occur at the agency and in its review process.

The Study Section

- Is constituted by scientific discipline or biomedical topic
- Provides initial *scientific review* of grant Applications
- Assigns numerical ratings (which are subsequently converted to priority scores by multiplying the average of the numerical ratings by 100)—based on scientific merit—to a percentage of the Applications that are within the range that may get funded
- Makes budget recommendations but no funding decisions
  —Funding decisions are the prerogative of each Institute or other NIH funding component, which has full discretionary powers
- Does *not* set program priorities
  —Program relevance is determined by the current priorities of the potential funding institute
- Has about 14 to 20 (or more) members, all scientists
- Is headed administratively by a Scientific Review Administrator (SRA) from the Center for Scientific Review (CSR)—but discussions about the scientific merit of Applications are led by a chairperson who is a **member** of the Study Section and is an active *scientist*
- Is only advisory

Council

The second level of review is by the **Advisory Council or Board** of the potential awarding component (Institute, Center, or other unit).

The Council

- Evaluates Applications against program priorities and relevance
- Concurs with or modifies Study Section action on grant Applications—or defers the Application for further review
- Advises on policy
- Has 12 or more members
  —scientists from the extramural research community
  —public representatives
- Is only advisory
  —Council makes recommendations about funding to the Institute staff—but Council makes no decisions
  —Councils ensure that NIH gets advice in the process of deliberation and decision-making from a cross-section of the U.S. population

NOTE: **You can find the NIH National Advisory Council Rosters and the Meeting Schedule of NIH National Advisory Councils on the NIH Web site.**

Note that both the Study Section and the Council are only advisory bodies and officially have no decision-making powers.

THE TRAVELS OF AN NIH GRANT APPLICATION

A grant Application to NIH is
- Initiated by a Principal Investigator (PI)
- Submitted by her/his sponsoring institution to the NIH
- Received at NIH by the Referral Office of the Center for Scientific Review (CSR)

The Center for Scientific Review (CSR)

When a grant Application is sent to NIH, it goes first to the **Referral Office** of the *Center for Scientific Review (CSR)* where it is assigned to (a) a Study Section for initial review and (b) to a funding Institute, or other funding component, on the basis of administrative guidelines. (See list of NIH funding components in Appendix III.)

At the Referral Office, the grant is assigned a number, for example; 1 R01 EY 01234–01: Every part of this number has a meaning, as indicated in Table I.

The Center for Scientific Review (CSR)

- Is not part of any Institute
- Is a separate body that answers to the Director of NIH
- Is advisory to the Institutes
- Sets up both standing (chartered) and, when necessary, ad hoc, Study Sections to review Applications for Research Grants (R01) and certain other types of grants. (Contact NIH or visit the NIH Web site for specific types of Applications reviewed by the CSR Study Sections.) Applications submitted to NIH go first to the CSR Referral Section. The referral officers assign the grant Applications to specific Study Sections for Review. The PI of a grant Application may suggest 3 Study Sections that s/he deems appropriate to review the Application. In general, NIH is obliged to honor the PI's request.

Grant Application assignment to a Study Section

At CSR the Application is assigned for scientific review to one of more than 100 Study Sections. The number of Study Sections changes periodically as new areas of investigation emerge or the Application load in specific research areas increases.

In addition to the Initial Review Groups (IRGs) within CSR, there are also Initial Review Groups within the individual NIH Institutes. It is noteworthy that about half of NIH peer review is done outside CSR, by review units of the individual Institutes. The Institute IRGs review Applications for

Cooperative Agreements

Program Projects

Table I: Explanation of Number Assigned to NIH Grant Applications

1	R01	EY	01234	01	A1 or S1
Status of grant Application 1 = new 2 = renewal etc.	Type of grant Application R = research F = fellowship etc.	Proposed Funding Institute or other Component. See Appendix III for a list of acronyms for NIH funding components	ID number of the grant within the Institute.	Year of the project. (e.g., **01** means first year.) Note that a senior researcher who has been continually funded to work on the same project, with the same title, for 31 years would have a "31" in this place.	Sometimes there is a suffix following the "Year of project"; for example, A1 means "amended" (commonly referred to as "revised"); S1 means "supplement." Note that A2 would signify that the Application had been submitted for review 3 times: i.e., the original Application and 2 revised Applications.

> Center Grants
> Institutional Training Grants
> Contracts
> Responses to Requests for Applications (RFAs)

The Institutes also have Special Emphasis Panels (SEPs). In this book I will discuss primarily the review process at CSR.

- CSR has Referral Officers who assign Applications to specific Study Sections for review. The referral officers are generally scientists who have become Scientific Review Administrators and have had extensive experience running Study Sections.
- Referral Officers rely heavily on the title, project description (abstract), and specific aims of an Application to make Study Section assignments.
- The Referral Officers use specific guidelines to make assignments of grant Applications to Study Sections and may discuss the appropriateness of a Study Section with the SRA of the relevant Study Section.
- When electronic submission of grant proposals becomes the predominant mode of grant submission, Study Section assignment probably will be made by computer—using keywords assigned by the Principal Investigator.

You may suggest 3 Initial Review Groups that would be appropriate to review your Application.

- Attach such correspondence to the Application at the time of submission.
- **Suggestions will be considered, but the final determination will be made by the CSR.**

    —An important aside: Do not leave things to chance. Once NIH goes to totally paperless Applications, you should get an e-mail acknowledging receipt of your Application. If you are submitting an Application on paper, always attach a **self-addressed, stamped** postcard to the original of your Application. On the postcard write:

    > The title of your Application _____
    > By (your name) _____
    > Was received by _____
    > On (date) _____
    > Thank you.

    Mark your calendar! If you do not get acknowledgment of receipt of your Application within 2 weeks, call the relevant agency to determine whether your Application was received and logged in by the agency. If your Application does not arrive at the agency on time it is YOUR responsibility, not the agency's responsibility!

    —Information about Study Section membership—and the advice of colleagues who are "savvy" about the grants process—can be of great help in directing a proposal to the most suitable Study Section. If you go to

    http://www.csr.nih.gov/committees/rosterindex.asp

    you can access an alphabetical listing (*by acronym*) of the name and description of each CSR-chartered study section, a list of the members, e-mail addresses for the Scientific Review Administrators (SRAs) for each Study Section, and the Scientific Review Group meeting schedules. General information about CSR can be found at

    http://www.crs.nih.gov

- If you think there has been a serious error in the Study Section assignment of your Application, you may request corrective action by writing to the SRA of the Study Section.

Grant Application assignment to an Institute or other funding component

At CSR your proposal is also assigned for management and possible funding to one, or in some cases two (dual assignment), of the NIH funding components listed on the NIH Web site

http://www.nih.gov/icd/

NOTE: Not all the ICDs (which now seems to stand for Institutes, Centers, and Offices) are funding components. The above site also gives summaries of the missions of each of the ICDs as does the site below

http://www.nih.gov/icd/programs.htm

The Referral Officers use specific guidelines to make assignments of Grant Applications to Institutes (or other funding components). The assignment is made according to the *overall mission* and *specific programmatic mandates* and interests of the Institute or other funding component. In the future, assignment of potential funding component(s) will most probably be made by computer.

As is the case with Study Section assignment, you may suggest/request an NIH funding component that would be appropriate for your Application. Suggestions/requests about funding component assignment should go into the same letter as suggestions/requests about Study Section assignment.

- Attach such correspondence to the Application at the time of submission.
- Suggestions will be considered, but the final determination will be made by the CSR.

At the Institute the Application is assigned to a member of the Institute program staff who

- Is your primary Institute contact for all matters dealing with your grant Application before and after the review process
- Is responsible for administration of the grant if the Application is funded
- Is expected to attend the Study Section meeting at which the Application is reviewed—but only as an observer; i.e., s/he does not participate in the review and evaluation of the Application
- Is prepared to defend and elucidate the recommendations of the Study Section to Council

   The member of the Institute program staff assigned to your Grant Application acts as an ombudsperson for the Application with respect to procedures that affect the Grant Application/grant at NIH. It is the responsibility of that individual to respond to questions by the Applicant. These questions may relate to (1) priority scores, (2) items within the Summary Statement, (3) rebuttals, or (4) advice about the course of action to be taken when a proposal is not funded. In addition, s/he can be questioned about the relevance of potential research ideas—for future proposals—with respect to the research priorities of the funding Institute/component. The Institute program staff members are instructed to remain neutral in all dealings pertaining to Grant Applications/grants.

When assignment to a Study Section and a funding component is completed, the PI is informed of the assignments.

The Study Section (the first stage of NIH peer review)

Each Study Section is composed of about 14 to 20 (or sometimes more) scientists (including, when appropriate, research-oriented clinicians, community practitioners, ethicists, etc.) chosen by the SRA for their competence in particular scientific areas. One of these scientists is selected by the SRA to be the **chairperson** of the Study Section. The chairperson moderates the discussion of the scientific merit of the proposals during the Study Section meeting, whereas the SRA attends to all administrative and policy aspects of the proceedings. Each Study Section meets 3 times a year, usually for 2 to 3 days at a time, and reviews on the order of 40 to 120 Applications.

The Scientific Review Administrator (SRA)

- Is a Federal employee who is in charge of a Study Section
- Usually has a Ph.D. degree and was an active scientist prior to becoming an SRA

- Nominates Study Section members

  Sometimes solicits recommendations from retiring Study Section members
- Selects the chairperson for the Study Section
- Performs administrative and technical review of Applications
- Selects primary and secondary Reviewers and Readers (Discussants) for each Application
- Manages the administrative aspects of the Study Section meeting
- Prepares the Summary Statements

  The Summary Statements are sometimes still referred to as "Pink Sheets" although they have not been printed on pink paper for many years
- When requested, provides information about Study Section recommendations to

  Institute staff

  Advisory Councils

  PIs

Criteria for selections of Study Section members

- Scientific excellence

  As demonstrated by

  —doctoral degree or equivalent

  —grant and publication record
- Breadth of expertise
- Respect in the scientific community
- Demonstrated scientific expertise
- Mature judgment, fairness, and evenhandedness in review
- Balanced perspective and objectivity
- Willingness to do the work required
- Ability to work effectively in a group context
- Clarity of presentations and quality of participation at meetings
- Interest in serving on a Study Section

Other considerations for choice of Study Section members

- Members must represent a wide range of expertise related to main subjects reviewed by that Study Section.

  For example, selected areas of competence represented on the *Surgery, Anesthesiology and Trauma Study Section* include:

    —Biochemistry

    —Burn physiology and electrolyte metabolism

    —Cardiovascular and pulmonary physiology

    —Clinical anesthesiology

    —Drug metabolism (anesthetics)

    —General surgery

    —Immunology and transplantation

    —Nutrition

    —Pharmacology

> —Pulmonary embolism
> —Shock and trauma
> —Toxicology and anesthetic drugs
> —Urology
> —Vascular surgery

- There may be no more than 1 member from a given institution.
- Member may be on only 1 Study Section at a time.
- Member generally serves 4 years but may serve longer.

  The maximum service permitted is 2 *non-consecutive* 4-year terms (total of 8 years) in a 12-year period.

- No more than 25% of members may be Federal employees.

  In practice, CSR aims to have no more than 1 Federal employee per Study Section

- The membership must have representation—insofar as possible
  > —of both genders
  > —from diverse ethnic groups
  > —from a diverse geographic distribution

- Potential member usually has history of NIH funding

  See also **"Guidelines for Study Section Chairs"** at

  http://www.csr.nih.gov/events/guidelineschairs.htm

NOTE: Study Section members are expected to be familiar with NIH procedures and requirements for consultants (Reviewers) about confidentiality and avoidance of conflict of interest.

The NIH Web site

http://www.csr.nih.gov/Committees/rosterindex.asp

lists the following for every NIH Study Section:
- Members
- Chairperson
- Scientific Review Administrator

Ad hoc members may not appear on this site in a timely fashion. It's a good idea to call the SRA and ask whether there will be any ad hoc Reviewers at the Study Section meeting and, if so, who they are. **NEVER ask—or "fish" for information about—who the Reviewers for your Application are/were!!!**

It is wise to be familiar with the membership of the Study Section that will review your proposal. The Scientific Review Administrator of the Study Section assigns specific grants to particular Reviewers. Each Grant Application is assigned primary and secondary Reviewers who are responsible for its in-depth review. Sometimes a third Reviewer is assigned to an Application. Sometimes the SRA will send an Application out for additional reviews by mail.

The Reviewers study the Application carefully and sometimes do a great deal of "research" to determine the merits of the Application. See

http://www.niaid.nih.gov/ncn/grants/basics/basics_c2.htm

As with any group of individuals, the Reviewers who make up a Study Section tend to represent the range of personality types. Some are conscientious and/or compulsive; others may be more casual. How much homework or library work a given Reviewer will do in the course of reviewing a particular proposal will depend also, to some extent, on the pressures and time constraints of the Reviewer's own schedule (both at work and at home) at the time of review. Because it is generally not possible for you to predict the situation of your Reviewer, it is critical that your Application be clearly understandable on its own—without an Appendix—and without extensive trips to the library, or the Internet on the part of the Reviewers. See

http://www.niaid.nih.gov/ncn/grants/write/write_d1.htm

In addition to assigning two or three primary Reviewers to an Application, the Scientific Review Administrator also assigns two or more Readers (Discussants) to each Application. Readers, like primary Reviewers, are expected to (1) be very knowledgeable about the Applications to which they have been assigned and (2) participate actively in the discussion about that Application. But, unlike the primary Reviewers, the Readers are not required to prepare a written report about the Application—although some choose to do so. Some SRAs apparently ask Readers to turn in brief written comments about the proposals for which they are responsible.

The Scientific Review Administrators of Study Sections sometimes also enlists ad hoc members for specific meetings when additional expertise in a particular field is necessary. Like regular Study Section members, ad hoc Reviewers vote on the disposition of the Application and assign priority scores. The names of the ad hoc Reviewers are included in the roster of each Study Section meeting, though they may not be posted until close to or after the Study Section meeting.

The Scientific Review Administrators of Study Sections also may request "outside" opinions about an Application, by mail.

Each member of the Study Section is sent a copy of every Application to be considered at the meeting except those in which they may have a **conflict of interest**. To enable Study Section members to participate in the discussion and rating of all Applications, all members are expected to be familiar with all the Applications. The primary and secondary Reviewers are responsible for thoroughly evaluating—in writing (according to a set of guidelines provided by CSR)—the scientific merits of the Applications assigned to them. Reviewers must sign a Certification of No Conflict of Interest.

> **NOTE: You, the PI, will NOT be given, and should NOT ask for, the names of the primary and/or secondary Reviewers—or the Readers—of your Application!!!**

At the Study Section meeting

Study Section meetings are open to the public—limited by space available—for approximately 45 minutes at the beginning of the first session of the first day of each Study Section meeting during the discussion of administrative details relating to Study Section business. Thereafter, the meetings are closed and confidential. See

http://www.niaid.nih.gov/ncn/grants/basics/basics_d1.htm

The primary Reviewers come to the Study Section meeting with a written report in which they have assessed the Application, to the best of their ability, according to 5 criteria that were last revised in October 1997.

The review criteria are:

- **Significance**
  —Does the proposed research address an important problem?
  —If the aims of the Application are achieved, how will scientific knowledge be advanced?

- **Approach**
  —Are the conceptual framework, design, methods, and analyses adequately developed, well-integrated, and appropriate to the aim(s) of the project?

- **Innovation**
  —Does the project employ novel concepts, approaches, or methods?
  —Are the aims original and innovative?
  —Does the project challenge existing paradigms or develop new methodologies or technologies?

- **Investigator**
  —Is the investigator well-trained and well-suited to carry out this work?
  —What is the investigator's "track record"?

- **Environment**
  —Does the scientific environment in which the work will be done contribute to the probability of success?
  —Are the facilities suitable (including availability of resources and scientific ambiance) for carrying out the project?

NIH **Reviewers** are provided with a set of specific instructions, which they are asked to follow when they write their reports about each Application for which they are a primary or secondary Reviewer.

Although the **Readers** are not required to bring a written report to the Study Section meeting, they are expected to provide substantial discussion about an Application's major strengths and weaknesses. The Readers sometimes also help put an Application into final perspective for the Study Section to help assure that the best Applications are supported.

The **non-primary Reviewers**—who may have read a particular Application only cursorily, but who are nonetheless obliged to assign a numerical rating (later converted to a priority score) to each Application reviewed at the Study Section meeting—especially value the additional opinions provided by the Readers about Applications. Thus, **the Readers may have substantial influence on the numerical ratings assigned by non-primary Reviewers,** and, in some sense, may play a pivotal role in the review of an Application and its ultimate averaged priority score. Because the Readers' input is sometimes critical, the Scientific Review Administrator may—after review of an Application—ask a Reader to provide one or more written paragraphs of critique for inclusion into the Summary Statement. Some SRAs encourage Readers to arrive at the Study Section meeting with some written comments about the Application.

"Streamlined Review Process"

Beginning in 1994, with the move to "Re-invent Government," NIH was asked to make changes that would streamline the review process and save the time the Study Section spends in session.

In September 1994, a new procedure was adopted for review of R01 and certain other types of Applications. The procedure was initially referred to as "Triage," but was later renamed **"Streamlined Review Process."** This process gives assigned Reviewers the option to suggest which Applications, in their opinion, would score in the bottom 50% of priority scores for that review cycle. Essentially, Reviewers are asked to (1) arrange all the proposals (except those to be deferred for additional information) in order of merit and (2) suggest that the bottom 50% be "Streamlined out," that is, not be discussed (reviewed) during the Study Section meeting.

Most of the "Streamlining" is expected to occur prior to the Study Section meeting. But an Application may also be "Streamlined out" during the meeting. Any Application designated as "Streamlined out" may be recalled to full review **at any time** before or during the meeting **by any one member** of the Study Section. **Thus, such elimination of an Application from review by the whole Study Section must be unanimous.**

Applications that are "Streamlined out" are left "Unscored." However, although such Applications are not discussed at the Study Section meeting, they **do get a full review** by at least 2 reviewers. For an Application to be "Streamlined out," the primary reviewers must concur on this decision. Moreover, any other Reviewer on the Study Section may recall the proposal for full review; that is, **an objection from even a single member of the relevant Study Section brings the Application back for full review at the Study Section meeting.** Applications that are "Streamlined out" are not assigned a priority score and are referred to as the "Unscored" Applications.

Note that being "Streamlined out"/"Unscored" says nothing about the quality of an Application. For example, in theory, the Study Section might receive 100 superb Applications for review in a given review cycle. The members of the Study Section would be obliged to arrange the Applications in order of merit and the last 50 Applications, despite all being very meritorious, would be "Streamlined out." Given that the funding rate at NIH has been about 30% (averaged over all NIH funding components) for almost two decades, there is still a sizable buffer between Applications that are discussed at the Study Section meeting and those that are "Streamlined out."

> **A WORD OF CAUTION:** A disappointed PI (Dr. X) who may know someone on a Study Section should keep in mind the **inappropriateness** of berating the Study Section member for not recalling Dr. X's proposal for full review. It is the Study Section member's obligation to permit appropriate Applications to be "Streamlined out" unless there is a **very cogent, rational, non-personal reason** not to do so.

- The Summary Statements for **scored** Applications consist of the individual Reviewer's reports plus a summary of the discussion about the about the Application by the Study Section members.
- The Summary Statements for Applications that are "Streamlined out" (left "Unscored") consist of the individual Reviewer's reports plus a brief explanation of the "Streamlined Review Process."

"Unscored" Applications are not routinely forwarded to the relevant Advisory Council (the second level of NIH peer review). However, Council has a list of all Applications submitted to NIH for each submission deadline and may request to see any of the "Unscored" Applications.

It is important to reiterate that

- **An Application that is "Streamlined out" does not necessarily lack merit**

  If an Application is "Streamlined out"

  —It means ONLY that the Application *is not likely to be awarded in the current funding climate.*

  —It does NOT give the PI any information about what the Reviewers thought about the quality of the Application.

For Applications that have NOT been "Streamlined out"

- The primary and secondary Reviewers present their reports at the meeting.

  At some Study Sections, Reviewers read their reports verbatim; in others, Reviewers only summarize their reports. The pattern is determined by the SRA and/or the chairperson.

- Presentation of the formal report is followed by comments from the assigned Reader(s).

- Then there is general discussion, by the Study Section members, of the

  —merits and pitfalls of the proposal

  —qualifications of the principal investigator (PI)

  —appropriateness of the proposed staff

  All Study Section members are expected to

  —be familiar with the general substance of all of the Grant Applications to be reviewed

  —participate in the discussion

Administrators from the relevant NIH Institute(s) may be present at Study Section meetings. They may be asked to provide administrative information, for example, about the Applicant's grant history, but they do not participate in the general discussion.

Possible actions taken on Applications being reviewed

Anytime during—or at the end of—the discussion about an Application, which may take anywhere from 10 minutes to as long as an hour, a member of the Study Section can make a recommendation that the Application be designated as

- **"Unscored"**

  No numerical rating is assigned

  or

- **"Deferred for additional information"**

  The deferral mechanism is used when a basically good proposal is missing readily definable information that the Study Section members think the PI can provide by mail or—in some cases—via a project site visit. For Applications that are deferred, the Reviewers delineate for the SRA what additional information needs to be supplied by the PI to enable appropriate review by the Study Section. After the Study Section meeting, the SRA contacts the PI to convey this information. Deferred Applications are generally reviewed again at the next Study Section meeting (i.e., in about 4 months) if the PI has responded to the request for additional information in a timely manner.

If either of these recommendations ("Unscored" or "Deferred") is adopted, the Applications so designated are

NOT further discussed by the Study Section

NOT given priority scores

NOT considered by Council

"Scored" Applications

If an Application is NOT designated "Unscored" or "Deferred for additional information," the Application is

- informally referred to as a "Scored" Application
- assigned a numerical rating by each Study Section member
- the numerical rating is subsequently converted to a priority score

    Priority score = 100 × the average of the numerical ratings assigned by the individual Reviewers

For each Application that is to be scored, each member of the Study Section individually records, **by secret ballot**, a numerical rating that reflects her/his personal evaluation of the scientific merit of the proposed research. The primary Reviewers may suggest an appropriate priority score range or merit descriptor (Table II) for the Application at the end of their formal report about the Application and before the individual Reviewers are asked to assign a numerical rating for the Application. Reviewers by mail are also expected to recommend a merit rating or a merit descriptor for Applications that they are asked to review.

Table II: Numerical Ratings and Corresponding Merit Descriptors

Numerical Rating	Corresponding Merit Descriptor
1.0–1.5	Outstanding
1.5–2.0	Excellent
2.0–2.5	Very good
2.5–3.5	Good
3.5–5.0	Acceptable

Numerical ratings are assigned according to a scale of 1.0 (best) to 5.0 (worst), in increments of 0.1. As noted above, the numerical ratings are later averaged and multiplied by 100 to generate priority scores.

The research proposed in scored Applications is considered to be significant and substantial. The recommendation to assign a merit rating may be for

- the time and amount requested

or

- an adjusted time and amount

The budget is discussed *after* the individual Reviewers assign a **confidential** numerical rating for the Application on their scoring sheet. **In theory, the budget is not supposed to influence the Reviewers with respect to their assignment of a numerical rating for the Application.**

A site visit

Occasionally, the Study Section may recommend a project site visit to the principal investigator's laboratory. Because site visits are costly, they are now used sparingly—and primarily for the more complex Applications such as Program Project Grant Applications.

A site visit to a Principal Investigator's laboratory is recommended

- before a Study Section meeting if a primary Reviewer or the Scientific Review Administrator recognizes the need for additional information that cannot be obtained by mail or telephone. That is, when information needed to make a recommendation about an Application can be obtained only at the proposed research or training site.

- at a Study Section or Council meeting in conjunction with a "Deferral" action.
- when the Application involves complex coordination of individuals or institutions, for example, Program Project Grants and Training Grants.

The site visit is made by a special **Site Visit Committee.**

- The Scientific Review Administrator

  —selects the members of the project site visit team
  —accompanies the team
  —coordinates the proceedings during the site visit

  Typically, the site visit team (for an R01 Application) is composed of 3 or more members of the Study Section and, when necessary, ad hoc consultants who are experts in critical aspects of the proposed work. Representatives from the potential awarding Institute also attend the site visit as observers. The site visit team reports its findings and recommendations back to the Study Section in time to be considered at the next meeting of the Study Section.

Reverse Site Visit

In the past, site visits, as their name implies, have been to the PI's laboratory. Because of increasing budgetary constraints, the relevant PI and members of her/his laboratory may now be invited to come to the Bethesda/Washington, DC, area to meet with the site visit team. This is referred to as a "Reverse Site Visit."

Conference Call Reviews

NIH also occasionally does Conference Call Reviews—a sort of site visit by phone.

After the Study Section meeting

At the end of each Study Section meeting, the Scientific Review Administrator prepares a Summary Statement for each grant Application. **Summary Statements have a specific format.**

All Summary Statements contain the primary and secondary Reviewers' reports, i.e., critiques of the project proposed in the grant Application.

> Reviewers are expected to modify their written critiques during the review of an Application—for example, removing a criticism that was deemed to be invalid following group discussion.

Summary Statements for scored Applications also have a

- "Description of Project"
- paragraph summarizing the Study Section's discussion about the proposal (including budget recommendations, if appropriate)

Summary Statements for "Unscored" Applications

- contain an explanation of the "Streamlined Review Process" instead of the summary paragraph

Some Summary Statements contain notations about special points, such as

- a split vote

  A split vote refers to the situation at an NIH Study Section meeting when the members do not agree on a voting category for a particular grant Application. If there are 2 or more dissenting members, they are required to write a Minority Report explaining their reasons for dissenting. If only 1 member of the Study Section gives a dissenting vote, a Minority Report is optional. In this case the SRA may designate whether such a report must be written. If the SRA does not request a Minority Report, the dissenting member has the option of writing one.

- a potentially hazardous experimental procedure
- concerns about proposed human studies
- concerns about proposed use of vertebrate animals

In preparation for generating the Summary Statement

- The numerical scores assigned by the individual Study Section members for each scored Application are averaged and multiplied by 100 to provide a 3-digit rating for the proposal. This rating is known as the *priority score.*

  In the process of averaging the numerical scores, the SRA has both responsibility and latitude to ignore unsubstantiated outlying scores. This avoids the problem of an occasional low score given for the wrong reasons. A very low score assigned to an Application by a Reviewer who thinks the other Reviewers are missing a major fault in the Application is not considered an outlying score. If a probable outlying score comes to light during the discussion at the Study Section meeting, other Reviewers may adjust their scores to compensate. If the SRA discovers an unanticipated outlying score after the Study Section meeting, s/he may discard the score after discussion with a supervisor or may decide on a re-review if the issues are serious.

- Percentile ranks are calculated from the averaged Priority Scores.

  The Priority Scores and Percentile rankings are the primary, but not the only, determinants for funding decisions.

  Funding decisions are also

  —influenced by the assessment of the Application by Council
  —based on program considerations (program relevance and priorities)
  —determined by availability of funds

- Applications that are "Deferred for additional information" or left "Unscored" are not given Priority Scores or Percentile ranks.

What PIs should expect after the Study Section meeting

NOTE: The Priority Score and Percentile rank are sent to the PI, approximately 2 weeks after the Study Section meeting. See

http://www.niaid.nih.gov/ncn/grants/charts/timeline_review.htm

With the advent of electronic grants administration, the Priority Score and Percentile rank are now sent to the PI via e-mail.

- The Summary Statement has historically been sent to the PI about 6 to 8 weeks after the Study Section meeting. With the advent of electronic grants administration, the Summary Statement is sent via e-mail and generally gets to the PI in appreciably less time.

  —If your Application was "Unscored," you generally get your Summary Statement sooner than if it got scored.
  —Find out (from the NIH Web site) when the Study Section that will review your Grant Application is scheduled to meet.

—Mark the meeting dates for the Study Section on your calendar.

> If you have not received your Summary Statement by 4 to 6 weeks after the Study Section meeting, contact your SRA.

- The Summary Statements for scored Applications are generally also forwarded to the Council of the appropriate Institute (or other funding component) for further review and possible recommendation for funding.

  Applications that are "Deferred for additional information" or designated "Unscored" are NOT sent to the Council/Board.

  Some institutes do not routinely send all scored Applications for Council review. **However, Councils and Institutes have the flexibility to make special exceptions (based on program or policy considerations and may request to see certain Applications that were submitted to the Study Section for review (whether scored or not scored) that are NOT automatically sent to them.**

NOTE: All Applications reviewed, whether given a priority rating, or designated "Unscored," are included in the calculation of Percentiles.

The Council (the second stage of NIH peer review)

Each NIH Institute has a National Advisory Council composed of 12 to 16 individuals, approximately 25% of whom are lay people; the remaining members are scientists. The Scientific Review Administrator of a Study Section attends the Council meeting when a grant Application reviewed in her/his Study Section is discussed.

The Council considers the Summary Statements from each Study Section and adds its own review based on judgments of both scientific merit and relevance to the program goals of the assigned Institute. *In some cases, the program relevance can alter the ranking position of the Application for funding.* The Council then makes recommendations on funding. Consideration by the Council constitutes the second half of the peer review process.

Overall, and within the confines of availability of funds, the *awards are based on both scientific merit and program considerations*. Thus, it should not come as a great shock if an Application with a worse priority score (higher number) is funded in preference to an Application with a better priority score (lower number).

Keep in mind that both the Study Section and the Council are only advisory. Neither the Study Section nor the Council has the power to make funding decisions. Final decisions about funding are made by the Director of the relevant Institute or funding component.

For most Applications the minimum time from receipt of the Application to notification of award has historically been approximately 10 months. The initial scientific merit review by the Study Section generally takes place within 4 months of receipt of the Application, after which the results for most Applications recommended for funding by the Study Section are conveyed to the relevant Institute Advisory Councils. A copy of the Summary Statement for the Grant Application is usually sent by the Institute/funding component to the PI about one month before the Advisory Council meets. Council generally meets about 3 or 4 months after the initial review by the Study Section, and awards are made as early as within 1 month, or as late as 1 year, after the Council review. With the advent of electronic grants administration, the time taken for this process is expected to be reduced appreciably.

SOME GRANTSMANSHIP ADVICE

Before you work on your next grant Application, take a look at some of the **tutorials** at

> **http://www.niaid.nih.gov/ncn/grants/default.htm**

and at the **checklist** given on the NIH Web site

> **http://www.niaid.nih.gov/ncn/grants/charts/checklists.htm**

Know your Study Section

NIH Study Section members usually serve for 4 years. Members rotate on and off a Study Section in July in a staggered fashion that assures overlap between old and new members. Check the membership rosters on the NIH Web site

- Go to **http://www.csr.nih.gov/Committees/rosterindex.asp#A**
- Click on
  "CSR Regular Standing Study Section Rosters"
- In the middle column, find and click on the name of the Study Section of interest
- Under the name of the Study Section at the top of the page, click on "[Name of SS] Roster"
- Click on the second column from the left, "Membership Roster" to view the chartered membership roster, if available.

  For actual meeting rosters, click on the date for which you want to see the actual Study Section participants in the right-hand column called "Meeting Rosters."

  Current rosters are usually

  —posted 4 weeks before the Study Section meeting date

  —are only tentative

  —list all members present, whether permanent or *temporary*

  —provide the total scope of expertise that may be present at the meeting

---

NOTE: Because Web sites are not always updated in a timely fashion, you may want to call the SRA of the Study Section for the latest information on the membership roster of the Study Section meeting.

It is important to understand that if you submit an Application and subsequently submit a **revised** Application, your revised Application may or may not be reviewed by the same primary Reviewers and Readers. This might be because one—or both—of your original Reviewers may have completed their term of service on the Study Section since you submitted the previous Application.

The essence of the grant review process is reasonably consistent throughout all CSR Study Sections. However, the subtle factors that influence the review process, for example, the scoring of proposals, may differ from one Study Section to another and may change as the membership and workload of a Study Section changes. Each Study Section has a distinct "culture" (i.e., a set of unwritten but generally agreed upon policies) that is determined by the

- Scientific Review Administrator
- Chairperson

- Current membership (4–year staggered terms)
- Number of Grant Applications being reviewed
- Subject matter under review and the context

Information about the number of Applications reviewed and awarded by CSR may be found at the NIH Web site.

> **NOTE:** Do not be surprised to find that the NIH Web site information is not always as up-to-date as one might wish.

Think about the Reviewers' workload

The number of Grant Applications reviewed by CSR has increased by about 60% since 1975. This increase has created a tremendous increase in workload for Reviewers.

Grant Application writers should appreciate that Reviewers receive a small honorarium plus expenses (at the government rate) for attendance at the Study Section meetings (usually 2 or 3 days per meeting; 3 meetings per year). However, they receive NO financial compensation for the many hours of work they devote—prior to the meeting—to reviewing proposals in preparation for the meeting.

To be a successful Grant Application writer, it is important to think about the Reviewers as real people who have many important obligations in addition to reviewing your proposal.

It is to your advantage to make *your* Reviewers' job as easy as possible *before*—and *during*—the Study Section meeting. Give the Reviewer good cause to become your advocate rather than your adversary:

- "You never get a second chance to make a first impression."

  The Reviewer is likely to form a first impression within seconds of pulling your Application out of the carton. Be certain that it is a **good impression**. Your Application should look neat and should be responsive to *all* instructions provided by the agency either in the instruction packet or on the NIH (or other agency) Web site.

- Rarely will a Reviewer be able to read/review your Application from start to finish in one sitting.

  —Make it easy for Reviewers, who are likely to read your proposal in bits and pieces (and in odd times and places), to understand what you propose to do without having to do much backtracking.

  —Imagine yourself in the Reviewer's "place" and present information as you would like to have it presented if you were the Reviewer.

- When you write your proposal be

  —accurate

  —clear

  —concise

  —meticulous about following the instructions

- Never cause the Reviewer to have to guess what you plan to do or what you are trying to say.

  —Explain precisely and clearly what you plan to do.

  —Although some Reviewers may know more about a subject than the grantee, **never take it for granted** that the Reviewer will "know what you mean."

—Give all necessary information
    in the correct places
    in logical order
    according to the required format
    within the stipulated page limitations
—Don't make the Reviewer have to search the library/Internet to find out how you plan to do your experiments.

Dr. Jane Koretz, who has served as a member of the NIH Visual Science-A Study Section in past years said, "The heavy loads that Reviewers must cope with reduce their patience with poor writing, implicit assumptions about the expertise of the Reviewers, and poor layout. A good guideline for Applicants would be to assume that they are writing for a qualified scientist in a somewhat related field, rather than an expert directly in the PI's area."

Keep up to date

It is extremely important that you keep up to date with what is going on at NIH and at other agencies to which you might apply for funding. In the last decade of the twentieth century, NIH:

- adopted a "Triage" system (later renamed "Streamlined Review Process") in its Study Section review of grant Applications
- changed the nature of the Summary Statement
- began attempting to identify research that is "high risk" but is likely to have "high impact" on our knowledge base
- adopted a "chunk" system for grant budgets that were below $250,000 per year
- instituted a **"Just In Time"** program whereby Grant Applicants do not have to provide certain administrative details (which had previously been required in the Application) until the Application has been judged to be "likely to be funded."

Also, during this period, new directors were installed at both NIH and NSF.

Undoubtedly, the future will bring more changes.

It is your responsibility to watch for changes at NIH and other funding agencies that may be of interest to you, so that you will always be able to provide the potential funding agency with the information they ask for.

- Access the *NIH Guide for Grants and Contracts* weekly via computer
  You can have the Table of Contents e-mailed to you by contacting:
  NIHTOC-L@LIST.NIH.GOV
- Maintain contact with—and establish a good relationship with—the administrators of your funding Institute.
- Keep track of the funding situation—both nationally and within your NIH Institute.
- Understand current funding priorities for research relevance at your funding Institute—and at other organizations where you might seek financial support.
- Visit the Office for Grants and Contracts (sponsored research) at your institution.
  —Get to know the people and the resources.
  —Determine whether the office publishes a newsletter.
  —Ask whether the office searches the *Federal Register* for items of interest to members of the organization's research community.

—Ask whether the office alerts faculty members about appropriate funding opportunities.

- Subscribe to pertinent newsletters that publish news of available funding sources and grant submission deadlines, e.g., those published by various professional organizations.
- Get on the mailing list of funding agencies that may support your type of research.
- Always look for the revision date on the Grant Application form you use, and be sure you use the latest version.
- Always check the funding agency's Web site for possible recent changes in grant Application instructions.

For information about the review process at private foundations, see:

—Tips for Applying to Private Foundations For Grant Money, by L. Reif-Lehrer, in *The Scientist*; 1991; Sept. 16, p. 20.

—Appendix V.

RECAP FOR PART II: UNDERSTANDING THE REVIEW PROCESS

Understanding the review process will help you write a better Grant Application.

A fundable grant proposal requires that the PI have:

- A good research idea
- A well-focused, well-written research proposal
- A good "track record" and/or substantive preliminary results (pilot studies)
- A substantial percent effort
- A stable work group
- An ample number of substantial, preferably peer-reviewed, publications

NIH has a dual peer review system:

- Initial Review Group (Study Section)
- Advisory Council

The travels of an R01 Grant Application to NIH:

- Initiated by PI
- Submitted by PI's sponsoring institution
- Received by Referral Office at CSR
- Assigned a number, for example, 1 R01 EY 01234–01
- Assigned to a Study Section; PI may suggest 3 suitable Study Sections
- Assigned to an Institute or funding component (possible dual assignment); PI may suggest an appropriate funding component
- Assigned to a member of the Institute's program staff (this person is the Institute's contact for the PI)
- Study section and funding component assignments are sent to PI

About the Study Section:

- Supervised by a Scientific Review Administrator (SRA) who attends to administrative and policy aspects of proceedings.
- Membership consists of 14 to 20 (or more) scientists (chosen by the SRA according to certain selection criteria).
- One member is selected by SRA to be the chairperson. The chairperson moderates the discussion of the scientific merit of proposals.
- The Study Section meets 3 times a year.
- The SRA assigns specific Grant Application to particular Reviewers (primary and secondary) and Readers (Discussants) for in-depth review prior to the Study Section meeting.

Primary Reviewers' reports assess the:

- **Significance** of the proposed research
- PI's **Approach** to the project
- **Innovation** of the project
- Suitability and "track record" of the **Investigator**
- **Environment** and facilities available to the project

Actions on R01 Grant Applications:

- Left "Unscored"
- Deferred for additional information and/or site visit
- Assigned a scientific merit rating via secret ballot on a scale of 1.0 (best) to 5.0 (worst).

Numerical Rating	Corresponding Merit Descriptor
1.0–1.5	Outstanding
1.5–2.0	Excellent
2.0–2.5	Very good
2.5–3.5	Good
3.5–5.0	Acceptable

- Calculate a Priority score by multiplying the average of the numerical (merit) ratings by 100.

After the Study Section meeting:

- SRA prepares Summary Statements.
- Merit ratings are averaged and converted to priority scores.
- Percentile ranks are calculated.
- Priority score and Percentile rank are sent to the PI.
- Summary Statement is sent to the PI.
- Scored Applications are sent to the Council for further review and possible recommendation for funding.

About the Council:

- Each NIH Institute has a National Advisory Council.
- Each council has about 12 to 16 members (scientists + 25% lay-people).
- The SRA of the Study Section attends the Council meeting during discussion of grant Applications reviewed in her/his Study Section.
- The Council reviews the Application's scientific merit and relevance to the program goals of the assigned Institute.
- The Council makes recommendations on funding.

Basis of awards:

- Scientific merit
- Program considerations
- Amount of funding available

Be aware:

- **Both the Study Section and the Council are only advisory. Neither body has decision-making powers.**
- Final funding decisions are made by program staff at Institutes/funding components.
- Program relevance can alter the ranking position of a proposal for funding.
- The time from Application receipt to award used to be about 10 months. This time has been shortened since the advent of electronic aids to the grant Application review process.
- Keep up to date with funding/events/changes at NIH and other funding agencies. Get agency literature. Make frequent checks of the agency's Web site.
- Maintain contact with the potential funding agency.
- Get to know people/resources at your institutional office for sponsored research.
- Give the Reviewer good cause to become your advocate:
  - —Think about Reviewers' workload.
  - —Write accurately, clearly, and concisely.
  - —Follow instructions and page limits meticulously.
  - —Put information in correct places, in logical order, and in the required format.
  - —Write for the average Reviewer: a qualified scientist in a somewhat related field, not necessarily an expert in your field.

PART III

PARTS OF THE GRANT APPLICATION

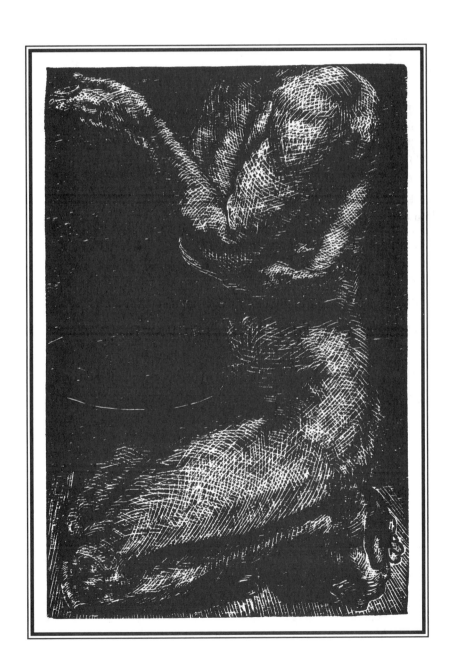

INTRODUCTION

The Application form for an NIH investigator-initiated Research Grant (R01) is Public Health Service (PHS) Form 398. This form is revised periodically, and the changes vary from minor to extensive. However, the general overall format has not changed dramatically in the more than 35 years that I have been writing proposals, except for: (1) introduction of page limits, and (2) discontinuing the requirement for submission of detailed budget pages for Applicants requesting less than a certain amount of funding.

You might find it helpful to begin by looking through the set of slides at

http://www.nichd.nih.gov/funding/apply_nih/sld001.htm

The PHS 398 form is now on the Internet and is no longer available in printed form.

> **NOTE:** NIH now provides fillable pages on its Web site. It is expected that in the not-too-distant future you will be able to transmit these forms electronically. Until then, applicants should fill out the pages on their computers, print out the forms, and submit them on paper by mail.

You should keep up to date with what's new at NIH with respect to electronic research administration by going to

http://grants.nih.gov/grants/era/era.htm

NIH also has a list of updates for instructions at

http://grants.nih.gov/grants/funding/phs398/phs398.html

Scroll to the bottom of the site for a dated list of recent changes to the NIH information. If you go to the following Web site,

http://grants.nih.gov/grants/funding/phs398/phs398.html

you will find directions for filling out an NIH grant Application. You should follow these instructions carefully. Scroll through the whole document and note the dates of the postings.

The PHS 398 and PHS 2590 Rich Text File (RTF) and Portable Document File (PDF) Form pages as provided are acceptable by NIH.

All other sections of the Application (e.g., Biographical Sketch, Introduction, if necessary, and the Research Plan) must conform to the following 4 requirements:

- The height of the letters must NOT be smaller than 10-point; Helvetica or Arial 12-point is the NIH-suggested font
- Type density, including characters and spaces, must be **no more than** 15 characters per inch (cpi)
- Vertical spacing should be **no more than** 6 lines of type within a vertical inch
- Margins, in all directions, must be at least 1/2 inch

You may substitute computer-generated facsimiles for government-printed forms; however, they must maintain the exact wording and format of the government-printed forms, including all captions and spacing. The PHS 398 and 2590 include Form Pages and Format Pages. The format pages are intended to assist you in the development of specific sections of the Application. Format Pages have been left "unprotected" to allow you to format text, and insert graphics, diagrams, or tables. Alternatively, you may create a page similar to the format provided and inclusive of the requisite information.

Be aware that NIH has a disclaimer on its Web site to the effect that

- the forms at the NIH Web site are NOT provided by NIH
- NIH is not responsible for the accuracy of the forms
- NIH cannot assure that the forms are the most current version required

It's a good idea to check out the NIH Grants Policy Statement occasionally. The NIH Grants Policy Statement can be accessed at

http://grants2.nih.gov/grants/policy/nihgps/nih_gps.pdf

It is also important that you read the weekly edition of the *NIH Guide for Grants and Contracts* (often referred to just as the *NIH Guide*) to access news about changes in submission guidelines and other news from NIH.

You can access the guide at

http://grants.nih.gov/grants/guide/index.html

From that site you can also subscribe to the weekly notifications, via e-mail, of the *NIH Guide* contents by using the **NIH Guide Table of Contents Notification LISTSERV service**.

In this book, I will use as an example—and discuss in detail—only the **NIH R01 (investigator-initiated Research Grant)** Application. However, many of the basic concepts presented in this book can be adapted to other types of Applications at NIH and also to Applications at other funding agencies.

If you

- know how to prepare a good NIH grant Application
  and
- understand the principles of responding to a set of instructions

you should be able to prepare a good Application to any other agency—or, for that matter, other similar types of proposal documents such as a **Business Plan**. A Business Plan is actually very similar to an NIH grant Application except that a lot more information about financial matters is required.

It is important for people who apply for grant funds to become familiar with the various sections of a grant Application and understand the purpose and importance of each.

The **parts** of the R01 Application from the PHS 398 can be accessed at

http://grants.nih.gov/grants/funding/phs398/phs398.html

The **instructions** for preparing your Application are given at

http://grants.nih.gov/grants/funding/phs398/section_1.html

Keep in mind that Web sites are subject to change. For information about the grants process at NIH, you can generally find what you need by starting your search at

http://grants.nih.gov

Be sure that you always use the **latest version** of the NIH forms and that you **read the instructions very carefully** before writing your proposal.

> NIH advises investigators to bookmark the Web site
>
> **http://grants.nih.gov/grants/funding/phs398/phs398.html**
> and check it for updated instructions and policy information prior to submission of an Application.

The PHS 398 Grant Application instructions are available electronically in (1) MS WORD and (2) Portable Document File (PDF) format on the NIH Web site. The Table of Contents on the Web site includes direct links to specific sections of the document, and text searches are also possible.

> For example, specific parts of the Application can be accessed more rapidly using more specific URLs, e.g.
>
> **http://grants.nih.gov/grants/funding/phs398/section_1.html#6_bios**
> will take you directly to information about Biosketches.

Also available on the NIH Web site are dynamic Web site links and cross-references, which enable you to navigate through sections of the PHS 398 document.

The PHS 398 forms have been modified to enable the fields to be filled in directly using word processing programs (MS WORD) or Adobe Acrobat Reader software (PDF)—but form pages prepared using PDF can be **saved only** if you have obtained the **full** Adobe Acrobat program.

NOTE: Form Pages and Format Pages have been renumbered and are thus different from the older printed pages. Among other items provided are

- format pages to be used for all (modular and other) research Grant Applications
- a *standardized format* for the **Biographical Sketch**, including a sample biographical sketch. Note that the biographical sketch **may not exceed 4 pages** for each key person. See further restrictions at the NIH Web site.
- a format page and specific instructions for preparing **Modular Grant Applications**

For sample Modular Budgets, go to

http://grants.nih.gov/grants/funding/phs398/phs398.html

and scroll down to access samples of
- Modular Budgets with the **same** dollar requests each year
- Modular Budgets with **Variable Modules**

Modular Grant Applications require
- a budget narrative regarding Key Personnel by
  - —position
  - —role
  - —level of effort

- a total cost estimate for any Consortium/Contractual arrangements
- additional budget justification "just-in-time" only in exceptional circumstances

ADMINISTRATIVE AND FINANCIAL INFORMATION

The first part of the NIH Grant Application asks for administrative and financial information about you and your institution—which you may or may not need to supply initially—or at all—depending on the size of your budget request and other factors.

You are also required to write a **Description (Abstract) of the Research Plan** that you submit. The Abstract is often limited to a certain number of words or, in the case of an NIH Application, to a certain area (i.e., space) using a **specified** range of type sizes and lines per vertical inch.

Face page

Title of Application (maximum of 56 spaces)

The title of an Application is quite important. It is the first introduction of your project to the Referral Officers and to the Reviewers and Readers and thus helps formulate their first impression about your Application. As an old proverb suggests, "You never get a second chance to make a first impression." Thus, the title of your Application deserves serious consideration. The title should

- be descriptive
- be specific
- be appropriate
- reflect the importance of your research project

The title may be used

- by the Referral Officers for routing the Application to an appropriate Study Section
- to assign the Application to an appropriate funding component if **you** have not designated/requested specific assignments

For example, an Application with a title about a particular study in animal cells might be assigned to the National Institute for General Medical Sciences for possible funding and would go to a Study Section that reviews a large number of Applications with subject matter relevant to that Institute.

In contrast, if the Principal Investigator (PI) specifies that the study will be done in retinal cells, the Referral Officer may route the proposal to a vision Study Section for review and to the National Eye Institute (NEI) for possible funding. The level of funding at these two Institutes may be quite different!!! A bit of research into the mandates and funding levels of the relevant bodies that may review and—perhaps—fund your Application, might mean the difference between support for your project or having to re-apply at a later date. Be aware that the major components of the NIH have Web sites that provide useful information for applicants. Check

http://www.nih.gov/icd/

to get a sense of the general subject matter that is reviewed by the various Study Sections. This information may help you "direct" your Application to the Study Section that is likely to be more interested in your project.

Another reason to be thoughtful about the title you give your Application is well-illustrated in a 1992 *Science* article (Richard Stone, "Peer Review Catches Congressional Flak," *Science*, Vol. 256, May 15, 1992, page 959) concerning "congressional flak" about some grant Applications with trivial sounding titles that had been funded by NSF and NIH. The article ends with a quote from Herb Simon, a Carnegie-Mellon economist and 1978 Nobel Laureate (now deceased): "We ought to learn that when we write down a title of a project, it should reflect the importance of the research."

Dates of entire proposed project period

NIH CSR Study Sections review R01 grant Applications 3 times per year. The review process at NIH has traditionally taken about 9 months. Thus, for example, if you apply for the February 1 deadline (new R01 or R29 Application), and are successful, the earliest starting date would be December 1.

Application Receipt Date	Study Section Meets	Council Meets	Earliest Possible Start Date
Feb. 1/Mar. 1	June/July	Sept./Oct.	Dec.
June 1/July 1	Oct./Nov.	Jan./Feb.	April
Oct. 1/Nov. 1	Feb./Mar.	May/June	July

Be aware that when electronic grants administration becomes totally integrated into the NIH system, the review process at NIH will undoubtedly take appreciably less time.

Check for possible recent changes with the

- Office of Sponsored Research or Office for Grants Administration at your institution
- CSR Grants Information Office

    —NIH: Tel: 301-435-0714

    —E-mail: grantsinfo@nih.gov

Direct costs and total costs for the first 12-month budget period and entire proposed project period will be in terms of the number of **$25,000 modules** you request—**unless** your annual budget exceeds $250,000. If you are a new proposal writer, it might be wise for you to get help/advice developing your budget from the Office of Sponsored Research or the Office for Grants Administration at your institution.

PI's signature

Be sure to sign and date the Application.

Signature of official signing for applicant institution

Have the person sign early; if you wait until the last minute, s/he may be out of town!

A responsible institutional official will not sign an Application that s/he considers incomplete. It is that person's responsibility to ensure that the entire content of the Application (aims/goals, budget, facilities available, regulated activities (assurances), etc.) is acceptable within the context of your institution's mission.

IMPORTANT NOTE: The person responsible for signing the Application is generally a knowledgeable grants officer at your institution and, if given enough time, may be able to help you improve your Application. Bringing your Application for signature at the last possible moment is unfair to yourself and to the official and undermines the official's ability to do her/his job properly. Although some officials responsible for signing the Application are lenient, I have heard about some who have refused to sign applications that did not arrive in the institutional grants office at the time requested. It is both courteous and wise to get your Application to your Office of Grants and Contracts on or before the deadline designated by that office.

Abstract page

The Abstract should be a brief description of your Research Plan. The Abstract serves several purposes:

- The Abstract may be used to route the Application to an appropriate Study Section.
- The Abstract is often the first thing read by the Reviewers. It tells the Reviewer what the proposal is about and helps to form the Reviewers' initial impressions of the PI and the Application.
- Reviewers are encouraged to use the Abstract of the Application to write the "Description" part of the Reviewer's Report. A well-written Abstract helps the Reviewers do their homework more easily. All other things being equal, happy Reviewers tend to be more favorable Reviewers.
- The Abstract is one of the major things read by members of the Study Section who are not primary Reviewers for that Application. Although NIH Study Section Reviewers are rarely asked to be primary or secondary Reviewers on more than 10 to 20 Applications, they may be involved in the review process for as many as 100 or more grant Applications. Because Reviewers also have full-time jobs, it may not be possible for them to read so many grant Applications completely and thoroughly in the allotted time (usually about 4 to 6 weeks). In my experience, conscientious Reviewers read very carefully the Applications for which they are specifically responsible and sometimes do many hours of homework before they write their reviews of the Applications. For the remaining numerous Applications, Reviewers have to pick, choose, and scan the Applications so that they can be sufficiently knowledgeable about the proposal to participate in the discussion during the Study Section meeting. The Abstract and the Specific Aims section of the Application are essential for this process. It is often on the basis of these two sections that the Reviewers decide what other parts of a grant proposal to read more carefully.
- The Abstract helps the Reviewer to remember what your grant is about at the time of the Study Section meeting. Often days, or even weeks, have passed between the time the Reviewer reads a grant proposal and when the Study Section meets. By the time of the meeting, the Reviewer has read a large number of Applications. Exceptionally good and extremely bad Applications tend to be better retained in the Reviewer's memory. For the remaining Applications, the Reviewer may rely on the Abstract to help her/him recall the contents of the

proposal. Underlining key words may also help the Reviewer remember the most important parts of your proposal. The Abstract should

—meticulously follow the instructions given by NIH (or other agency)
—be well thought out
—be clear
—be concise
—realistically represent the contents of the total grant Application

If you are submitting a Renewal Application, it is useful to specifically (but very briefly) point out/discuss the **importance** of findings you have made in the prior project period. This is especially useful for members of the Study Section who are not primary Reviewers for your Application.

- The Abstracts of all funded research grant Applications are sent to the **National Technical Information Service (NTIS)**, U.S. Department of Commerce.

  NTIS uses the information for

  —dissemination of scientific information
  —scientific classification
  —program analysis
  —public access to information about funded proposals

Note that the NIH instructions for the Abstract specify that you

- state the **Broad, Long-Term Objectives of the proposal**
- state the **Specific Aims**
- make reference to the **Health-Relatedness** of the project
- describe the **Research Design and Methods** concisely
- avoid summaries of past accomplishments
- do **NOT** use the first person

  Note: Not using first person applies ONLY to the **Abstract**. It is acceptable and advisable to use first person in the Research Plan section of an NIH Application.

- do not exceed the space provided/suggested
- The Abstract "should serve as a succinct and accurate description of the proposed work [even] when [the Abstract is] separated from the Application."

It is easiest to satisfy the instructions and save yourself time by writing the Abstract as follows:

> "The *broad, long-term objectives* of this proposal are .... The *Specific Aims* are 1.)...; 2.)...; 3.).... The *Health-Relatedness* of the project is.... The *Research Design* is.... The *Methods* to be used are...."

In keeping with the instructions:

- do **NOT** begin the Abstract with a sentence such as "For the past 5 years I have been studying...."
- do **NOT** try to fit more words into the permissible space by changing to a smaller or more condensed font

  —NIH may return your Application without review if the type sizes used are not in keeping with NIH instructions.
  —Use 10- or 12-point letters and be sure the text does not exceed the dimensions permitted for the Abstract.
  —Use the strategies in Appendix II to help you shorten your Abstract.

—It is not necessary to fill the allowed space! When you have nothing more to say, stop writing!

When should you write the Abstract for your Grant Application?

Write the Abstract of the Research Plan LAST!!! —after you have finished writing the FINAL draft of the rest of the grant proposal. This will help ensure that the Abstract is both an accurate summary of—and an appropriate introduction to—the *final draft* of the proposal.

What's special about the Abstract?

The PHS makes information about **awarded** grants available to the public, including the title of the project, the grantee institution, the Principal Investigator, and the amount of the award. The Description (**Abstract**), on Form Page 2 of a funded research grant Application is sent to the National Technical Information Service (**NTIS**), U.S. Department of Commerce, where the information is used for the dissemination of scientific information and for scientific classification and program analysis purposes. The Descriptions (**Abstracts**) of **all funded** Applications are available to the public from the NTIS.

CRISP Database

CRISP (**C**omputer **R**etrieval of **I**nformation on **S**cientific **P**rojects) is a searchable database of **Current and Historical Awards**. The database includes federally funded biomedical research projects conducted at universities, hospitals, and other research institutions. Users, including the public, can use the CRISP interface to

- search for scientific concepts
- find out about emerging trends and techniques
- identify specific projects
- identify specific investigators

Release of research data

By regulation (45 CFR 74.36), grantees that are institutions of higher education, hospitals, or non-profit organizations are required to release research data first produced in a project supported in whole or in part with Federal funds that are cited publicly and officially by a Federal agency in support of an action that has the force and effect of law (e.g., regulations and administrative orders). The term, "Research Data" is defined as the recorded factual material commonly accepted in the scientific community as necessary to validate research findings.

"Research Data" does **NOT** include:

- preliminary analyses
- drafts of scientific papers
- plans for future research
- peer reviews
- communications with colleagues
- physical objects (e.g., laboratory samples, audio or video tapes)
- trade secrets
- commercial information
- materials necessary to be held confidential to a researcher until publication in a peer-reviewed journal
- information that is protected under the law (e.g. intellectual property)

- personnel files, medical files, and similar files, the disclosure of which would constitute an unwarranted invasion of personal privacy or information that could be used to identify a particular person in a research study

These requirements do not apply to

- commercial organizations
- research data produced by state or local governments

However, if a state or local governmental grantee contracts with an educational institution, hospital, or non-profit organization, and the contract results in covered research data, those data are subject to these disclosure requirements.

Key personnel

List all individuals, at the applicant institution or elsewhere, who will participate in the scientific execution of the project whether or not salaries are requested, including

- Principal Investigator
- collaborating investigators
- individuals in training
- support staff

For **each** individual, **list:**

—Name
—All degrees
—Social Security number (optional)
—Position title (within her/his own organization); e.g.,
  - assistant professor
  - staff researcher
  - predoctoral student
  - postdoctoral researcher
—Date of birth
  - month
  - date
  - year
—Role on project; e.g.,
  - principal investigator (PI)
  - consultant
  - graduate research assistant

Table of contents

Fill in the page numbers on this form in the last draft of the proposal. If there is an Appendix, list the Appendix items in the space provided.

> **NOTE:** A **separate** table of contents for the Research Plan, listing all subheadings, helps the Reviewer find topics quickly in an Application that is long and/or complex. The stringent page limitations of the NIH Application form will, in most cases, officially preclude the use of such an additional Table of Contents for the Research Plan of NIH applications. However, in discussions with a number of SRAs at NIH, I have been assured that inclusion of such **an additional Table of Contents on a separate sheet WITHOUT A PAGE NUMBER,** is unlikely to disturb anyone and would, indeed, be helpful to Reviewers. An extra Table of Contents for the Research Plan may also be useful for grant proposals to other agencies.

Subheadings in a Table of Contents should be informative:

> *Do* **Not** *write simply:* "Experiment 1"
>
> *Do write a* **descriptive** *subheading:* "Testing the effects of substance X on cell viability."

Detailed budget for initial budget period (usually the first 12 months)

At NIH a detailed budget is required only for Grant Applications requesting more than $250,000 per year. Read carefully the NIH (or other agency) instructions for presenting the budget for the initial budget period.

> **NOTE** the following caution on the NIH Web site at
>
> **http://grants1.nih.gov/grants/funding/phs398/section_1.html#4_detailed**
>
> *"Applicants are required to seek agreement from Institute/Center staff at least 6 weeks prior to the anticipated submission of any Application requesting $500,000 or more in direct costs for any year. If staff is contacted less than 6 weeks before submission, there may be insufficient time to make a determination about assignment prior to the intended submission date. If the requested dollars are significantly greater than $500,000, then approval should be sought even earlier. This policy does not apply to applications submitted in response to RFAs or in response to other Announcements that include specific budgetary limits. However, such applications must be responsive to any budgetary limits specified, or they will be returned to applicants without review."*

If you do have to submit a budget, the budget should be

- reasonable
- believable
- well-researched
- superbly justified
- developed *after* you have planned the project so that you can calculate to a good approximation what you will need to carry out the proposed work

Be sure the budget accurately reflects the proposed research.

> **Don't "underbudget."**
>
> Don't try to give NIH a bargain; Reviewers will think you're naïve.
>
> **Don't "overbudget."**
>
> Don't be an opportunist or a "thief." Reviewers spot "padded" budgets.
>
> Keep in mind that if all PIs ask for only the amount of funding that is really needed to carry out their project, more investigators can get funding!!!

Discuss with the appropriate personnel at your institution which items are considered direct costs as opposed to indirect costs.

Be aware of budgetary guidelines and restrictions imposed by

- your institution
- the funding agency

For example, NIH imposes a cap on the amount of salary that can be charged to a Grant Application or contract proposal for a given individual. Check with your Office for Grants and Contracts or with NIH.

Insert footnotes after budget items on the budget page, and match these footnote numbers with the relevant explanations in the Budget Justification section (see the example on the sample budget page, Fig. 3-1).

DD   Principal Investigator/Program Director *(Last, first, middle):*   Scientist, Jane X.

DETAILED BUDGET FOR INITIAL BUDGET PERIOD — DIRECT COSTS ONLY   FROM 12/01/93   THROUGH 11/30/94

PERSONNEL *(Applicant organization only)* (1)

NAME	ROLE ON PROJECT	TYPE APPT. *(months)*	% EFFORT ON PROJ.	INST. BASE SALARY	SALARY REQUESTED	FRINGE BENEFITS	TOTALS
Jane X. Scientist (a)	Principal Investigator						
"	"	9	25	$40,837	$0	$0	$0
John Y. Tech (b)	Senior Lab Technician	3	100	$13,612	$13,612	$3,811	$17,423
Tom Z. Grad (c)	Graduate Lab Ass't	12	100	$18,727	$18,727	$5,712	$24,439
Ann W. Help (d)	Undergrad Lab Ass't	12	100	$14,009	$14,009	$4,378	$18,387
		12	100	$ 6,650	$ 6,650	$0	$ 6,650
SUBTOTALS →					$52,998	$13,901	$66,899

CONSULTANT COSTS

EQUIPMENT *(Itemize)* (2)   Inverted microscope with DIC, epifluorescence, & photo capabilities ($32,140) (a); Leitz micromanipulator ($8,540) (b); New Brunswick G76 water bath($3,425) (c); JAIO rotor (1/2 share = $2,330) (d) $46,435

SUPPLIES *(Itemize by category)* (3)

Photo supplies	(a)	$2,465	Enzymes (b)	$3,150
Radioisotopes	(c)	$2,280	Chem reagents (d)	$2,880
Media	(e)	$1,990	Disposable supplies (f)	$4,270
Miscellaneous	(g)	$3,500		

$20,535

TRAVEL (4)   2 National research conferences; PI will present research results. ABC Mtg., Washington, DC. TDY Conf., San Francisco, CA $ 2,225

PATIENT CARE COSTS   INPATIENT / OUTPATIENT

ALTERATIONS AND RENOVATIONS *(Itemize by category)*

OTHER EXPENSES *(Itemize by category)* (5) Publication costs, $500 (a); photocopying and laser printing, $500 (b); Computer connection/services, $1,000 (c) $ 2,000

SUBTOTAL DIRECT COSTS FOR INITIAL BUDGET PERIOD $138,094

CONSORTIUM/CONTRACTUAL COSTS   DIRECT COSTS $ INDIRECT COSTS $ TOTAL →

TOTAL DIRECT COSTS FOR INITIAL BUDGET PERIOD *(Item 7a, Face Page)* → $ 138,094

PHS 398 (Rev. 9/91)   (Form Page 4) Page ___   DD
Number pages consecutively at the bottom throughout the application. Do *not* use suffixes such as 3a, 3b..

FIG.3-1 Detailed Budget for initial budget period (Form page 4 from PHS-398 grant Application packet)

Personnel

- List the **names and types of appointment** of all Applicant organization employees to be involved in the project during the 12-month budget period.

  Check with NIH (or other funding agency administrators) as to whether and which type of staff members and employees of the Applicant's institution may be listed as paid consultants on the Applicant's Grant Application.

  —List the Principal Investigator first
  —Next, list all Collaborating Investigators
  —Then list individuals in training
  —List support staff last
  —List personnel even if no salary is requested
- For each person listed, specify the person's role in the project; e.g.,
  —Principal Investigator
  —Consultant
  —Graduate research assistant

> **NOTE:** Although the terms "co-principal investigator" and "co-investigator" are commonly used by grant Application writers, NIH does not officially recognize these titles. It is preferable to refer to individuals in such positions as "Investigators" or "Collaborating Investigators."

- Type of appointment (months)

  List the number of months per year for which the individual has a contractual appointment at the Applicant organization; if there is no contractual appointment, specify the number of months for which a salary is being requested.

  NIH assumes that the appointments are full-time for that period. If this is not the case, type an asterisk (*) after the number of months, and explain the extent of the appointment (e.g., $\frac{1}{2}$ time or $\frac{1}{4}$ time) in the Budget Justification section.

  If the 12-month year is divided into academic and summer periods, identify and enter on separate lines the type of appointment for **each** period.
- Percent effort on the project

  For each individual, specify the percentage of the appointment at the Applicant institution to be devoted to **this** project. Note that if an investigator has other institutional responsibilities, such as teaching, the *total percent* devoted to *all* research activities must be *less than* 100%.
- Institutional base salary

  For each individual, list the annual compensation from the Applicant organization regardless of the individual's activity, but excluding income that the individual is permitted to earn outside of duties to the Applicant organization.

  You may leave this column blank in the Application, but NIH may request this information before making an award.
- Salary requested

  Multiply the base salary by the percent effort on the project. If a lesser amount is requested for any position, explain it in the Budget Justification.

  For information about "salary caps" (upper limits for salaries):

—Ask your Office for Grants and Contracts

—Check the NIH Guide for Grants and Contracts

—Ask the NIH/DRG Grants Information Office

For non-contractual appointments, contact NIH.

- Fringe benefits must be calculated in accordance with the existing rate agreement at your institution for each position and must be treated consistently with respect to all sponsors.

- Consultant costs

—Provide names and affiliations of consultants even if no costs are involved.

—Except under very particular circumstances, staff members and employees of the Applicant's institution may not act—or be listed—as paid consultants on the Applicant's Grant Application.

—Exclude consultants involved in consortium/contractual arrangements.

—Include physicians who consult on patient care and people who serve on external monitoring boards or advisory committees to the project.

Describe briefly in the Budget Justification:

Services to be performed

Number of days of consultation anticipated

Rate of compensation

Other related costs, e.g., travel and per diem

Provide Biographical Sketches for each consultant on the project. Place the Biosketches with those of other participants in the project. Consultants with major involvement in the proposed project may be considered as "Key personnel."

Provide letters from consultants attesting to their willingness to work on the project. These letters should contain sufficient detail to convince the Reviewers that the consultant

—understands your project

—understands and agrees to her/his specific role in the project

Place letters from consultants at the end of the Research Plan.

Equipment

- Be aware of the "Buy American" provision, which states that equipment purchased with grant funds should be American-made whenever possible. (See *NIH Guide for Grants and Contracts*, Vol. 23, No. 7, February 18, 1994, page 2.)

- List separately each item of equipment requested that has a unit acquisition price of $500 or more and justify the need for the item in the Budget Justification.

- **Include the shipping costs** with the price of the item, and specify this in the Budget Justification. Shipping costs may be substantial for large pieces of equipment.

If you need—and request funds for—an expensive piece of equipment:

—Get a written cost estimate from the manufacturer or distributor and include the written cost estimate with the Budget Justification.

—If appropriate, try to split the cost of an expensive piece of equipment with

- another funding agency
- a colleague
- another department
- some other entity

—Consider applying for a Shared Instrumentation Grant

—If you must ask for the full cost of the equipment, write a very cogent and well-thought-out justification
- List (under "Other Expenses") the cost of any necessary service agreements/contracts
- Check that items you request in the budget are not contradictory to items listed on the Resources page under "Facilities" or "Major Equipment" (see example under Budget Justification below).

Supplies
- Itemize supplies in separate categories such as glassware, chemicals, radio-isotopes, etc., if the category total exceeds $1000.
- Categories for which you request amounts less than $1000 should be combined as "Miscellaneous Supplies."
- For animals, give

    —species
    —number to be used
    —unit purchase cost
    —unit care cost
    —number of care days

NOTE: Purchase, housing, and disposal costs for animals are usually also listed under "Supplies." However, depending on the grantee institution's accounting practices, these charges may be listed under "Other Expenses."

Travel
- On the budget page, specify:

    —number of trips
    —number of persons who will travel
    —total costs
- For each trip, specify in the Budget Justification:

    —person(s) who will travel
    —purpose of travel, e.g.,
      - will you present a paper/poster about your research?
      - What do you expect to gain/learn as a result of the travel?
    —destination

  Professional organizations generally know 3 to 5 years in advance where their annual meetings will be held. Call your professional organization(s) and determine where and when the annual meetings will take place.
- Estimated cost

  Travel agents can provide approximate costs to specific destinations. For expensive trips, it's a good idea to get a "quote" letter from the travel agency; ask the agency to specify—on a written estimate—the agency's "best estimate for inflation"; i.e., what the price is likely to be by the time of travel.

  Reviewers are less likely to recommend travel budget cuts if it seems obvious that the PI has carefully researched the travel plans rather than just filled in some "guestimate" figure ending in 3 zeros.

Patient care costs
See instructions on the NIH Web site.

Alterations and renovations
See instructions on the NIH Web site.

Other expenses
Itemize by category and unit cost:
- Publication costs
  —Drafting
  —Photographs
  —Page charges
  —Reprints
- Books and professional journals
- Computer charges
- Rentals and leases
- Equipment maintenance
  —Service contracts
  —Repairs
- Fees for services
- Office supplies
- Postage

> **NOTE:** NIH has restrictions on the "Other Expense" category.
>
> • For reimbursement for tuition remission that is given in lieu of all or part of salary for students who work on the project, provide details in the Budget Justification.
>
> • For reimbursement for expenses incurred by human subjects who participate in the project, provide details in the Budget Justification. Note that this category is different from *patient care costs* listed above.

Consortium/contractual costs
See instructions on the NIH Web site, and consult your grants office.

Budget for total project period
- Account for (i.e., include and justify) annual raises for personnel (cost-of-living, merit, promotion) and predictable changes in fringe benefit rate. Check guidelines at your institution's Office for Sponsored Research and/or at NIH to determine appropriate percentages to use to calculate these increases.
- Think about new expenses that may arise in later years of the project, e.g.:
  —Repairs
  —Replacements
  —Beginning new experiments that require new supplies or additional personnel
- On the "Budget for entire proposed period of support," identify with an asterisk (*) any significant increase or decrease in any category, including personnel

effort, over the initial budget period. For example, for experiments that you propose to start in year 3, you will need a new instrument and a technician to run and maintain the instrument. Explain such changes in the Budget Justification.

Budget justification

Justify *everything* in the Budget that is not obvious, keeping in mind that what is obvious to you may not be obvious to the Reviewers!!! The Reviewers will be in a better mood if they do not have to puzzle over things such as unexplained changes in the Budget for subsequent years. Any changes should be specifically pointed out. It is to your *disadvantage* if the Reviewers think that you are trying to "pull a fast one" by slipping extra items into future year Budgets.

Dr. Jane Koretz, Professor of Biology & Biophysics at Rensselaer Polytechnic Institute, who has served as a member of the NIH Visual Science-A Study Section, says, "The Budget Justification is crucial. It is essential that each expense be well-justified, even if the need for something or someone appears to have already been implicitly justified in the Research Design and Methods section. Items will be cut by the Study Section or Council in the absence of appropriate justification."

> **NOTE:** A PI should also consider that the care illustrated in the writing of the Budget Justification tells the Reviewers a great deal about the care and conscientiousness with which the PI approaches her/his work and also is indicative of the PIs awareness of—and sensitivity about—good resource management.

Over the years, NIH has from time to time changed the rules about page limits for the Budget Justification section. When you are ready to write a Grant Application, and if you have to submit a detailed budget because you are requesting more than $250,000/year, always check with NIH (or other agency) to determine whether there are page limits for the Budget Justification.

If you do have to submit a Budget and Budget Justification, write the Budget Justification section:

- (a) *concisely*
- (b) in clear **outline form**
- (c) underline key words to make them stand out
- (d) use appropriate formatting, such as indentation, to delineate secondary information (for example, details about how you arrived at the final figures). Appropriate formatting gives Reviewers the opportunity to choose what to read and what to ignore

The Budget discussion at the Study Section meeting occurs **after** the members have **confidentially** assigned priority scores on their individual scoring sheets. During the budget discussion, Reviewers, for the most part, should not have to refer to sections of the proposal other than the Budget and Budget Justification; nor should they have to waste time doing arithmetic—do it for them. Show your work, not just the answer, and be sure it is correct (but do not include absurd levels of detail). There may be one Reviewer in the room who pulls out a pocket calculator and checks the math; incorrect calculations detract from your credibility!

An indented format makes it easy for Reviewers to find increasing levels of detail in the Budget Justification.

— — — — — — — — — — — — — —
— — — — — — — — —
— — — — —

For example:

(4) **Supplies:**		$10,856
(a) Animals		$ 7,950
z Rats	$ xxx	
x/wk for y weeks for the __ experiments		
x Rabbits	$ yyy	
y/wk for x weeks for the __ experiments		
(b) Chemicals		$ 1,006
Compound A, 3 g per month		
for x months at $y/g	$ 3xy	
Compound B, 7 g per month		
for y months at $z/g	$ 7yz	
(c) Glassware		$ 1,900

Justify everything!

Footnote budget items on the Budget pages and use corresponding numbers for explanations in the Budget Justification section.

Justify all personnel.

- The personnel category is likely to be the largest item in your budget.

  Justify it accordingly!

- Specify what *unique* role each person will play in the execution of the research.

  —Describe each person's specific functions in the project.
  —Show how the person's qualifications match her/his role in the project.
  —Give the Reviewers good reasons to invest funds in this individual.

- Try to avoid using "To be named."

  If you must use "To be named," explain what qualifications you will look for in the individual to be recruited:

  —field of expertise
  —specialty within the field
  —years past BA/BS, MA/MS, or PhD
  —years of work experience

Explain and justify annual increases in budget items/categories

If you request a piece of equipment in the Budget, explain why this equipment is necessary for this project.

Explain, in **brief** detail, why the equipment is **critical** for the experiments.
Do not just say that it will let you do an experiment better or faster.

If a piece of equipment is to be shared—or made available to other investigators for their work—it is sometimes helpful to mention this. However, you should give good reasons why *you* are requesting the total cost (rather than sharing the cost).

Check Equipment requests against the list of Resources you have listed as being available to your project to be sure they are not contradictory. Justify *particularly well* equipment you have listed under "Resources." For example, if you say that your institution has 5 centrifuges (because you want to convince the Reviewers about what a good facility it is!!!), you must present a very strong argument for requesting funds to purchase a sixth centrifuge.

Justify and explain new equipment requests in later budget years
- If you are requesting a Model XYZ Microscope in the third-year budget and under "Resources" you write that you have access to a Model XYZ microscope, you should explain why you need another microscope. For example, the microscope that you now use belongs to Dr. X, who will be moving to another university in the third year of your project period and she has been given permission to take the microscope with her. Therefore, you will need a new microscope at that time.
- If you ask for a piece of equipment in the third year and justify the request by saying that there is no such equipment available at your institution, you should explain why you're not asking for it in the first year. For example, the project for which you need the piece of equipment is not scheduled to begin until the third year.

Although YOU may plan to continue your research for many years, there is no assurance that your future Applications will get funded. Thus, Study Section members are highly **unlikely** to recommend that you purchase an expensive piece of equipment **in the last year of a project period** unless you provide a very cogent argument for why you need the item in question at that time.

For expensive equipment, it's a good idea to provide a ***written quote*** from the company. This is especially important if the item is large and/or expensive. Ask the company to estimate **what the price is likely to be at the time the item is likely to be purchased.** Remember, at least a year may elapse between the time you obtain the quote and the time the grant is funded!

Justify supplies that you request
It helps to include receipts of previous purchases or other proof of price and/or actual usage for major supplies categories. Be especially careful to justify:
- Supplies that cannot be obtained via readily available catalogs
- Supplies for which there has been a recent major price increase
- Items for which you are requesting a very large sum of money or a large quantity of a particular item

  Reviewers sometimes forget about inflation. It pays to provide them with proof of the facts. **Whether or not you have to submit a budget,** a little Internet, telephone, or library research toward creating a realistic budget is time well spent.

Justify all travel
- Specify
  —who will travel
  —for what purpose

- Attend a conference
  Specify whether or not the person traveling will present a paper.
- Learn a new technique in another location

■ Estimate expenses based on actual meeting places. For conferences, find out where meetings will be held and how much it costs to get there.

Keep in mind that many professional organizations know several years in advance where their annual meeting will be. It pays to call and get this information to help you formulate a realistic travel budget for your grant Application.

Asking for $1,000 in travel expenses for each year of the project period to go to the annual XYZ meeting does not "sit" well with the Reviewers if someone on the Study Section is aware that in the second year of your project period, the XYZ meeting is in your own home town!!!

■ Unless you are a fairly senior investigator (i.e., over approximately age 50!!!) you would be wise to specify that costs are based on:

—shared room
—tourist class train
—advance purchase airfare
and provide other indications that you are using the agency's money thoughtfully and wisely.

Although important for information exchange and education of younger researchers, travel sometimes is not considered a very high-priority budget item. Some Reviewers consider one meeting per year per investigator reasonable. Other Reviewers consider the norm to be only one to two trips per year per lab group. If you are requesting money for travel, it is imperative that you justify why it is important for each individual to go to specific meetings, and why and how you think she/he will benefit from attendance. It helps to get travel money if, for example, the Reviewers feel assured that the person in question will give a good talk at a meeting for which you are requesting travel funds.

Justify ALL other expenditures
Justify consortium and contractual (subcontract) costs thoroughly both here and in the section of the Research Plan about "Consortium and Contractual Arrangements."

Justify the budget for the total project period
■ Justify any significant increases in any category over the first 12-month budget period. *Identify such significant increases* with asterisks next to the appropriate amounts.

■ Specify, for example: "'Other Expenses' is increased by an extra $1000 (above the annual X% increase) in year 03 to pay for a routine, but major, expensive service of the XYZ instrument purchased in year 01."

■ Or state, for example, "No additional equipment is requested in subsequent years."

■ Never give the Reviewers the opportunity to think you are trying to "slip something through" or, in any other way, "put one over" on them.

Sample Budget Justifications are given in Appendix III.

Biographical sketches (Biosketches)

See **http://grants.nih.gov/grants/funding/phs398/section_1.html#6_bios**

You must provide Biographical Sketches for all **key** personnel including consultants. In your Application, place the Biosketches in the same order in which they are listed on the "Abstract" (Project Description) page.

A sample Biographical Sketch is provided at

http://grants.nih.gov/grants/funding/phs398/phs398.html

Scroll down to "Biographical Sketch **Sample**" and click on either MS WORD or PDF format.

Scroll down to get to the filled-in sample.

Use the sample format on the "Biographical Sketch Format Page" to prepare this section for all grant Applications (Modular and other).

NOTE: The Biographical Sketch has specific page limits:
- The Biographical Sketch may not exceed 4 pages.
- Items A and B (together) may not exceed 2 of the 4-page limit.

Complete the educational block at the top of the format page, and complete sections A, B, and C, as indicated below and in the "Biographical Sketch **Sample**" given on the NIH Web site.

(A) Positions and Honors.
> —List, in chronological order, previous positions you have held.
> Conclude with your present position.
> —List any honors.
> Include present membership on any Federal Government public advisory committee.

(B) Selected Peer-Reviewed Publications.
> —**List them in chronological order.**
> —List only articles that have been published or are "in press."
> —Do **NOT** include publications **submitted** or in **preparation**.

(C) Research Support.
> —List selected ongoing or completed (during the last 3 years) research projects.
> —Include federal and nonfederal support.
> —Begin with the projects that are most relevant to the research proposed in this Application.
> —Briefly indicate the overall goals of each project and your role (e.g., PI, Co-investigator, Consultant) in each research project.
> —*Note:* Do NOT list award amounts or percent effort on projects.

> **NOTE:** Information on "Other Support" beyond that required in this Biographical Sketch should NOT be submitted with the Application.
>
> Failure to comply with this requirement will be grounds for the PHS to return the Application without peer review.
>
> "Other Support" information is required for all Applications that are to receive grant awards; however, NIH will request complete and up to date "Other Support" information from Applicants at an appropriate time after peer review. The awarding Institute's scientific program and grants management staff will review this information prior to the award.

Provide a Biosketch for the Principal Investigator and **all other key professional personnel** listed on the "Abstract" page. **Note that postdoctoral training should be listed under "Education" and not under "Research and Professional Experience."** Be sure that all the Biosketches provided are in the *same format*, including the publications.

List of Publications for the Biographical Sketch:

Incorrect	Correct
Your publications list should **NEVER** look like the list below.	Your publications list should look like the list below. **Note that all entries have a uniform style.**
Reif-Lehrer, Liane, Promoting Yourself Is Key To Climbing Academic Ladder. 1992; Jul. 20, p. 20, The Scientist.	Reif-Lehrer, Liane, Promoting Yourself Is Key To Climbing Academic Ladder. *The Scientist*; 1992; Jul. 20, p. 20.
Technological and Cultural Impediments Slow Electronic NIH Grant Submission by Liane Reif-Lehrer. 1995; The Scientist, Apr. 3, p. 1, 8-9.	Reif-Lehrer, Liane, Technological and Cultural Impediments Slow Electronic NIH Grant Submission. *The Scientist*; 1995; Apr. 3, pp. 1, 8–9.
The Scientist; 1995; Getting Funded: It Takes More Than Just A Good Idea; Aug. 21, p. 14, by Reif-Lehrer, Liane.	Reif-Lehrer, Liane, Getting Funded: It Takes More Than Just A Good Idea. *The Scientist*; 1995; Aug. 21, p. 14.
Following Instructions Is Critical To Success Of A Grant Application. The Scientist; 1996; Liane Reif-Lehrer, Mar. 4, pp. 15-16.	Reif-Lehrer, Liane, Following Instructions Is Critical To Success Of A Grant Application. *The Scientist*; 1996; Mar. 4, pp. 15–16.
Agencies, Institutions Progress Toward Electronic Grant Administration. The Scientist; 1996; Jul. 8, pp. 3-5, by Liane Reif-Lehrer.	Reif-Lehrer, Liane, Agencies, Institutions Progress Toward Electronic Grant Administration. *The Scientist*; 1996; Jul. 8, pp. 3–5.

Research and professional experience includes:

- Previous employment—in chronological order (present position last)
- Experience
- Honors
- Present membership in any federal government Public Advisory Committee

- Give complete references (including titles) to:
  —*All* publications *of the past 3 years*
  —*Representative* earlier publications that are **pertinent** to this Application
  —Note that **Item A plus Item B of the Biosketch may not exceed 2 pages of the 4-page limit.**
  —Follow the formats and instructions on the NIH Web site.
  —Because there is a page limit, **choose publications wisely.**
  List the best and most recent publications **that are relevant to the subject of the proposed project.**
  —*List the publications in chronological order.*
  —If you are a **new** Applicant with few publications, list **all** of your publications (assuming the list will not exceed the page limit).
  In the list of publications, underscore (or use bold type for) your name to make your name clearly apparent when there are multiple authors on publications.

> **NOTE:** Your own publications should appear in 3 places:
> - Biosketch
> - Progress Report
> - Literature Cited
>
> In an elegant, carefully prepared Application, references in all 3 bibliographies—including the Biosketches—are presented in an identical format.

Avoid the temptation to simply collect Biosketches from collaborating investigators and insert them in your proposal without reworking them into the same format—and (if you are submitting on paper) without changing the name of the Principal Investigator at the top of the Biosketch page.

Instead, ask collaborating investigators to send you their Biosketch on a diskette or via email and reformat all the Biosketches to the same format.

Other support

As noted earlier, information on "Other Support" beyond that required in the Biosketch should **NOT** be submitted **with** the Application. Failure to comply with this requirement will be grounds for the PHS to return the Application without peer review. Note that **"Other Support" information is required only for applications that are scheduled to receive grant awards.** NIH will request "Other Support" information from applicants at an appropriate time after peer review and will review this information prior to award.

If you are asked to provide information about "Other Support," *list all* active or pending sources of project-specific support to the **Principal Investigator** and **other key personnel** on the project, *whether related to this Application or not.*

Consider:
- Current active support
- Applications pending review or funding
- Applications planned or in preparation

Include:
- Federal
- Nonfederal

- Institutional support
- All types of
  —Grants (research, training, etc.)
  —Cooperative agreements
  —Contracts
  —Fellowships
  —Gifts
  —Prizes
  —Other means of support
- Support administered through another institution

Resources

Read carefully the instructions about "Resources." There is no "Form Page" for Resources. Follow the sample format and instructions on the "Resources Format Page" when completing information on Resources available for the project. If there are multiple performance sites, then Resources available at **each** site should be described.

Facilities

- List the facilities available at the Applicant organization.
- Indicate the capacity of the facilities.

  For laboratory, office, and other spaces, give the total number of square feet available to the project.

  —Explain pertinent capabilities of the facilities.
  —Describe relative proximity of the facilities to your main workspace.
  —Detail the extent of availability of the facility to your project.
- Under "Other," describe support services and to what extent these services will be available to the project:

  Machine shop

  Electronics shop

  Etc.

Major equipment

- List major equipment available to the project (remember to compare these items to budget requests!!!).
- Note the location and pertinent capabilities of each item.
- Specify the extent of availability of such equipment for use for the project described in your Application.

THE RESEARCH PLAN

Introduction

The Research Plan is the **main** (that is, the science) part of the grant Application and the most important part for the review process.

Writing the Research Plan for an NIH Application—or any other type of grant Application—requires much planning and care. It is imperative to allow yourself plenty of time to take each of the steps described below. This will enhance your chance of getting funded. It is also wise—especially if you are a first-time Applicant—to contact Institute program personnel before you begin to write, and discuss with them:

- The Application process
- The relevance of your project in relation to the mandates and program priorities of that Institute
- What help the Institute personnel might be able to provide in the Application process

The instructions in earlier versions of the NIH instructions stated, "Reviewers often consider brevity and clarity in the presentation to be indicative of a focused approach to a research objective and the ability to achieve the Specific Aims of the project." This piece of good advice may be even more pertinent as pressures on scientists and other researchers increase.

You are expected to include sufficient information in the Research Plan to permit an effective review without reference to any previous Application. However, you should be aware that, in the case of renewal and revised Applications, wise Reviewers are almost certain to ask to see the Summary Statement for the previous Application and may also have requested NIH to send a copy of the complete previous Application.

New proposers/new proposals

Reviewers tend to make certain allowances for **first-time** applicants. The Reviewers understand that novices generally do NOT have track records or a substantial list of publications. However, in the current funding climate, at least some **substantive pilot experiments and good preliminary data are essential** to convince the Study Section members that you really can do the project. Likewise, one or more **good papers**—in well-respected journals—on which you are the sole—or at least first—author are a big plus.

If you are a seasoned investigator applying for a *new* grant, Reviewers will want to know why you are expanding into new areas or changing direction. If appropriate, explain/emphasize relatedness between projects—**but assure the Reviewers that there is NO overlap.** Include a few sentences of rationale in the "Background and Significance" section and have ample and substantive preliminary data for the new project. If the new project is in addition to an ongoing project for which you are funded, make it very clear in the Application—and in the Budget Justification, if you have to submit one—that you have the time and personnel to do the work for both projects—and do it well.

Renewals

Even when Study Section review criteria remain unchanged, there may be subtle differences in the expectations of the Study Section members for first renewals (the second Application to the same agency to continue a given project) compared to second renewals (the third Application to the same agency to continue a given project). A first renewal that shows somewhat expanded horizons and new Specific Aims related to those of the initial proposal may be acceptable if the Principal Investigator has made sufficient progress in the form of substantive original research publications and new preliminary data. By the time of the second renewal, Reviewers may look for somewhat more than just "linear" progress. The Principal Investigator would do well, at this stage, to demonstrate some maturity of outlook in the form of:

—a realistic assessment of whether the project is worthy of a long-term study or is perhaps in need of a more effective new direction

—awareness—and incorporation—of appropriate new technology, perhaps from other fields of science

—new approaches to the problem

—a broader conceptual base

—a more encompassing hypothesis

Collaborators

In the past several decades, NIH, NSF, and other agencies generally have not been anxious to spend their limited resources for training investigators in new fields after the investigators have finished their postdoctoral training. Thus, for example, if you are a biochemist and your project requires some electron microscopy, it would NOT be wise to write that you will take a year off to learn electron microscopy. **Get a Collaborator,** who already is a known expert in electron microscopy, to work on the project with you!!! As mentioned earlier in this book, be sure to provide:

>—a letter confirming the Collaborator's willingness to work on the project
>—a Biographical Sketch for the Collaborator

General instructions for the Research Plan

Even if you are using electronic transmission to submit your Application, print the Research Plan using a type size that is acceptable to NIH (or other agency to which you are applying)—or preferably, a larger type size. Try to put yourself in the Reviewers' place. Is the font size you are using one that you would be happy to read at 2 AM if you

>—had worked all day
>—were presbyopic (far-sighted)
>—were tired
>—had several more proposals to read that evening

Of course, with an electronic file, the Reviewer can change the type size on her/his own computer. But it is your responsibility

>—to follow the instructions
>—to make sure that the format is OK
>—not to create any additional chores (be they ever so small) for the busy Reviewer.

Also be aware that

- Every part of your Application must have the Principal Investigator's name on it in the following format: *"Last name," first, then "First name," then "Middle name or initial"*

- You are asked to insert your Social Security number in certain places (however, providing this information is optional)

- You must stay within the margins indicated by NIH

- It is important to use an **easy-to-read font style** and a **permissible font size**

The paragraph below is copied verbatim from

http://grants.nih.gov/grants/funding/phs398/phs398.html

NOTE: Applicants who encounter problems with the forms or print margins due to printer settings are advised to use the individual files for Forms/Format Pages below. Alternatively, applicants may select "Unprotect Document" under "Tools" to make necessary modifications. Be aware that you can add Page numbers by un-protecting the document and double-clicking in the "footer." Applicants are advised that TYPE SIZE AND FORMAT SPECIFICATIONS MUST BE FOLLOWED OR THE APPLICATION WILL BE DESIGNATED AS **INCOMPLETE** AND WILL BE RETURNED TO THE APPLICANT ORGANIZATION WITHOUT PEER REVIEW.

Page limits

There is a *25-page limit* for the 4 major components of the Research Plan:

- Specific Aims
- Background and Significance
- **Preliminary Studies** (for **new** Applications) or **Progress Report** (for **renewal** Applications)
- Research Design and Methods

Applicants must resist the temptation to use the Appendix to supply information that they were unable to accommodate within the page limits for the Research Plan. The Application—exclusive of the Appendix—must be able to stand on its own. Making the Application **complete and clear within the imposed page limits** is one of the obligations of—and challenges to—the writer of the Grant Application. The Appendix should be limited to material that is **supportive** of the Application, not integral to it.

The 25 pages of the Research Plan must include copies (which may be reduced in size) of all items (other than reprints/publications) that you provide in the Appendix. Items should be submitted in the Appendix only because you can supply better reproductions in a larger (easier to read/ easier to see detail) or glossy (better detail) format in the Appendix; this may apply, for example, to:

> tables
>
> charts
>
> electron micrographs
>
> photographs of gels

Your Application may be returned without review if you

- exceed the page limits

    Proposals have been returned for being as little as a half page over the allowed limit

- *have not used permissible* fonts and font sizes

You may use any page distribution within the 25-page overall limit for the 4 parts of the Research Plan, but NIH recommends:

Part of Research Plan	# of pages recommended by NIH for this part of the Research Plan
Specific Aims	1 page
Background and Significance	2–3 pages
Progress Report/Preliminary Studies	6–8 pages for the narrative portion*
Research Design and Methods	25 pages minus the number of pages used for the other 3 items above (i.e., 13–16 pages)

*To indicate what you have already accomplished in the subject of your Grant Application, you may submit a maximum of 10 manuscripts in the Appendix.

Parts of the Research Plan

Note: If you go to

http://grants2.nih.gov/grants/forms_faq.pdf

you will find answers to some general questions related to the PHS 398 and PHS 2590 Forms and Instructions. You might find some of these helpful.

Optional additional Table of Contents for the Research Plan

In addition to the Table of Contents provided for the Application by NIH, it is sometimes desirable to provide an **additional Table of Contents**—specifically for the Research Plan. This additional Table of Contents should include all **subheadings** within the Research Plan. The Reviewers can use this detailed Table of Contents to quickly locate specific items

- when they are reviewing your Grant Application before the Study Section meeting
- during the discussion at the Study Section meeting

> **NOTE:** The *extra* Table of Contents is not useful for proposals with severe page limitations (if you are short of space)—unless you can get permission from the funding agency to include this extra Table of Contents as an un-numbered page for the convenience of the Reviewers. If you get permission to include a more detailed Table of Contents with your NIH proposal, put this extra Table of Contents *before* the Research Plan and **mark it "For convenience of Reviewers,"** and **do not number this page**!

Subheadings in a Table of Contents should be informative:

> *Do* **Not** *write simply:* "Experiment 1"

>> The subheading "Experiment 1" may mean something to you, but it conveys nothing to the Reviewer, except perhaps that it was the first experiment that you did.

> *Do write, for example:* "Testing the effects of substance X on cell viability."

Abstract (Summary)

This is a summary of the general information you have presented in the 4 previously mentioned parts of the Research Plan for an NIH Application.

> In addition to an Abstract (Summary), the type of information shown in the table below is required in an NIH grant Application and is also generally required—in some form—in many other types of grant Applications.

Part of Research Plan	Required information
Introduction	At NIH, this section is required only for revised and supplemental applications (see below)
Specific Aims	What you intend to do?
Background and Significance	What has already been done in the field? What are the "gaps" and unsolved problems in the field? Why is the work important?
Preliminary Studies or Progress Report	What you have done already on this project?
Research Design and Methods	How you will fulfill the aims? How you will do the work?

Introduction

In an NIH Application, the Introduction is limited to 3 pages and is required only for Revised or Supplemental Applications.

- Introduction for a **Revised** Application

Do not exceed 3 pages

—Respond to *every* criticism in the Summary Statement for the previous Application.

—Summarize all significant changes you have made in the Application.

—Be polite and direct.

—Be careful not to use an adversarial tone.

> Whether your proposal is returned to the **same** Reviewers or to different Reviewers, a "sour grapes" or "cry baby" response to the critique in the Summary Statement will probably elicit a negative response from Reviewers and may hinder your chance to improve your priority score.

—Highlight changes made in the text of the revised Research Plan by use of

- brackets
- indents
- different typography

> Do *NOT* use shading or underlining to highlight changes.
>
> Be aware that failure to highlight changes creates an unnecessary burden on Reviewers and may irritate them!

—Incorporate into the Progress Report/Preliminary Studies a description of any work done—and results obtained—since the prior version of your Application was submitted.

> A **Revised** Application *will be returned if*:
>
> - it does not address criticisms in the previous Summary Statement
> - an Introduction is not included
> - substantial revisions are not clearly apparent

■ Introduction for a **Supplemental** Application

Do not exceed 1 page

—Explain the significance of the supplemental work proposed with respect to the original proposal.

Specific Aims

Recommended maximum: 1 page

> All other things being equal

- ■ a proposal that is **hypothesis-driven** is likely to be more favorably received than one that is not
- ■ "fishing expeditions" are unlikely to be funded
- ■ proposals referred to by the Study Section members as being primarily "descriptive" are also not likely to get good scores unless they are biotechnology projects

To write the Specific Aims section:

> Although the instructions for the **Specific Aims** section ask only for the items described below, some successful grant getters begin this section with a **brief** paragraph that provides a context ("mini-background") for the Specific Aims. This is a good idea as many Reviewers will not see the Background for the Application until after they have read the Specific Aims. A brief cogent "introduction" to the Specific Aims can be immensely helpful to put the Specific Aims in context for the Reviewers.

The instructions for the **Specific Aims are:**

- ■ State the broad, long-term objectives of the proposal.

- Describe concisely and realistically

   —what the specific research described in the Application is intended to accomplish (**Specific Aims**)

   —any hypotheses to be tested, or clear, specific questions to be addressed.

   Webster's Third New International Dictionary defines a hypothesis as "a proposition tentatively assumed in order to draw out its logical or empirical consequences and so test its accord with facts that are known or may be determined."

   Be aware that simply placing the phrase "The hypothesis is..." before a string of words does not make the statement a hypothesis!!!

   A hypothesis generally states a problem in a form that can be tested and also generally predicts a possible outcome. A good hypothesis will generally suggest—to someone who is knowledgeable in the field—experiments that will test the hypothesis. Generally, the hypothesis is: If we do XXX, we predict that YYY will happen.

   For a more extensive discussion of the nature of a hypothesis, see:

   > Locke, L. F., Spirduso, W. W., and Silverman, S. J., *Proposals That Work: A Guide for Planning Dissertations and Grant Proposals*, 3rd ed., Sage Publications, 1993. Sage Publications, 2455 Teller Rd., Thousand Oaks, CA 91320-2218 (Out of print)
   >
   > Or
   >
   > Locke, L. F., *Proposals That Work: A Guide for Planning Dissertations and Grant Proposals*, 4th ed., Sage Publications, 1999. Sage Publications, 2455 Teller Rd., Thousand Oaks, CA 91320-2218
   >
   > ISBN: 0761917071 (Paperback)
   >
   > ISBN: 0761917063 (Hard Cover)

   See also: Locke, L. F., *Reading and Understanding Research*, 2nd ed., Sage Publications, 2004.

- Avoid grandiose designs.

   —If appropriate, state the hypotheses—or questions to be addressed—in the form of short bulleted statements rather than narrative paragraphs.

   —"To study the effect of substance X on system Y" is not a good Specific Aim! The statement is too vague.

- Understand the difference between the

   —*broad, long-term objective(s)*.

   For example, "Eradicate diabetes" (hard to quantify progress)

   and

   —*Specific Aims*.

   For example, "Develop a method to continuously measure blood sugar levels" (something that can be crossed off a list of n items—which are necessary to accomplish the broad, long-term objectives—at the end of one, or possibly 2 project periods; i.e., perhaps 4 to 8 years).

- Be careful not to include Methods as Aims unless the major goal of the proposal is to develop a new method/technique. But keep in mind that a proposal whose primary aim is to develop a new method/technique may not be as well-received or funded as a hypothesis-driven proposal—unless it is a biotechnology proposal or subsequent aims within the proposal involve using the method once it is developed.

NOTE: Keep in mind that a Specific Aim that, if not successfully accomplished, prevents successful completion of the rest of the proposed project, is a **dangerous Specific Aim!** In general, it is better to **avoid having Specific Aims that are overly interdependent**.

Background and Significance

Recommended maximum: 2–3 pages

1. *Briefly* sketch the *Background* for the proposal.
2. Critically *evaluate* the existing knowledge in the field.
3. Specifically **identify the *gaps*** the project is intended to fill.
4. State *concisely* the importance of the research (**Significance**) by *relating* the Specific Aims to the broad, long-term objectives.
5. **Provide ample references** in this section (especially in the Background).
   - Unless you are a first-time Applicant, these references will probably include papers about your own work.
   - The references go into the "Literature Cited" section of the Research Plan.

Use the Research Design and Methods section of the Grant Application to
   —demonstrate your understanding of the subject
   —justify the need for the proposed research

- Do not simply delineate the Background (any clever high school student can probably do that!), but **evaluate** the existing knowledge (a clever high school student probably does not have sufficient experience in the field to do that!).
- State clearly why the information to be obtained is useful; that is, explain what you will/can do with the information after you get it.
- If appropriate, explain the clinical relevance of your proposed research.
- In the Background section, make it clear which previous work was done by others and which was done by you, the PI.

Background discussions should avoid fanning the flames of scientific controversies. Someone on the Study Section may have a strong bias in the debate that may not coincide with yours. Discuss all sides and aspects of the issue, remain strictly scientific and unbiased, and let the data speak for you. If you are certain that your conclusions are correct, do ***not*** compromise your position, but state your position politely and with respect for the opinions and publications of others. They may be your Reviewers!

References that are **cited by author and year** in the text of your Application—and listed in alphabetical order (and numbered!) in the bibliography—are more meaningful to Reviewers than references cited by number in the order of being cited.

References cited only by number cause the Reviewer to have to frequently flip back to the bibliography pages to determine what the reference is. In contrast, author/year citations generally have meaning to people in the field without having to see the particulars of the reference.

However, the author/year method of citation takes up valuable space in the context of stringent page limitations. In addition, the author/year method of citation can interrupt the flow of text for the Reviewer/Reader, especially when there are multiple citations at a given place in the text. You will have to make a judicious decision about the best way to cite references in your Application, considering the positive and negative aspects of each method. The decision may vary with the precise nature of the particular subject and the particular Grant Application.

Help the Reviewers

- The Reviewer may want to check a statement without taking the time to search through a long article to find it. Therefore, if you refer to a long article (for example, a review article), put a note in the text to the effect that "discussion pertinent to the XYZ subject may be found on pp. 15–18, 29–32, and 56 in Abbott and Woods, 1959 (reference 43)."
- If an article that you cite is not readily available, ask the SRA for permission to provide photocopies of the article—or at least the pertinent pages of the article for the Reviewers. If permission is granted, ask the SRA how many copies you should send and where in the Application they should be placed. (See the section on Bibliography below).

Preliminary Studies

- Recommended maximum: 6–8 pages for the narrative portion.
- The page limit does NOT include the list of publications.

New **Applicants** may use this section of the Application to provide information that will help to establish their experience and competence to pursue the proposed project. Thus, a new Applicant may discuss past projects that may not be directly related to the current project but may serve to assure the Reviewers about the Applicant's experience in research and general competence in the field. Discussion of work not directly related to the subject matter of the Grant Application in question is an opportunity that is generally not available in a renewal Application!!!

It is imperative that you provide preliminary data that show that your project is feasible—and do-able by you. The chances of a new Grant Application without any preliminary data getting funded are pretty remote. I once heard a member of a Study Section remark, "Preliminary data in a new Grant Application are about as optional as breathing."

- Discuss preliminary studies *by the Principal Investigator (PI)* that are pertinent to the Application.

- Provide any other information that will help to establish the experience and competence of the *Principal Investigator* to pursue the proposed project. **Note** that NIH is asking for 2 separate things here:

  —experience
  and
  —competence

  Also Note that it is possible to:
  - have a great deal of experience but not be very competent
  - be very competent but have little or no experience

- List the titles and complete references to all:

  —publications such as journal articles, books, and book chapters
  —manuscripts accepted for publication
  —patents
  —other published materials that have resulted from the project since it was last reviewed competitively

Submit 5 copies each *of no more than 10* such items in the Appendix. If you are submitting on paper, submit the Appendix items as collated sets with a cover sheet. The cover sheet should be labeled with:

—your name

—the title of your Grant Application

—a list of the Appendix items attached

Do NOT include/list manuscripts that have been submitted, but have not yet been accepted, for publication.

Provide any relevant preliminary data you have collected. The data do not have to be in final format, but they

- must have a clear connection to the proposed work
- should be clearly and neatly presented

Any evidence that your project is realistic and/or that the proposed experiments will work in your laboratory is valuable. Data that indicate that your basic premises—your hypotheses—are correct are especially helpful for bridging the credibility gap for new applicants. A photocopy of a graph from even a single experiment that you have carried out successfully is better than no preliminary data, but be sure that the data are comprehensible to the Reviewers.

- Label the coordinates properly
- Give the figure a title
- Explain what is in the figure by providing a good figure legend

Keep in mind that a curve derived from an "in-house" experiment, labeled with "lab jargon" with which you are familiar, may not be easily understood by someone not familiar with the "lingo" of your laboratory.

Be careful about including preliminary data in this section of the Application that pre-empt experiments that you have proposed to carry out in the forthcoming project!

Do NOT include preliminary data that have no relevance to the project described in the Application!

> **NOTE:** In renewal Applications, the "Preliminary Studies" section is replaced by the Progress Report.
>
> ### PROGRESS REPORT
>
> - Recommended maximum: 6–8 pages for the narrative portion.
> - The list of professional personnel and list of publications do not count towards the page limit.

A Progress Report is required (in lieu of Preliminary Studies) for Competitive Renewal and Supplemental Applications.

The Progress Report is a very important part of the proposal because it lends credibility to what you proposed in the previous Application and helps the Reviewers decide whether you did a good job.

- Give the beginning and ending dates of the period covered since the last competitive review

  (i.e., the date your funding began, to the date of submission of the proposal for which you are writing this Progress Report)

NOTE: These dates do not coincide with project period dates. Remember that you are reapplying about a year before the present project period is up. Also, the beginning date for the Progress Report will be the day after the ending date for the previous Progress Report.

- List all personnel who have worked on the project in this period and give the following information for each:
  —Name
  —Title
  —Birth date
  —Social Security number (optional)
  —Dates of service
  —Percentage of appointment devoted to this project
- Summarize the Specific Aims of the **preceding** Application, and provide a succinct account of progress (published and unpublished) toward achievement of these aims. Make it easy for the Reviewers to find the information they want by using a format like the one that follows:

Specific Aim (1)

> Summary of Specific Aim (1) of the previous proposal
>
> Summary of progress made toward achieving Specific Aim (1):
>
>> "SA (1) has been accomplished in that . . . and a publication describing the results appeared in . . ." (give reference).

Specific Aim (2)

> Summary of Specific Aim (2) of the previous proposal
>
> Summary of progress made toward achieving Specific Aim (2):
>
>> "SA (2) was not pursued after we did X initial experiments because we ran into an unexpected, serious experimental difficulty that did not show up in our preliminary experiments." (State briefly what the difficulty was.)

Specific Aim (3)

> Summary of Specific Aim (3) of the previous proposal
>
> Summary of progress made toward achieving Specific Aim (3):
>
>> "SA (3) was started in the Xth year of the project period. One publication has resulted (give reference), but the project has evolved into a more extensive one than we had originally anticipated. We plan to use a new method, described in the current proposal, to further evaluate . . ." (Then, in the "Specific Aims" section of the renewal Application, one Specific Aim would be related to the continuation of this work.)

Specific Aim (4)

> Summary of Specific Aim (4) of the previous proposal
>
> Summary of progress made toward achieving Specific Aim (4):
>
>> "Work relating to SA (4) was begun X months ago. Figure Y, below, shows the results of the first 3 experiments and indicates . . . We expect this aspect of the project to be complete by the end of the current project period."

—Number items in the Progress Report to correspond to numbers of the Specific Aims of the *preceding* proposal so that the Reviewer can easily follow along in the preceding Application.

—The NIH instructions specify that you "include sufficient information in the Progress Report to facilitate an effective review *without* reference to any previous Application." However, Reviewers are generally provided with the Summary Statement for the PI's previous proposal and may also, depending on the "habit" of the SRA, be sent the entire previous proposal. Reviewers may also specifically request to see the previous proposal if it is not sent to them.

■ Summarize the **importance** of the findings.

Do not just list the findings! This is very important for the Reviewers.

■ Discuss any **changes** in original Specific Aims. Clearly note which of the original Aims of the previous proposals have been accomplished, which have not, and why (as illustrated above).

—Do not simply gloss over or fail to discuss a Specific Aim on which you have made NO progress.

—*You should account for* **every** *Specific Aim listed in the original Application*!

—A budget cut is a common reason why a Specific Aim was not accomplished. If that is the case, be sure to explain this.

■ List the titles and complete references to all publications that have resulted since the last competitive review:

—*published* manuscripts

—manuscripts *accepted* for publication

—patents

—invention reports

—other printed materials

■ Clearly distinguish between

—peer-reviewed original papers (research reports)

—reviews

—books

—abstracts

NOTE: Group publications into the above categories. When you list your publications in the Progress Report (within the category of peer-reviewed original papers), it is a good idea to list first the papers on which you are the sole author.

Submit—as collated sets—in the Appendix, 5 copies each of no more than 10 articles that have been **published** or **accepted for publication**.

If you are the **sole** author or **first** author on only a few papers—or have only a few publications—and if you have a valid reason for this lack of publications, explain why.

■ An enforced move to another laboratory, a long illness, or an equipment supplier who went out of business before delivering your order, may be acceptable explanations.

■ Problems with techniques or staff turnover are likely to make the Reviewers wonder about your ineptitude or lack of good public relations and are, thus, better left unsaid.

- If you must explain low productivity, think carefully about how you present the situation and try to find an experienced grant Reviewer to read your explanation for tone and impression.

Study Section members are generally unhappy with PIs who
>—suffer from "apublishanemia" (a term that was used frequently in the Study Section on which I served)
>or
>—have a high A:P ratio, where "A" stands for "abstracts," and "P" stands for "peer-reviewed publications" (terminology that was used in the Study Section of a colleague)

Clearly, you must think about your publication record long before it is time to write your Renewal Application. The current NIH instructions ask that only papers that have been published or accepted for publication be listed. However, if you have only a small number of publications, but have a paper that you have submitted for publication or that is in preparation but is essentially complete, call your SRA and ask for permission to submit copies. For each such paper listed, submit preprints in the Appendix, and indicate in the list of publications that the preprint is provided in the Appendix.

Research Design and Methods

You have on the order of 13–16 pages for this section of the Research Plan (i.e., the limit of 25 pages minus the number of pages used for the first 3 parts of the Research Plan).

The Research Design and Methods section is an important part of the Research Plan. In the Specific Aims section, you have delineated what you propose to do; in the Research Design and Methods section you tell the Reviewers **how** you propose to do what you described in the Specific Aims.

- Explain why the particular approach that you describe was chosen to address the problem that you plan to research.
- Convince the Reviewers that you are capable of doing what you propose to do:
  —That you have the requisite experience
  —That you have access to the necessary equipment
  —That you have access to the necessary space and facilities
  —That you have the necessary laboratory help/personnel

It is especially important to be very **focused**—and very **clear**—in this section of the proposal. Many Grant Application writers, totally absorbed in their own project and, thus, forgetting the needs of the Reviewers and the funding agency, begin this section of the Research Plan with a "shopping list" of methodologies they plan to use—without providing a context within which these methods will be used. This is a major problem for Reviewers and is well illustrated by the *New Yorker* cartoon reproduced on page 86. The 1986 change in the title of this section of the PHS-398 Form from "Methods" to "Experimental Design and Methods," and the further change in the 1991 revision of the PHS-398 Form to "Research Design and Methods" should send a message to Grant Application writers that NIH was not getting what they wanted in this section; i.e., they were not getting adequate descriptions of the Research Design in proposals submitted to the agency.

You should restate—or at least summarize—the relevant Specific Aim at the beginning of each sub-section of the Research Design and Methods section. In addition, providing a one- or two-sentence rationale for each aim (without including extensive Background or Progress Report material) also helps the Reviewers. A brief introductory or closing paragraph, indicating the relationship of the Specific Aims to each other as well as to the over-

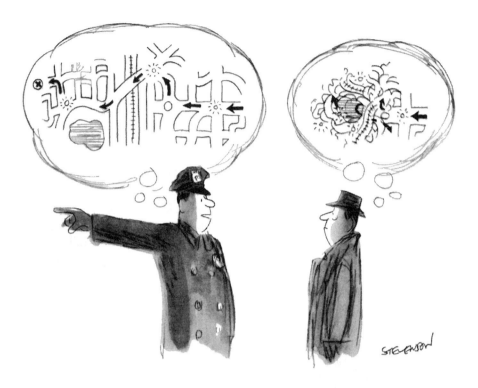

Misunderstood directions.

all objective of the proposed work also helps to focus the point of the work in the mind of the Reviewers/Readers.

- Outline the Research Design **AND** the Methods to be used to accomplish the Specific Aims of the project.
- Number the Research Designs and the Methods in this section to *correspond* to the numbers of the Specific Aims in ***this*** proposal.
- Use sub-numbering within this section when describing several methods applicable to the same Specific Aim. But do not overuse sub-numbering, and be sure that the numbering system is very clear and does not confuse Reviewers by overlapping with numbers used in a different section of the proposal.
- *Distinguish between the overall Research Design and the specific Methods:*
  First, repeat or summarize the Specific Aim in question.
  Then have separate sub-heads for Research Design and Methods. For example:
  Research design for SA (1):
  Methods for SA (1):
  A.) Techniques for …
    1. XXX
       Reference and/or describe the method briefly.
    2. YYY
       Reference and/or describe the method briefly.

B.) Determination of …
  1. XYZ
     Reference and/or describe the method briefly.
  2. ZYX
     Reference and/or describe the method briefly.

- *Do* **NOT** *repeat* identical procedures that apply to more than one Specific Aim. Describe such procedures once, and then refer the Reader back to that section—or group such procedures at the end of the "Methods" section—in a section entitled, "General Procedures," and refer to the procedures as necessary.

- Describe and/or reference protocols.

  —Reference, but do NOT describe in detail, **well-known** procedures.
  "Cookbook" repetitions of techniques copied from published papers do not convince Reviewers of your expertise. If you find it necessary to detail such a technique, describe it in the context of your specific research problem and experiments.

  It is a wise idea to have an experienced proposal-writer—or a colleague who has served as a Reviewer—advise you about how much detail to present.

  —Describe and reference procedures that are new or unlikely to be known to Reviewers.

  If in doubt, reference a paper that describes the methodology in detail, and ask the Scientific Review Administrator for permission to provide 3 copies of the reference (a reprint or a photocopy of the article) in the Appendix for use by the primary Reviewers/Readers. Providing reprints for Reviewers is especially important if the source of the original paper is not readily available.

- If you propose using a new method, explain why the new method is better than the existing method(s) that other workers in the field are using.

  —Try the proposed Method and provide preliminary data to show that the Method works in your laboratory under the specified conditions.
  —Alternatively, discuss a possible "Plan B" that you will use if your primary proposed method does not work as expected.

- Discuss/describe all applicable *control* experiments.

  Do not assume that the necessary control experiments will be obvious to the Reviewers! It is **your responsibility** to explain what types of control experiments you plan to do.

- For all data sets, explain how the data are to be:
  —Collected
    Explain how you will actually carry out the experiments.
  —Analyzed
    Do not simply say, "We will use ANOVA." Explain how the statistical analyses will be carried out. If necessary, get a statistician to help you formulate this aspect of the proposal.
  —Interpreted
    An explanation of how the data will be *interpreted* is a very important part of a good Grant Application, and is, in my experience, often omitted from proposals.

Describe *briefly* what might be expected in a given set of experiments. For example: "If the data come out thus and so, then it means…and we will do…; on the other hand, if the data turn out to be…, it might mean…and we will proceed as follows:….” Don't speculate on experimental outcomes for which you can propose no further experimental progress.

Convince the Reviewers that you have really thought through all aspects of your project and the possible interpretations of the data that you are likely to collect.

- Discuss:

    —*potential difficulties* of the proposed procedures

    —*possible limitations* of the proposed procedures

    A discussion of the *difficulties* and *limitations* of the procedures you have proposed is very important—as can be discerned from the excerpts, shown below, from Summary Statements (SS) for 3 NIH Applications.

    SS1: A major potential problem in this research, the contamination of material from…is serious. The principal investigator is fully aware of such criticism and has diligently attempted to deal with it. This is a major strength in the proposal. Nonetheless, questions remain. In particular, the separation…may require further analysis. The principal investigator might be encouraged, insofar as possible, to carry out…analysis on the material obtained by the…procedure of…. The alternative mode of preparation of…is an important complementary method. This should ensure more complete….

    SS2: A problem of the previous Application was that there was concern about several limitations of the proposed methodology. However, the investigators have added a substantial amount of text indicating that they are well aware of these limitations and do, in fact, have a great deal of insight into the ways of solving any potential problems that arise. It is now clear that the research will provide a substantial amount of new and important data.

    SS3: In any investigation which requires the use of…, the question of…introduced by…always arises. Dr. … is keenly aware of potential pitfalls, and is prepared to deal with them.

> **NOTE,** in SS3, that the PI's ability to point out possible problems to be encountered in the project is an asset rather than a liability. If YOU don't call attention to the problems and don't explain how you will deal with these problems, the Reviewers will find the problems and wonder how you will deal with them! That is, try to think of objections the Reviewers might raise and respond to them in your Application.

However, be careful not to sound too "NEGATIVE" by over-assiduously pointing out every little possible glitch for every proposed experiment. The Aim is to convince the Reviewers that you:

    —REALLY understand your system

    —REALLY understand the experiments you propose to do

    —are aware of areas that may present problems

- *Alternative approaches* to achieve the Specific Aims of your project

    A discussion of *alternative approaches* can sometimes save your proposal if a Reviewer is not convinced that your primary approach will yield the desired results. Grant Application writers should also be aware that Reviewers, who are generally chosen because they are established investigators in their field of research, may have access to very up-to-date, as yet unpublished, and unreported information about developments in your field. Thus, they may know about data that may put your approach into question. Discussion of alternative approaches to your project may rescue your proposal under these circumstances.

Having experts in the field of your Application review and critique a fairly complete draft of the Application is also a good safeguard to assure that your Application is well-thought-out and well-presented.

- Point out:
  —procedures
  —situations
  —materials

  that may be *hazardous* to personnel and describe *precautions* to be exercised to protect personnel.

- Convince the Reviewers that you really understand how to deal with every aspect of your research problem.

  Some years ago, I asked a Program Officer at one of the NIH Institutes what he would say to proposal writers about preparing a good "Methods" section. He responded: "Try to convince the Reviewer that you have not merely gone to the library, but that you really understand and know how to carry out the research and are familiar with the techniques and their shortcomings."

- Provide a **tentative** *sequence* or *timetable* for the project.

  Be realistic, not exact.

  In many cases, this timetable deserves no more than 1/3 to 1/2 page. Reviewers do NOT want a blow-by-blow account of what you will do when (assuming that you are funded) on a week-by-week basis for the duration of the grant period. They want:
  —assurance that you have really thought through the project
  —some indication of approximately when various aspects of the project will be started and finished

  Some applicants use diagrammatic or tabular formats to present the necessary information.

- Document any proposed collaborative arrangements with letters from the individuals with whom you propose to work.

  The letters should **demonstrate that the Collaborators understand your project** and should **define** what **role** the **Collaborator(s) will have** in the project.

As a courtesy:
  —write a draft of the letter of collaboration for your Collaborator.
  —assure the Collaborator that she/he should feel free to change the letter as she/he finds appropriate.
  —ask the Collaborator to print the letter on her/his own letterhead and send it to you.

The letter should be very specific about what the Collaborator role in your project will be, i.e., what the Collaborator will do to help your project progress/succeed.

  A letter that simply says something such as, "I will be happy to help you with your project," is useless.

The letters of collaboration should be placed at the end of the Research Plan.
  Biographical Sketches must be obtained from all Collaborators.

The Biographical Sketches should be placed with the Biosketches of the Principal Investigator and other key personnel.

You, the PI, should edit the form of the Biosketches to be sure they are **all in the same format** and that all Biosketches have all the required information in the correct part of the Biosketch.

Human subjects (no page limit; be as brief as possible)

See: **http://grants.nih.gov/grants/funding/phs398/section_3.html#human_subjects**

Definitions of the terms:
- Human subject
- Intervention or interaction with a human subject
- Identifiable private information

and the regulations governing the **inclusion** and **protection** of human subjects in research may be found at the above NIH Web site or by calling NIH. Below is some information, as well as some Web sites and telephone numbers that might also be helpful:

Research on transplantation of human fetal tissue

Office of Recombinant DNA Activities Web site
http://www4.od.nih.gov/oba/

In signing the Application Face Page, the duly authorized representative of the Applicant organization certifies that if research on the transplantation of human fetal tissue is conducted, the Applicant organization will make available, for audit by the Secretary, DHHS, the physician statements, and informed consents required by the Public Health Service.

Women and minority inclusion in clinical research policy

http://grants.nih.gov/grants/guide/notice-files/NOT-OD-02-001.html

Women and members of minority groups and their sub-populations must be included in all NIH-supported biomedical and behavioral research projects involving human subjects in clinical research, unless there is a clear and compelling rationale and justification not to do so.

A description of the proposed outreach programs for recruiting women and minorities as participants is useful.

Inclusion of children policy

It is the policy of NIH that children (defined as individuals under the age of 21) must be included in all human subjects' research, conducted or supported by the NIH, unless there are scientific and ethical reasons not to include them. This policy applies to all NIH conducted or supported research involving human subjects, including research that is otherwise "exempt" in accord with Sections 101(b) and 401(b) of 45 CFR 46—Federal Policy for the Protection of Human Subjects. The inclusion of children as subjects in research must be in compliance with all applicable subparts of 45 CFR 46 as well as with other pertinent federal laws and regulations. Therefore, **proposals for research involving human** subjects must include a description of plans for including children. If children will be excluded from the research, the Application or proposal must present an acceptable justification for the exclusion. In the Research Plan, the investigator should **create a section titled, "Participation of Children."** This section should provide either a description of the plans to include children and a rationale for selecting or excluding a specific age range of child, or an **explanation of the reason(s) for excluding children** as participants in the research. When children are included, the plan must also include a description of the expertise of the investigative team for dealing with children at the ages included, of the appropriateness of the available facilities to accommodate the children, and the inclusion of a sufficient number of children to contribute to a meaningful analysis relative to the purpose of the study. Scientific Review Groups at the NIH will assess each Application as being "acceptable" or "unacceptable" with regard to the age-appropriate inclusion or exclusion of children in the research project, in addition to evaluating the plans for conducting the research in accord with these provisions.

Investigators should be familiar with the guidelines about inclusion of children that can be obtained from NIH staff or accessed via the NIH grants Web site under the *NIH Guide for Grants and Contracts*

http://grants.nih.gov/grants/guide/notice-files/not98-024.html

Research using human embryonic stem cells

http://www.nih.gov/news/stemcell/index.htm

In signing the Application Face Page, the duly authorized representative of the Applicant organization certifies that if research using human embryonic stem cells is proposed, the Applicant organization will be in compliance with the "Notice of Extended Receipt Date and Supplemental Information Guidance for Applications Requesting Funding that Proposes Research with Human Embryonic Stem Cells."

http://grants.nih.gov/grants/guide/notice-files/NOT-OD-02-006.html

Vertebrate Animals (no page limit; be as brief as possible)
Go to

http://grants.nih.gov/grants/funding/phs398/section_3.html#human_subjects

and scroll down to "Vertebrate animals."

If your studies involve vertebrate animals you should assure the Reviewers that your animal experiments are

- necessary
- well-thought-out
- scientifically sound

A PHS award for research involving vertebrate animals will be made to an Applicant organization only if that organization is operating in accordance with an approved Animal Welfare Assurance, and provides certification that the Institutional Animal Care and Use Committee (IACUC) has reviewed and approved the proposed activity in accordance with the PHS policy.

NIH will not complete the processing of your Application without certification of IACUC approval. Check with the appropriate office at your institution to find out—before you begin to write your Grant Application—the
- procedures
- amount of time required to get approval to conduct vertebrate animal studies

Consultants/Collaborators
- List all Consultants and Collaborators, whether or not salaries are requested.
- Provide, in this section, a letter from each Consultant and/or Collaborator, confirming her/his role in the project. **Do NOT put the letters in the Appendix.**
- Provide a Biosketch for each Consultant and/or Collaborator. Place these Biosketches with those of other participants in the project.

Consortium/Contractual Arrangements
- **Justify** consortium and contractual (subcontract) costs thoroughly both **here and in the Budget Justification.**
- Provide a detailed explanation of the arrangements between the Applicant and collaborating organization:
    —Programmatic
    —Fiscal
    —Administrative
- Provide a statement that the Applicant and collaborating organization have established—or are prepared to establish—written inter-organizational agreements that will ensure compliance with all pertinent Federal regulations and policies.
- Provide copies of written agreements or letters (signed by the Applicant PI and an authorized official of the collaborating organization) confirming inter-organizational agreements.
- If the majority of the work is NOT being done at the Applicant organization, explain why the Applicant organization should be the grantee. That is, assure the Reviewers that the Applicant organization intends to have a substantive role in the project.

Literature Cited (Bibliography)
- NO page limit.
- Be concise and select only those literature references pertinent to the proposed research.
- The reference list should be limited to relevant and current literature.
    —List ALL **pertinent** references.
    It is important that you demonstrate good judgment in the references that you choose to list. Research proposals do not fare well when applicants fail to reference relevant published research. Make wise decisions about when to list original papers and when to list Review articles. Refer to the literature thoroughly and thoughtfully but not to excess. Hundreds of references are likely to be too many! The publication list need not be exhaustive. As a guideline, unless there is a good reason to have more, think in terms of listing about 100 of the most relevant citations.
    —Include, but do not replace, the list of publications required in the Progress Report for competing continuation Applications.

—Each reference must include:
- Title of publication
- Names of all authors (do NOT use "et al."!)
- Title of book or journal
- Volume number (if appropriate)
- Page numbers (beginning and ending)
- Year of publication

■ Acknowledge the work of others, including that of your competitors.

Do not let the Reviewers think that you are biased or arrogant.

■ Reviewers are interested in how up to date you are.

A grant Application submitted in November 200X in which the latest reference cited is from March 200(X-1) does not sit well with the Study Section members unless you can specifically point out that no publications have appeared in the field in the interim.

■ Make life easy for the Reviewers.

If your bibliography contains obscure or foreign journal references that you went to a lot of trouble to obtain and that are unlikely to be readily available to the Reviewer—and if the reference is important in the context of the proposal—you may wish to get permission from the Scientific Review Administrator of the Study Section to provide (with your Grant Application) copies of the article—or at least, the (English) summary of the article—for the primary Reviewers/Readers. If permission is granted, ask the SRA how many copies to send.

■ Use a consistent format throughout the "Literature Cited" section. This format should also be the same as that used in the list of publications in ALL the Biographical Sketches AND in the "List of publications" in the Progress Report.

■ Be sure every citation in the text is listed in the bibliography.

■ Be sure every citation in the bibliography is referred to in the text.

■ Do not scatter citations throughout the text.

—List them in this section of the Research Plan.
—Even if you use the author/year method of citation, list the **complete citation** in the "Literature Cited" section.

■ The "Literature Cited" section may include, *but not replace*, the list of publications in the Progress Report.

Choose wisely what you include in the "Literature Cited" section. Your inclusions should be selective rather than exhaustive. Your choice of citations tells the Reviewer about your

—quality as a scientist
—ability to evaluate the work of others
—ability to distinguish the important from the mundane

TO REITERATE: Although there is no page limit for the "Literature Cited" section, it is important to be concise and to select only those literature references pertinent to the proposed research. See

http://grants.nih.gov/grants/funding/phs398/section_1.html#8_research

Method of citation

Advantages of the author/year citation

The use of the author/year citation system in the text is much more meaningful to Reviewers than number citations and saves Reviewers the time it takes to flip back to the bibliography whenever they come to a numbered citation.

If you use the author/year citation system, you should

- present the references in alphabetical order (by surname of first author) in the bibliography ("Literature Cited" section)
- number the articles in the bibliography

    The numbers make it easier for Reviewers to refer to specific references during the discussion at the Study Section meeting (e.g., "Doesn't Homenflof have more recent references on…than those cited at numbers 37 to 41?").

Disadvantages of the author/year citation

The disadvantages of the author/year system are

- it takes up more space (not a trivial matter when there are stringent page limits!)
- multiple citations cause a long interruption in the text. This may break the Reviewer's train of thought and can thus be annoying or confusing to the Reviewer.

APPENDIX

NOTE: Applicants must NOT use the Appendix to circumvent the page limitations of the Research Plan.

NOTE: Unlike the rest of the proposal, the Appendix is not duplicated by NIH. The SRA gives a copy of the Appendix, in the original form that the PI submitted, to selected members of the Study Section, usually only the two or three primary Reviewers and the Readers. The remaining copies are available at (or before) the Study Section meeting for other members who may request to see the Appendix. Perhaps when complete electronic grant administration (including transfer of figures and photos) is achieved, the Appendix will be sent electronically to all the Reviewers on the Study Section.

NOTE: When you consider what to put into the Appendix for an NIH Application, keep in mind that there is a good chance that only a few of the Reviewers will see the Appendix section!!! Proposals must be comprehensible without reference to the Appendix!

The following types of Applications may include an Appendix:

- New Applications
- Revised Applications
- Competing Continuation Applications
- Supplemental Applications

If you include an Appendix and you are submitting an Application on paper:

- Provide **5 collated sets** of the complete Appendix
- Place the Appendix in the same package with the Application
- Place all the Appendix sets following all 6 copies of the Application

- Identify each Appendix item with the name of the Principal Investigator
- **Do not intermingle Appendix materials with the Application**

The following materials may be included in the Appendix:

- Up to 10 of the following (staple as sets):
  —Publications
  —Manuscripts (accepted for publication)
  Manuscripts **submitted** for publication should NOT be included
  —Abstracts
  —Patents
  —Other printed materials directly relevant to this project
- Any of the following (if on paper, staple as sets):
  —Surveys
  —Questionnaires
  —Data collection instruments
  —Clinical protocols
- Any of the following **provided that** a photocopy (that may be reduced in size) is also included within the 25-page limit of Items a-d of the Research Plan:
  —Original glossy photographs
  —Color images of gels
  —Micrographs
  —Original work that does not reproduce well in black and white or grey scale or does not photocopy well

Photographs and color images may be included in the Appendix **ONLY if they are also represented** (in reduced form) within the page limits of the first 4 parts of the Research Plan.

Graphs, diagrams, tables, and charts that do not need to be in a glossy format to show detail should NOT be included in the Appendix. **An Application that does not observe these limitations will be returned. These Appendix limitations may not apply to specialized Grant Applications.** Request and follow the additional instructions for those Applications.

If you have other items that you wish to submit with the Application, contact the SRA of your Study Section or a Program Officer to **ask permission**. Such items might include:

- Questionnaires
- Oversized documents
- Other materials that do not reproduce well
- Materials intended to help the primary Reviewers by saving them a trip to the library. These reprints or abstracts need only be submitted in triplicate—unless the SRA requests otherwise.
- *New* Applicants may provide similar Background materials to document preliminary studies.

How to prepare the Appendix for the final draft

- Be sure each Appendix item is referred to in the text of the Application.
- Be sure each Appendix item referred to in the text of the Application is provided in the Appendix and entered in the list of Appendix items.
- Identify each Appendix set—and each item within each Appendix set—with the name of the Principal Investigator/Program Director, Social Security number (optional), project title, and title of item.

- Individual manuscripts within the Appendix should be stapled; the rest of the Application should NOT contain staples.
- Provide a list of Appendix items in 2 places:
  —At the bottom of the Table of Contents
  —On a separate sheet at the front of each collated Appendix set
- Do not number Appendix pages.
- Send the Appendix with the rest of the Application. Do not send the Appendix separately.

> **NOTE:** An Application may be returned if the Appendix fails to observe the limitations on content.
>
> **http://grants1.nih.gov/grants/funding/phs398/section_1.html#9_appendix**

CHECKLIST

See

http://grants.nih.gov/grants/funding/phs398/section_1.html#10_checklist

and

http://www.niaid.nih.gov/ncn/grants/charts/checklists.htm

The Checklist is a form page for the NIH PHS 398 Application that can be accessed with instructions via the first of the above Web sites. You can also access just the fillable form, in RTF or PDF format, directly from

http://grants.nih.gov/grants/funding/phs398/phs398.html

The Checklist requires you to provide information about:

- Inventions and Patents

  (Competing Continuation Applications Only)

  NIH has developed an optional on-line Extramural Invention Information Management System, known as "Edison," to facilitate grantee compliance with the disclosure and reporting requirements of 37 CFR 401.14(h). The Internet address for this system is **http://s_edison.info.nih.gov/iEdison/**

  Information from these reports is not available to the public.

- Program Income
- Assurances/Certifications

> **NOTE:** Much of the information about ASSURANCES AND CERTIFICATIONS is taken verbatim from the following Web site
>
> **http://grants.nih.gov/grants/funding/phs398/section_3.html#g_assurance**
>
> I have omitted certain details that the reader can find at the Web site, if necessary. I have also occasionally changed the wording to either shorten or clarify a statement. I will assume that readers who are involved with policies listed below will go the Web site to read the relevant NIH mandates/instructions.

Each Application to the PHS requires that the assurances and certifications listed below be verified by the signature of the Official Signing for the Applicant Organization on the Face Page of the Application.

The assurances listed may not all be applicable to your project, program, or type of Applicant organization.

There are also a number of additional public policy requirements with which applicants and grantees must comply. You should check with your institution's research grant administrative office or with the *NIH Grants Policy Statement* that is available at

http://grants.nih.gov/grants/policy/policy.htm

In signing the Application Face Page, the duly authorized representative of the Applicant organization certifies that the Applicant organization will comply with the following policies, assurances, and/or certifications:

- **Human Subjects**

  See page 91
- **Research on transplantation of human fetal tissue**
- **Women and minority inclusion in clinical research policy**

  The current amended Guidelines can be found at

  http://grants.nih.gov/grants/guide/notice-files/NOT-OD-02-001.html

  Awards will NOT be made if the research project does not comply with this policy.

  In addition, awardees must report annually on enrollment of women and men, and on the race and ethnicity of research participants in the "5/01 **Inclusion Enrollment Report Format Page** (<u>RTF</u> or <u>PDF</u>)."
- **Inclusion of children policy**

  See

  http://grants.nih.gov/grants/guide/notice-files/not98-024.html

  Note that NIH defines "children" as individuals under the age of 21.
- **Research using human embryonic stem cells**

  See

  http://www.nih.gov/news/stemcell/index.htm

  and

  http://grants.nih.gov/grants/guide/notice-files/NOT-OD-02-006.html
- **Vertebrae animals**

  The PHS Policy on Humane Care and Use of Laboratory Animals requires that Applicant organizations proposing to use vertebrate animals file a written Animal Welfare Assurance with the Office for Laboratory Animal Welfare (OLAW), establishing appropriate policies and procedures to **ensure the humane care and use of live vertebrate animals** involved in research activities supported by the PHS.

  All institutions are required to comply, as applicable, with Federal statutes and regulations relating to animals. These documents are available from:

  Office for Laboratory Animal Welfare
  National Institutes of Health
  Bethesda, MD 20892
  Tel: 301-496-7163

- **Debarment and suspension**

  Before a grant award can be made, the Applicant organization must certify that the primary participant nor any research personnel are not (among other things) presently (nor in the 3-year period preceding) debarred, suspended, proposed for debarment, declared ineligible, or voluntarily excluded by any Federal department or agency.

- **Drug-free workplace**

  People receiving grants from any Federal agency must certify to that agency that they will maintain a drug-free workplace.

- **Lobbying**

  Title 31, United States Code, Section 1352, entitled "Limitation on Use of Appropriated Funds to Influence Certain Federal Contracting and Financial Transactions," generally prohibits recipients of Federal grants and cooperative agreements from using Federal (appropriated) funds for lobbying the Executive or Legislative Branches of the Federal Government in connection with a specific grant or cooperative agreement. Section 1352 also requires that each person who requests or receives a Federal grant or cooperative agreement must disclose lobbying undertaken with non-Federal (non-appropriated) funds. These requirements apply to grants and cooperative agreements exceeding $100,000 in total costs. DHHS regulations implementing Section 1352 are provided in 45 CFR Part 93, "New Restrictions on Lobbying."

  The complete Certification Regarding Lobbying is provided below.

  "The undersigned (authorized official signing for the Applicant organization) certifies, to the best of his or her knowledge and belief that:

  No Federal appropriated funds may be used for Lobbying Activities."

  Standard Form LLL, "Disclosure of Lobbying Activities," its instructions, and continuation sheet are available from GrantsInfo, National Institutes of Health, e-mail: GrantsInfo@nih.gov, (301) 435-0714.

- **Non-delinquency on federal debt**

  Organizations and individuals indebted to the United States are NOT eligible to receive a Federal grant.

- **Research misconduct**

  An institution that receives or applies for a research, research training, or research-related grant must agree to report possible misconduct in Science and to protect Research Misconduct "Whistleblowers."

  "Misconduct in Science" and "Research Misconduct" are defined by the Public Health Service as "fabrication, falsification, plagiarism or other practices that seriously deviate from those that are commonly accepted within the scientific community for proposing, conducting or reporting research. It does not include honest error or honest differences in interpretation or judgments of data."

  Further information is available from:

  Office of Research Integrity
  Division of Education and Integrity
  Rockwall II, Suite 700
  5515 Security Lane
  Rockville, MD 20852
  Phone: (301) 443-5300
  Fax: (301) 594-0042 or (301) 445-5351

- **Assurance of compliance**
  —Civil rights
  —Handicapped individuals
  —Sex discrimination
  —Age discrimination
  Before a grant award can be made, a domestic Applicant organization must certify that it has filed with the DHHS Office for Civil Rights: an Assurance of Compliance (Form HHS 690) with regard to prohibition of discrimination based on any of the 4 categories mentioned above.

  The Assurance of Compliance Form HHS 690 is available from:
  >   GrantsInfo
  >   E-mail: GrantsInfo@nih.gov
  >   Tel: 301-435-0714

- **Financial conflict of interest**
  To promote objectivity in research, NIH requires grantees and investigators (except Phase I SBIR/STTR applicants) to ensure that there is no reasonable expectation that the design, conduct, or reporting of research funded under PHS grants or cooperative agreements will be biased by any conflicting financial interest of an investigator.

- **PHS metric program**
  PHS policy supports Federal transition to use of the metric system for measurement in all grants, cooperative agreements, all other financial assistance awards, reports, publications, and other communications regarding grants.

- **Smoke-free workplace**
  See

  http://grants1.nih.gov/grants/funding/phs398/section_3.html

  and scroll down to:
  >   "SMOKE-FREE WORKPLACE"

  The PHS strongly encourages all grant recipients to provide a smoke-free workplace and to promote the non-use of all tobacco products. In addition, Public Law 103-227, the Pro-Children Act of 1994, prohibits smoking in certain facilities (or in some cases, any portion of a facility) in which regular or routine education, library, day care, health care, or early childhood development services are provided to children. This is consistent with the PHS mission to protect and advance the physical and mental health of the American people.

- **Prohibition on awards to 501(C)4 organizations that lobby**
  Organizations that engage in lobbying are not eligible to receive grant/cooperative agreement awards.

- **Government use of information under privacy act**
  The Privacy Act authorizes discretionary disclosure of certain information within the Department of Health and Human Services and outside the agency to the public, as required by the Freedom of Information Act and certain other purposes.

- **Information available to the principal investigator**
  Principal Investigators
  —may request copies of records pertaining to their Grant Applications from the PHS component responsible for funding decisions

—are given the opportunity under established procedures to request that the records be amended if they think the records are inaccurate, untimely, incomplete, or irrelevant. If the PHS concurs, the records will be amended.

■ **Information available to the general public**

Information about **awarded** grants is available to the public, including:

—Title of the project
—Grantee institution
—Principal Investigator
—Amount of the award

The Description (Abstract) of a **funded** research grant Application is available to the public from the National Technical Information Service (NTIS), U.S. Department of Commerce.

The Freedom of Information Act requires release of certain information about grants, upon request, irrespective of the intended use of the information. Trade secrets and commercial, financial, or otherwise intrinsically valuable information that is obtained from a person or organization and that is privileged or confidential information may be withheld from disclosure. Information, which, if disclosed, would be a clearly unwarranted invasion of personal privacy, may also be withheld from disclosure. **Although the grantee institution and the Principal Investigator will be consulted about any such release, the PHS will make the final determination.** Generally available for release, upon request, except as noted above, are:

—all **funded** Grant Applications including their derivative funded noncompeting supplemental Grant Applications
—pending and **funded** noncompeting continuation Applications
—progress reports of grantees
—final reports of any review or evaluation of grantee performance conducted or caused to be conducted by the DHHS
—Grant Applications (initial, competing continuation, and supplemental) for which awards have NOT been made
—evaluative portions of site visit reports

Summary Statements of findings and recommendations of review groups are generally **NOT** available for release to the public.

■ **Access to research data**

Grantees that are institutions of higher education, hospitals, or non-profit organizations are required to release research data first produced in a project supported in whole or in part with Federal funds that are cited publicly and officially by a Federal agency in support of an action that has the force and effect of law (e.g., regulations and administrative orders). **"Research data" is defined as the recorded factual material commonly accepted in the scientific community as necessary to validate research findings.** "Research data" does **NOT** include:

—preliminary analyses
—drafts of scientific papers
—plans for future research
—peer reviews
—communications with colleagues
—physical objects (e.g., laboratory samples, audio or video tapes)
—trade secrets
—commercial information

—materials necessary to be held confidential to a researcher until publication in a peer-reviewed journal

—information that is protected under the law (e.g., intellectual property)

—personnel and medical files and similar files, the disclosure of which would constitute an unwarranted invasion of personal privacy

—information that could be used to identify a particular person in a research study

These requirements do not apply to commercial organizations or to research data produced by state or local governments. However, if a state or local governmental grantee contracts with an educational institution, hospital, or non-profit organization, and the contract results in covered research data, those data are subject to these disclosure requirements.

■ **Recombinant DNA and human gene transfer research**

The *National Institutes of Health Guidelines for Research Involving Recombinant DNA Molecules (NIH Guidelines)* apply to NIH-funded and non-NIH-funded gene transfer projects that are conducted at or sponsored by an institution that receives NIH support for recombinant DNA research—and apply to both basic and clinical research studies.

Recombinant DNA molecules are either:

(1) molecules which are constructed outside living cells by joining natural or synthetic DNA segments to DNA molecules that can replicate in a living cell

or

(2) DNA molecules that result from the replication of those described in (1)

Specific guidance for the conduct of human gene transfer studies is available at

http://www4.od.nih.gov/oba/rac/guidelines/guidelines.html

or from

NIH Office of Biotechnology Activities

6705 Rockledge Drive, Suite 750

Bethesda, MD 20892

Tel: 301-496-9838

See also: Recombinant DNA Activities Web site at

http://www4.od.nih.gov/oba/

■ **Information resources**

A list of the NIH program guidelines and other publications is available at

http://www.nih.gov/index.html

and from

http://grants.nih.gov/grants/index.cfm

Applicants may also contact GrantsInfo:

E-mail: GrantsInfo@nih.gov

Tel: 301-435-0714

■ **Facilities and Administrative (F&A) Costs**

Indicate the Applicant organization's most recent F&A cost rate established with the appropriate DHHS Regional Office, or, in the case of for-profit organizations, the rate established with the appropriate PHS agency cost advisory office.

Special Instructions for Modular Applications

Applicant institutions should calculate the F&A costs using the current negotiated F&A rate, less exclusions, for the initial budget period and all future budget periods. It is NOT necessary to list the exclusions on the Checklist or anywhere in the Application.

Other items about which you should be aware:

The Web site

http://grants.nih.gov/grants/funding/phs398/section_3.html#human_subjects

also contains:

- Definitions for the following terms used by NIH:
  —AIDS Related research
  —Applicant Organization Types
  —Small Business Concerns
  —Socially and Economically Disadvantaged Small Business Concerns
  —Women-Owned Small Business Concerns
  —Children
  —Clinical Research
  —Clinical Trials
  —Co-Investigator
  —Commercialization
  —Consortium or Contractual Agreement
  —Consultant
  —Consulting fees
  —Cooperative Agreement
  —Essentially Equivalent Work (i.e., "scientific overlap")
  —Feasibility
  —Foreign Component
  —Full-Time Appointment
  —Gender
  —Grant
  —Human Subjects
  —Innovation
  —Institutional Base Salary
  —Key Personnel
  —Principal Investigator, Program Director, or Project Director
  —Program Income
  —Prototype
  —Research or Research and Development
  —Research Institution
  —Significant Difference (not to be confused with "statistically significant difference")
  —Socially and Economically Disadvantaged Individual
  —Subcontract
  —United States
  —Valid Analysis (i.e., an unbiased assessment)
- Information about "Other support"
  —Budgetary overlap

—Commitment overlap
—Scientific overlap
—Resolution of overlap

> **NOTE: Submit information about other support ONLY when requested by the NIH institute/center (I/C)**
>
>   Follow the sample format on the "Other Support format page" for guidance regarding the type and extent of information requested.

- Instructions for selected other items
  - Project Number
  - Source of support
  - Major Goals
  - Dates of Approved/Proposed Project
  - Annual Direct Costs
  - Percent Effort
  - Overlap with active or pending projects and the current Application in terms of the science, budget, or an individual's committed effort
- Personnel Report
  - Form page (RTF or PDF)
  - Only for Competing Continuation Applications
  - Use only when requested by the awarding component
- Grant solicitations
  - Specific Program Announcements (PAs)
    Program Announcement: A formal statement about a new or ongoing extramural activity or mechanism. It may serve as a reminder of continuing interest in a research area, describe modification in an activity or mechanism, and/or invite Applications for grant support. Most Applications in response to PAs may be submitted for any appropriate receipt date and are reviewed with all other Applications received at that time.
  - Requests for Applications (RFAs)
    Request for Applications: A formal statement that invites grant or cooperative agreement Applications in a well-defined scientific area to accomplish specific program objectives. The RFA indicates the estimated amount of funds set aside for the competition, the estimated number of awards to be made, and the Application receipt date(s). Applications submitted in response to an RFA usually are reviewed by an SRG convened by the awarding component that issued the RFA.

  PAs and RFAs are published in the
  - *Federal Register*
  - *NIH Guide for Grants and Contracts*
    For information about obtaining the *NIH Guide for Grants and Contracts* go to
    http://grants.nih.gov/grants/guide

■ Guidelines for some popular NIH programs

Note that

Institutional National Research Service Awards

and

Individual National Research Service Awards

both have the same abbreviation: **NRSA**

—Extramural program guidelines NIH National Research Service Award Individual Postdoctoral Fellowship (F32) guidelines

http://grants.nih.gov/training/nrsa.htm

—NIH National Research Service Award Senior Fellowship (F33) guidelines

http://grants.nih.gov/training/nrsa.htm

—NIH National Research Service Award Institutional Grant (T32) guidelines

http://grants.nih.gov/training/nrsa.htm

—NIH National Research Service Award Short-Term Training for Students in Health Professional Schools (T35) guidelines

http://grants.nih.gov/training/nrsa.htm

—Research Grants to Foreign Institutions and International Organizations

http://grants.nih.gov/grants/policy/nihgps/part_iii_5.htm#awardsforeign

—K Awards-Research Career Program Awards

http://grants.nih.gov/training/careerdevelopmentawards.htm

For scientists with clear research potential who need additional experience in a productive scientific environment to prepare for a career in independent biomedical research.

—Academic Research Enhancement Award (Area, R15) guidelines

http://grants.nih.gov/grants/funding/area.htm

For scientists at eligible domestic institutions who want to do small-scale health-related research projects, such as pilot research projects and feasibility studies; development, testing, and refinement of research techniques; and similar discrete research projects that demonstrate research capability. This award is directed toward faculty members at smaller public and private colleges and universities that provide undergraduate training for a significant number of U.S. research scientists.

■ Applications available from other offices

—Fogarty International Center
International Research Fellowship Award
Application (NIH 1541-1)
Tel: 301-496-1653

—Health Resources and Services Administration
Non-research Training Grant Application (PHS 6025)
Tel: 301-443-6960

—Substance Abuse and Mental Health Services Administration (SAMHSA)
Health Services Project Application (5161-1)
Tel: 301-436-8451

- Other useful information/Web sites
  - —Publications about NIH extramural research and research training programs
    http://grants.nih.gov/grants/oer.htm
  - —Telephone number for NIH staff
    http://directory.nih.gov
    Tel: 301-496-4000 (the NIH locator)
  - —NIH Extramural Research and Research Training Programs
    (general information)
    http://grants.nih.gov/grants/oer.htm
    E-mail: GrantsInfo@nih.gov
    Tel: 301-435-0714
  - —For information about a specific Application, before review, telephone or
    e-mail the Scientific Review Administrator (SRA) named on the "notification
    of assignment."
  - —To check on receipt and referral of an Application, contact:
    Division of Receipt and Referral Center for Scientific Review
    Tel: 301-435-0715
    Fax: 301-480-1987
  - —For information about Human Subject Protections, Institutional Review
    Boards, or related assurances (Office for Human Research Protections):
    http://ohrp.osophs.dhhs.gov/index.htm
    Tel: 301-496-7041
  - —For animal welfare and related regulations and assurances contact Office of
    Laboratory Animal Welfare (OLAW)
    http://grants.nih.gov/grants/olaw/olaw.htm
    Tel: 301-496-7163

SOME IMPORTANT CONSIDERATIONS

Incomplete Applications
An Application will be considered incomplete and *returned to the Principal Investigator if:*
- It is illegible
- It does not conform to the instructions
- The material presented is insufficient to permit adequate review

Simultaneous submission of Applications
You may NOT simultaneously submit **identical** Applications to different agencies within
the PHS or to different Institutes within an agency except as follows:
- Research Career Development Award Applications may propose work identical
  to that proposed in an Individual Research Grant Application.
- An Individual Research Grant Application may propose work identical to a sub-
  project that is part of a Program Project or Center Grant Application.

> **NOTE:** The PI must **fully disclose simultaneous submissions** under "Other support," *in
> both Applications.*

Sending additional information after submission of the proposal
(See also the Section of this book called "Tracking the Application")
You **may send additional or corrective material** pertinent to an Application after the submission deadline (specified Application receipt date). You may do this as late as 4 weeks *prior to* the Study Section meeting, but *only* if it is **specifically solicited—or agreed to—** by prior discussion with an appropriate Public Health Service staff member, usually the Scientific Review Administrator of the pertinent Study Section. Be sure that the SRA concurs that the material you plan to send is acceptable and that the time of submission is acceptable. Some SRAs have cutoff dates for acceptance of additional materials.

If permission is granted, ask the official how many copies to send. If it is not long after the Grant Application submission deadline, you will probably need to send 5 or 6 copies. If it is only a few weeks before the Study Section meeting, you should offer to send 25 copies of the item so the SRA does not have the bother of getting copies made. Once complete electronic submission of Grant Applications becomes a reality, the issue of sending multiple copies may no longer apply.

Any materials you send should be **addressed to the Scientific Review Administrator** of the Study Section to which your Application has been assigned and should always be accompanied by a **cover letter**. (Your materials are likely to get lost if you address them simply to "Center for Scientific Review.")

Enclose a self-addressed, stamped postcard with a note asking that the postcard be returned to you to acknowledge that the materials you sent were received by the Scientific Review Administrator. Call the SRA if you do not get your postcard back within 2 weeks.

At the same time, **send copies** of the letter and the item(s) **to the Institute program staff ombudsperson** for your Application. Indicate that the materials are "For your information."

Use and availability of information contained in Grant Applications
- NIH may use the information contained in proposals for
   —reviewing Applications
   —monitoring grantee performance
   —identifying candidates to serve as regular or ad hoc Reviewers for Study
      Sections, Councils, etc.

Analyzing costs of proposed grants
- The Privacy Act of 1974 allows certain disclosures and permits Principal
   Investigators and Program Directors to request copies of records pertaining to
   their Grant Applications from the NIH component responsible for funding decisions. Established procedures permit Principal Investigators and Program
   Directors to request correction of inaccurate records. NIH will amend such
   records if the agency concurs that the records are incorrect.
- NIH makes information about *awarded* grants available to the public, including
   the
   —title of the project
   —grantee institution
   —name of Principal Investigator or Program Director
   The Abstracts of all funded research Grant Applications are sent to the National
   Technical Information Service (NTIS), U.S. Department of Commerce, and *are
   available to the public from NTIS.*

- The Freedom of Information Act and implementing DHHS regulations require the release, upon request, of certain information about **grants that have been awarded**, irrespective of the intended use of the information. For information about the types of information that are generally available and *not* available for release, contact NIH. *Final determination about information release is made by NIH.* The Principal Investigator or Program Director of the grant in question is consulted and/or informed about any such release of information.

A Word of Caution

Considering the above regulations, it seems obvious that if you are unable to obtain a good example of a successful Grant Proposal/Application (to use as a "model") from colleagues, you can search NTIS files for an Abstract of a proposal in your field—or in a field related to yours—and then request to see the relevant proposal. Although this is a way to get a successful proposal to read, reading another scientist's current proposal is fraught with ethical dilemmas, so one should use this method **ONLY AS A LAST RESORT**. To point out just one problem: the human brain, unfortunately, does not have a "delete" key. Once you read someone else's good idea(s), it is not possible to delete the information from your brain. Thus, if you use the mechanism described above to obtain a sample proposal to study and perhaps use as a model, you must **be extremely careful not to inadvertently "borrow" ideas from the proposal**. Moreover, the Principal Investigator of the proposal that you have requested to see will be informed that you (Dr. X at University of XYZ) requested her/his Application, and s/he may have misgivings about your request. If you decide to obtain a proposal in this manner, it is wise to get an older, rather than a current, proposal so that the Principal Investigator is likely to have had an opportunity to publish some of her/his work and establish her/his foothold in the field.

NON-COMPETING CONTINUATION APPLICATIONS

NOTE that as of late 2002 the NIH notification of the Progress Report due date has been sent by electronic communication.

In 1994, an announcement in the *NIH Guide for Grants and Contracts* (Volume 23, Number 38) introduced a **streamlined** non-competing continuation award process for certain types of NIH research grants and career awards. This notice provided clarification and guidance for submitting the **streamlined** non-competing continuation Application (PHS Form 2590) for the grants covered by the process. NIH grant recipients are expected to use the guidelines when submitting the **streamlined** non-competing continuation Application for R01, R03, R13, R15, R18, R21, R24, R25, R29, R37, R42, R44, or the "K" series mechanisms. See:

SUPPLEMENTAL GUIDANCE ON THE NIH STREAMLINED NON-COMPETINGCONTINUATION PROCESS

NIH GUIDE, Volume 24, Number 2, January 20, 1995
accessed at

http://grants2.nih.gov/grants/guide/notice-files/not95-027.html

For questions about competing Applications procedures call the:

Referral Office
Division of Research Grants
Tel: 301-435-0715

Throughout a funded project period, non-competing continuation Applications must be submitted annually, 2 months before the beginning date of the next budget period. Information and forms for the NON-COMPETING GRANT PROGRESS REPORT, PHS 2590 (REVISED May 2001) - Updated: 06/28/2002 are available at

http://grants.nih.gov/grants/funding/2590/2590.htm

Read and follow the PHS 2590 instructions carefully, and prepare the Application accordingly, following the outline and numbering system prescribed in the PHS 2590. PHS 2590 contains some of the same parts as the PHS 398. Unless you are submitting electronically, be sure that you submit the completed original continuation Application and the number of copies requested—signed by both the PI and the official signing for the institution—directly to the awarding component that is funding the grant. Some help for filling out PHS 2590 is available at

http://grants.nih.gov/grants/forms_faq.pdf

When you go to this Web site, you will find multiple pages of questions and answers about the PHS 398 and PHS 2590 Forms and Instructions under the following headings:

- General Questions
- RTF (Rich Text Format)
- PDF (Portable Document Format)
- Questions Related to Form Pages
- Questions Related to the PHS 2590
- SBIR/STTR Applications
- Other Helpful Hints

See also

http://grants.nih.gov/grants/funding/2590/section_2.html#snap

If you submitted a detailed budget with your initial Application, you must be careful not to exceed the amount shown on the "Notice of Grant Award" for the year about which you are reporting. If funding requirements have changed since the award notice, you should discuss such changes with your Program Officer at the awarding Institute.

Provide Biographical Sketches for any **NEW key personnel and Consultants/ Collaborators** who have joined your research group since you submitted the original Application.

Progress Report Summary

The **Progress Report Summary** is the record of your accomplishments in the preceding year and serves as the basis for continuing support for the project. Write the Progress Report Summary so that it assures the agency that their money is being well spent. Contrary to commonly held beliefs, the non-competing Applications are read by the staff at the awarding agency and should be prepared carefully and with attention to the needs of the Readers at the awarding agency.

The **Progress Report Summary** is also used by the awarding component staff to:

- Prepare annual reports
- Plan programs
- Communicate scientific accomplishments supported by the agency

Therefore, the language used in the **Progress Report Summary** should be readily understandable by a biomedical scientist who may *NOT* be a specialist in your project—or even in your general research field. Aim for the style used in articles in Scientific American.

Parts of the Progress Report Summary

- Specific Aims (maximum of 250 words)

    —Summarize the Specific Aims of the project as *funded*.

    —Unless otherwise specified, the budget awarded is based on the assumption by the awarding agency that the funds provided are adequate to accomplish the Specific Aims of the original proposal. In some cases, however, Study Section or Council recommendations or budget modifications (usually reductions) made by the awarding component may require a change in the scope of the Aims compared to those in the original competing Application.

- Studies and results (maximum of 750 words)

    Discuss any significant negative results and/or technical problems that you have encountered.

- Significance

    —No page limit specified; this part probably deserves about half a page.

    —Use lay language.

    —Discuss the potential impact of your findings on health.

- Plans

    —No page limit specified; probably deserves 1-2 pages.

    —Summarize plans for the next budget year to address the aims listed in Specific Aims.

    —Discuss any modifications to your original plans for the project.

The total of the aforementioned 4 parts of the PHS 2590 Progress Report Summary should be no longer than the equivalent of about 5 single-spaced $8^{1}/_{2} \times 11$ inch pages (using NIH-approved font styles and sizes). If you wish to submit any major inclusions (such as large data sets, figures, tables) pertinent to your progress, consult the Institute program staff person responsible for your Application, and ask about the appropriateness of the intended submission.

- Publications

    —Report only publications (accepted for publication or published) not reported previously, which have resulted directly from this grant.

    —Provide 1 copy of each such manuscript or publication.

- Inventions and patents
- Checklist

    —There is a 1-page Checklist that **must be filled out and included as the *last* page** of the renewal Application. This Checklist deals with:

    assurances and certifications

    program income

    indirect costs

RECAP FOR PART III: PARTS OF THE GRANT APPLICATION

Application form for NIH grants: PHS 398
- For Research Grants (R01) and many other types of grants
- Has historically been revised about every 3 years
- **Is no longer available in paper form**

Other funding agencies have different Applications and instructions. If you know how to prepare a good NIH Grant Application and understand the principles of responding to a set of instructions, you should be able to prepare a good Application to any funding agency.

PARTS OF THE GRANT APPLICATION

Administrative and financial information
For additional specific instructions go to

   http://grants.nih.gov/grants/funding/2590/section_2.html#snap

and scroll down to **"B. SPECIFIC INSTRUCTIONS"**

Face page
- Title of Application
     56 spaces
     descriptive
     specific
     appropriate
- Dates of entire proposed project period
- Direct costs and total costs
     Unless you are requesting a budget that exceeds $250,000 per year, you are required to submit a **Modular Grant Application** and request an appropriate number of $25,000 modules
- PI's signature
- Signature of official signing for Applicant institution

Abstract page
   Abstract of Research Plan
     Broad, long-term objectives
     Specific Aims
     Health-Relatedness
     Research Design and Methods

To save time and ensure that your Abstract **accurately reflects the final proposal, write the abstract AFTER** you have printed the **FINAL** draft of the rest of the Application and are certain that you will not change any of the Research Plan.

   Make life easy for yourself and the Reviewers: Write the Abstract as follows: The broad, long-term objectives are: (1)...; (2).... The Specific Aims are (1)...; (2)...; (3).... The Health-Relatedness is.... The Research Design is.... The Methods to be used are (1)...; (2)...; (3)...; (4)...; (5)....

Be sure to read the other instructions for the Abstract.

Key personnel (bottom half of Abstract page)

Fill in the requested information.

Table of Contents

- Fill in the page numbers **in the final draft** of the Application.

  Consider including a **separate** Table of Contents for the Research Plan **on a sheet without a page number**. Mark this sheet, "For the convenience of the Reviewers." This additional Table of Contents should list all the sub-headings in the Research Plan with the corresponding page numbers.

- List Appendix items (Each Appendix item should have a number and a Title/Description)

  —Number of the Appendix item

  —Title/Description of the Appendix item

If total budget for first year is over $250K:

Detailed budget for first 12 months should be:

- Reasonable
- Believable
- Well-researched
- Superbly justified
- Developed **AFTER** the project is completely planned

Budget for total project period

- Research the budget carefully.
- Provide quotes for large equipment.
- Include costs of service contracts and shipping.

Budget Justification

- Justify everything that is not obvious.
- Justify significant increases in future years.
- Be aware that the care demonstrated in writing the Budget Justification tells reviewers about the care and conscientiousness of the PI's research and resource management.
- Use an outline form.
- There are *no* page limits—but be brief.

Biographical sketches

- Photocopy a form for **each** key professional person.
- Put Postdoctoral training under "Education."
- Give complete references (including titles) to

  —*all* publications of the past 3 years

  and

  —representative earlier publications *pertinent* to the Application

- There is a 4-page limit per person. NIH gives specific instructions about what information is required and how to apportion the space! Follow the NIH instructions!

Other support
- Provide information about *all* active or pending support to the PI or other key personnel, whether or not it is related to this Application.
- Incomplete/inaccurate/ambiguous reporting may delay review and/or funding.
- Report to the potential funding agent any changes in support (e.g., from other funding agencies) that occur after proposal submission.

Resources and environment
- Facilities
- Major equipment
- Work environment
- Support services

The Research Plan
The Research Plan is the main **science** part of the Application. It consists of the following sub-sections:

Introduction	At NIH, an Introduction is required only for revised and supplemental applications (see below).
a. **Specific Aims**	What you intend to do?
b. **Background and Significance**	• What has already been done in the field? • Why the work is important?
c. **Preliminary Studies or Progress Report**	What *you* have already done on this project?
d. **Research Design and Methods**	• How you will fulfill the Aims? • How you will do the work?

There is a 25-page limit for parts (a) through (d) of the Research Plan. This 25-page limit must include tables/charts and reduced versions of Appendix materials other than reprints/publications.

Include sufficient information for effective review without reference to a previous Application.

Use collaborators for aspects of the project that are outside your field of expertise.

a. Specific Aims (1 page)
- State the broad, long-term objective(s).
- Describe what research is intended to accomplish.
- State the hypotheses to be tested.

b. Background and Significance (2–3 pages)
- Sketch the Background leading to the Application.
- Evaluate the existing knowledge.
- Identify the gaps that the project is intended to fill.
- State the importance of research, i.e., explain why the proposed work is worth doing.

- Cite appropriate references and list them in the "Literature Cited" section. Although the "Literature Cited" section has no page limit, be reasonable; cite important and pertinent references—not ALL possible references.

c. Preliminary Studies/Progress Report (6–8 pages)

New Applications:
Discuss **Preliminary Studies** and other information that will help establish the **experience** and **competence** of the PI. List publications and manuscripts that have been **accepted** for publication.

Renewal Applications:
Require a Progress Report
- Provide an account of progress for Specific Aims of the **preceding** Application.
- If you did not complete—or at least make progress with respect to—one or more of the Specific Aims of the preceding Application, explain why without "making excuses."
- Summarize the importance of the findings you have made in the previous project period.
- List publications and manuscripts accepted for publication.

d. Research Design and Methods (13–16 pages)
- Summarize the Specific Aims for the current proposal.
- Give a one- or two-sentence rationale for each Aim.
- Describe the Research Design for each Aim.
- Describe and/or reference the Methods to be used to accomplish each of the Aims.
- Explain why the proposed approach was chosen.
- Convince the Reviewers that you can do what you have proposed. If possible provide them with evidence in the form of Preliminary Data.
- Indicate the relationship of the Specific Aims to each other and to the overall objective(s).
- Discuss:
  —Control experiments
  —How data will be
  - Collected
  - Analyzed
  - **Interpreted**
  —Potential difficulties and limitations of proposed procedures
  —Alternative approaches to achieve the Specific Aims
  —Hazardous procedures/situations/materials and precautions to be exercised
  —Tentative sequence/timetable for project

Human subjects:
- Requires IRB approval
- Address all the points specified in the NIH Instructions (see NIH Web site)

- If appropriate, assure the Reviewers and the Funding Agency that experiments involving human subjects are
  —necessary
  —well-thought-out
  —scientifically sound
- Indicate how many patients per year will be available for studies, and demonstrate that this number is sufficient to provide a statistically significant answer to your questions

Vertebrate animals:
- Requires IACUC approval
- Address all points specified in NIH Instructions (see NIH Web site)
- Assure Reviewers that animal experiments are
  —necessary
  —well-thought-out
  —scientifically sound

Literature Cited
- List all pertinent references
- Use a **consistent** format
  The format should be the same as that used for the list of publications in the Progress Report.
- The list may include—but may NOT replace—the list of publications required in the Progress Report
- Each reference must include the
  —title of the article
  —names of **ALL** authors
  —title of book or journal in which the article is published
  —volume number
  —page numbers
  —year of the publication
- The references should be thorough but limited to relevant and current literature. Although there is NO page limitation, it is important to be concise. Choose wisely and list only those literature references **pertinent** to the proposed research.
- If you list critical references that are difficult to access, ask for permission to provide copies in the Appendix.

Consortium/contractual arrangements:
- Justify and explain arrangements (programmatic, fiscal, administrative)
- If consortium/contractual activities represent a significant portion of the overall project, explain why the Applicant organization, rather than the ultimate performer of the activities, should be the grantee.
- Establish the necessary inter-organizational agreement(s)
- Provide copies of written agreements

Consultants/Collaborators:

- List whether or not salaries are requested
- Provide a letter from each **Consultant** and/or **Collaborator**, confirming her/his role in the project
- Provide a Biosketch for each **Consultant** or **Collaborator**

Appendix:

- Questionnaires
- Graphs, diagrams, tables, charts, oversized documents, photographs, and/or other materials that do not reproduce well (however, reduced copies must also appear **within** the Research Plan)
- Maximum of 10 publications/manuscripts or other documents resulting from the project
- Materials that save primary Reviewers time (must first get permission from SRA to submit such items)
- Do NOT use the Appendix to circumvent the page limits for the Research Plan.
- Proposal must be comprehensible without reference to Appendix

Checklist

The CHECKLIST FORM PAGE in either <u>MS WORD</u> or <u>PDF format</u> is available directly from

http://grants.nih.gov/grants/funding/phs398/phs398.html

and also, with directions, from

http://grants.nih.gov/grants/funding/phs398/section_1.html#10_checklist

The CHECKLIST requires the Applicant to provide information about:

Type of Application

Inventions and Patents (Competing Continuation Applications Only)

NIH has developed an optional online Extramural Invention Information Management System, known as "Edison," to facilitate grantee compliance with the disclosure and reporting requirements of 37 CFR 401.14(h). Information from these reports is not made publicly available.

Program Income

Assurances/Certifications

Assurances and certifications listed on the Checklist must be verified by the signature of the official signing for the Applicant organization on the Face Page of the Application.

Facilities and Administrative (F&A) Costs

Indicate the Applicant organization's most recent F&A cost rate established with the appropriate DHHS Regional Office, or, in the case of for-profit organizations, the rate established with the appropriate PHS agency cost advisory office. See additional instructions at Web site.

Special Instructions for Modular Applications

Applicant institutions should calculate the F&A costs using the current negotiated F&A rate, less exclusions, for the initial budget period and all future budget periods. It is not necessary to list the exclusions on the Checklist or anywhere in the Application.

Smoke-Free Workplace

Follow the instructions on the Checklist. Response to the question has no impact on the review or funding of this Application.

Some additional information

- Incomplete Applications may be returned **without review**.
- Simultaneous submission of Applications to NIH is not permitted (except for certain types of Applications; call NIH for information). Simultaneous submission of Applications to 2 or more agencies may or may not be acceptable. Call both agencies to ask. In any case of simultaneous submission of Applications, be sure to make full disclosure of simultaneous submission under "Other support," in *both* Applications.
- Sending additional information after a proposal has been submitted is permitted at NIH *only* if solicited—**or agreed to**—by the SRA. **Always call to request permission before sending additional information/materials.**
- For information about use/availability of information contained in Grant Applications, contact NIH.
  —Information about awarded grants is available to the public from NTIS.

NON-COMPETING CONTINUATION APPLICATIONS AT NIH

- Must be submitted annually throughout a funded project period
  Use the PHS 2590 form on the NIH Web site.
- Do not exceed the budget amount shown on the "Notice of Grant Award" for the year for which you are submitting the PHS 2590 unless agreed to by Program Officer at the awarding Institute.
- Provide Biographical Sketches for any **new key personnel and Consultants**
- Submit a **Progress Report Summary** (5 single-spaced pages for Parts 1–4). Include publications not previously reported, and provide one copy of each (a) published paper and/or (b) manuscript accepted for publication.
- List inventions and patents
- Complete the required Checklist

PART IV

PLANNING THE RESEARCH PLAN

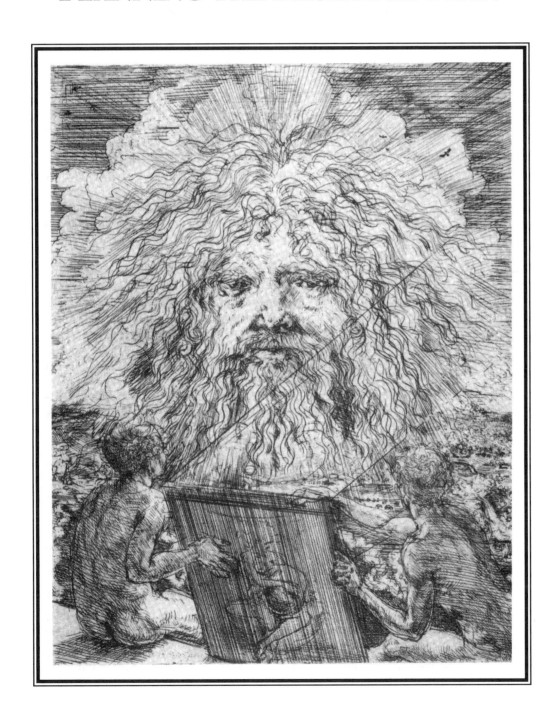

INTRODUCTION

The most important part of any grant Application is the Research Plan. It is the basis—or major subject and content—of the proposal.

The Research Plan should
- be innovative
- be timely
- have obvious (or clearly explained) significance
- have a clear rationale
- be focused
- be well-thought-out
- address a specific problem—or set of related problems—that can be solved by a logical sequence of experiments

NOTE: Do **NOT** try to incorporate **every idea you have** about all interesting topics into one grant proposal.

For Applications to NIH and other organizations that are primarily committed to solving problems related to health, clinical relevance is important. But avoid inventing an artificial, overly tenuous, or circuitous health-relatedness for the proposal.

Understanding the "Lingo"
If you plan to apply to NIH for funding, it is important that you understand certain NIH terminology. Likewise, if you plan to apply to another agency, you should familiarize yourself with the terminology used by that agency.

At NIH, **Success Rates** indicate the percentage of reviewed research project grant Applications that receive funding. This is computed on a fiscal year basis. The Success Rate is derived by dividing the number of competing Applications that are funded by the total number of competing Applications that were reviewed. Applications that have one or more amendments/revisions in the same fiscal year are only counted once. Success Rates for all activities are included. See

http://grants2.nih.gov/grants/award/success.htm

Data about NIH competing research project Applications by type of grant for fiscal years 1970–2002 are given at

http://grants2.nih.gov/grants/award/success/srbytype7002.htm

It is important that you are aware that **Success Rates** are generally greater than the "percentile pay-line," which varies from one Institute to another and also varies over time (see the above Web site). At NIH the variability depends on
- the difference in appropriations for the various NIH funding components
- how much of the funding is obligated for non-competing renewals committed to in prior years

- how each funding component chooses to use its funds

  For example, NIH funding components that fund many large programs, such as Program Project Grant Applications, fund fewer R01s and other smaller Grant Applications, and vice versa.

Consult the funding agency that you think may have an interest in your project to determine whether your ideas are considered to have a high priority in the view of that agency. Some NIH Institutes publish documents that indicate their research priorities. For example, the National Eye Institute has periodically published a 5-year plan (1983–1987; 1994–1998) of its program priorities. A variety of NIH publications, many of them free of charge and others now available at (and only at) the NIH Web site, including the *NIH Guide for Grants and Contracts*, are also good places to get an idea of current interests at NIH.

The *NIH Guide for Grants and Contracts* is the official document for announcing the availability of NIH funds for biomedical and behavioral research, research training, and disseminating NIH policy and administrative information.

Each week the NIH transmits via a LISTSERV e-mail the Table of Contents (TOC) information for that week's issue of the *NIH Guide for Grants and Contracts*. Associated with each TOC entry is the Internet address (URL) for each *NIH Guide* article.

It's a good idea to request to have the Table of Contents for the *NIH Guide* sent to you via **e-mail** on a regular basis. There is no charge.

To subscribe to the Guide TOC Notification LISTSERV service, send an e-mail to

listserv@list.nih.gov

In the first line of the e-mail **message** (NOT in the "Subject" line) type:

subscribe NIHTOC-L your name

where "your name" is the name you wish to use. Your e-mail address will be automatically obtained from the e-mail message you send to the LISTSERV.

Start building a reputation

Although it is important that you have expertise (a "**track record**") in your proposed field of research, **do not be discouraged** if you are a new entrant into the field.

You stand a good chance of getting funded **if** your

- training was good
- proposal idea is good
- Application contains substantive data from some significant pilot studies
- proposal plan is well-thought-out
- proposal plan is well-presented/clearly written

Presentation of pilot experiments and preliminary experimental results are imperative. Be aware that some agencies provide small grants that support pilot projects.

For example,

NIH has a Small Grants Program (R03)

http://grants2.nih.gov/grants/funding/r03.htm

and

NSF has a **Small Grants for Exploratory Research (SGER) Program.**

In addition to the SGER program, NSF has numerous other programs that may be of interest. Some of these programs are listed at

http://www.nsf.gov/od/lpa/news/publicat/nsf0203/cross/ocpa.html#section1

For small businesses, various government agencies have a **Small Business Innovation Research Grant Program (SBIR)** that provides Phase I funding for pilot projects.

Think carefully about what you will write.

A clear, concise, but adequately detailed description of the **Research Design and Methods** to be used to achieve the proposed research goals (**Specific Aims**) of your project is an essential part of the Research Plan of the Application. Do NOT plunge the Reviewer into a long "shopping list" of Methods that you plan to use without providing a context (Research Design) within which you will use these methods.

Don't present a global set of experiments.

- Experiments should be feasible and designed such that
    —they answer specific questions
    —one experiment leads logically to the next
- It must be clear to Reviewers that the proposed experiments can be **successfully completed**
    —with the proposed budget
    —within the time requested
- It is **critically important** to provide the Reviewers with **alternative procedures** to be used to achieve the Specific Aims, in case your primary approach turns out to be unfruitful.

    Having **preliminary data** from experiments that you propose to do is a good way of assuring Reviewers that your **proposed experiments will yield useful results.** Nonetheless, presentation of **alternative procedures** is useful for convincing the Reviewers that you have a good overall command of the project you plan to pursue.

- If the experiments you propose in your Application are sequentially dependent on each other, describing **alternative approaches** becomes even more important.

> **A CAUTION:** If a project hinges, for example, on one **early** experiment, the outcome of which any Reviewer might possibly question, and no alternative approaches are given, the project is **NOT** likely to be funded.

You must clearly indicate to the Reviewers that you have a realistic grasp of

- what will be required to do the project
    —personnel
    —equipment
    —supplies
- how much can be accomplished in the requested time

A reasonable **budget** reflects your knowledge and thoughtfulness about the costs associated with your research. Reviewers may consider you

- **"naïve" if you under-budget**
- **"greedy" if you over-budget**

Likewise, **Reviewers become wary** if you

- propose 10 years of work in a 3-year Grant Application (a common problem with junior investigators!!!)

or

- attempt to draw a 1-year project out to fill 3 years of time

Note taken from

http://grants1.nih.gov/grants/funding/phs398/section_1.html#8_research

> "Starting with the October 1, 2003 receipt date, investigators submitting an NIH Application seeking $500,000 or more in direct costs in any single year are expected to include a plan for **data sharing** or state why data sharing is not possible." See

http://grants.nih.gov/grants/guide/notice-files/NOT-OD-03-032.html

Schedule for Preparing the Research Plan

A **concise schedule** (placed at the end of the Research Design and Methods section) indicating the aspects of the project planned for each of the proposed years of support is a help to the Reviewers. But a detailed analysis of what you will do week by week, or month by month, is unnecessary. Moreover, exaggerated detail often provides—to your disadvantage—comic relief for the Reviewers and detracts from your credibility as an experienced, professional scientist.

For detailed instructions, see

http://grants1.nih.gov/grants/funding/phs398/phs398.html

THINGS TO THINK ABOUT BEFORE YOU WRITE THE RESEARCH PLAN

Writing a **good** Grant Application is a long and painstaking process. Before you devote any effort to this task, be sure that the idea that is the basis of your Application is

- a viable/do-able idea
- a GOOD idea
- of interest to the funding agency to which you plan to apply for support

Although bad writing can easily undermine a good idea, even the best writing will **NOT** turn a poor idea into a funded proposal. Likewise, a well-written proposal about a superb idea will probably not be funded by an agency that is not interested in the project. Targeting a proposal to the wrong agency wastes both your time and the precious time of the Reviewers! Thus, you may save hours of valuable time if—**before** you write the proposal—you discuss your ideas with

- more established and experienced colleagues
- administrators from the potential funding agency, for example, staff of the NIH Institute to whom your Application is likely to be assigned.

The agency staff can sometimes also provide helpful comments and advice about the general approach for preparing an Application to that agency. **However, do NOT expect them to help with the science aspects of the Application.** NIH encourages Applicants to contact staff of the relevant Institute.

One way to determine who might be a helpful person to talk to at NIH is to ask a more senior colleague who does research in an area similar to yours. If that is not convenient, or there is no appropriate person available, find an initial staff contact at the appropriate agency or Institute within the NIH at the NIH Web site, or contact:

Grants Information Office
Tel: 301-435-0714
E-mail: GrantsInfo@NIH.GOV

NOTE FOR APPLICANTS TO PRIVATE FOUNDATIONS: Personnel at some private foundations will **work with you** to help you develop your proposal if they consider that your idea is good and appropriate to the mandate of the agency.

Get help from colleagues and mentors

Having colleagues and mentors critique your Application—**after you have written a fairly good complete draft**—is a critical part of the Application preparation process and can help you

- avoid pitfalls in your logic or science
- test for clarity in your presentation
    —You understand your subject very well and know what you want to say; but do others perceive what you intend them to perceive from your writing?
    —It's important to remember that there can be no communication when there is a gap between the intention of the writer (or speaker) and the perception of the reader (or listener).
    —A communication gap generally implies that the proposal-writer is not thinking clearly. Your Reviewers are likely to conclude, "Muddy writing indicates muddy thinking." Make it difficult for the Reviewers to reach such a conclusion about your Application.

Plan to have **at least 3 people** review your Grant Application **before** you create the final draft:

- Someone who understands your specific research—to check for **accuracy**.
- Someone who understands science and research but does *not* know about your specific research (the "Intelligent Non-Expert")—to check for **clarity** and **consistency** of thought.
- Someone who is a good editor—to make sure that
    —your exposition is **consistent** throughout the whole proposal
    —**everyone who reads the Application will know exactly what you mean to say**
    —the Readers get a good impression of you

Make an appointment with **appropriate** Readers **early** in the process of working on your Application. This

- gives the Readers a chance to block out a specific time to devote to reading your proposal
- forces you to create—for yourself—a convenient **pre-deadline target date** by which to finish **a good second draft** of your proposal

Leave yourself ample time to do a good job!

As a courtesy to your Readers (Colleagues), ask **THEM—way ahead of time**—how much time they would like to have to read and critique your proposal. Even if they say they only need a few days, plan to give the Readers at least 2 to 4 weeks to read your proposal, and allow yourself at least 2 to 4 weeks (4 weeks is preferable!)—after they return your proposal—to implement their suggestions.

Before you plan your project—and again before you begin to write your grant proposal—carefully read the instructions for completing the Application. The instructions are given on the NIH Web site. Be aware that some aspects of the instructions are changed occasionally by NIH. There are special alerts about such changes/new developments on the NIH Web site. These changes are sometimes also announced in the *NIH Guide for Grants and Contracts*. Some of these changes are important. Therefore, it is important to

- keep up to date with the *NIH Guide for Grants and Contracts*
- check the NIH Web site frequently

Do not assume that you know the instructions by remembering them from the last time you submitted an Application.

Whatever instructions you are following, be they from NIH or another agency, it is wise to make a detailed outline of

- the information to be provided
- the order in which the agency wants you to provide the information

After you have read the instructions for preparing an NIH (or other agency) Grant Application—but before you begin writing your own proposal—read one or more well-written, **successful** Applications that have received good priority scores (remember that at NIH the best score is 100; the worst score is 500) and have been funded for 3 or more years. You should be able to find such proposals at many research institutions. Perhaps the PIs will allow you to read not only the proposals, but also the corresponding Summary Statements, i.e., the Reviewers' critiques about the proposal. Reading these documents will give you a better idea of

- what the instructions mean
- how to respond to the instructions
- what Study Section members look for in proposals
- what Study Section members DO and DO NOT like to find in proposals

Careful reading of the depersonalized Summary Statements in Part VII of this book will also give you a sense of what Reviewers look for when they review grant Applications. If you cannot find a good model proposal to read at your institution, contact NIH for information about use/availability of funded Grant Applications via the "Freedom of Information Act."

OTHER PRELIMINARY CONSIDERATIONS

The NIH instructions for the Research Plan specify:

The Research Plan should include sufficient information needed for evaluation of the project, **independent of any other document**. Be specific and informative, and avoid redundancies. Organize [the 4 parts of] the Research Plan to answer the questions in the last column of the table below:

Part #	Heading	What NIH wants you to describe in this part of the Application
a.	**Specific Aims**	What do you intend to do?
b.	**Background and Significance**	What has already been done and why is the work important?
c.	**Preliminary Studies/Progress Report**	What have **YOU** already done?
d.	**Research Design and Methods**	How are you going to do the work?

NOTE: In the list I have compiled below of things to think about when you are **preparing** to write a Grant Application, I have put in bold type the items I want to emphasize, including each of the 4 items listed in the above table.

ASPECTS OF PROPOSAL PREPARATION

Think about each of the following aspects of proposal preparation:

- Decide what you are going to do/propose
- Do a feasibility analysis. Consider
  - —facilities
  - —resources
  - —institutional support for the project
- Decide where (to what agency) to apply for funding
- Make contact with the funding agency
  Determine whether—and to what extent—the agency is interested in—and has funds available for—your project
- **Plan** the project **meticulously**
- If appropriate, arrange for appropriate
  - —Collaborators
  and/or
  - —Consultants
- Do preliminary (pilot) studies
  Collect sufficient good preliminary data to convince the Reviewers that your proposed **Research Plan** stands a good chance of yielding useful information.
- Describe **what you plan/intend to do** (i.e., outline—and then write the proposal)
- Develop a **realistic** budget
  - —Develop a reasonable budget **EVEN if you are not required to SUBMIT a detailed budget with your Grant Application!**
  - —Do NOT just guess/estimate how much money you will need to do the project described in your Application.
    - Determine what you will need to carry out the project
    - Find out how much the necessary items will cost
    - Determine which items you will need at what stage of the project
  - —For requests to NIH that are less than $250,000 per year, calculate how many modules of $25,000 each you will need per year.
  - —Be sure that you have checked the NIH (or other funding agency) guidelines concerning the most recent updated information about salary limitations.

Write down the answers to the following questions:
- What is to be done?
  What is the hypothesis to be tested or question(s) to be answered?
- Is the work original?
  Have you done a thorough library or computer search?

- Are you and your team aware of what has already been done in this and related fields?
    - —Have you fully researched the background of the project?
    - —Have you checked the literature in related fields?
    - —Have you checked the literature in countries outside of the U.S.?
      Remember that good research is also being carried out in other countries!
- What is the significance of the project?

  Why is the work important? That is, why is it worth doing?
- What is the **long-range goal** of the project?

  The long-range goal is
    - —the "carrot at the end of 'your' stick"
    - —what you are/will be working toward
    - —what you are **unlikely** to accomplish in 1 or 2 project periods
    - —what you **may perhaps accomplish** in the next 15 to 20 years
- What are the **Specific Aims/Objectives** of your research?

  This is what you hope to accomplish in the project period for which you are requesting funding.
- Do the Specific Aims/Objectives lead toward accomplishment of the long-range goal(s)?
- **How are you going to do the work?**

  Is the methodology **innovative**—or at least "state-of-the-art?"

    If the methodology you are proposing to use is novel, explain why it is better than the methods used by others in the field.
- Who will do the work?
    - —**To what extent is the PI involved** in the day-to-day planning and execution of the experiments?
    - —What is the **reputation** of the PI and her/his team?
    - —Who else may be able to help with the project?
- Why should the granting agency let *YOU* do the project?
    - —What are **YOUR capabilities** and unique **qualifications**?
    - —What is your "**track record?**"
    - —How does the proposed work **relate** to work you have done previously?
    - —If you are new to applying for grant funds, what evidence can you provide that will convince the Reviewers that you will do good work and are likely to get meaningful results; i.e., that you will **use** the funding agency's **money wisely**?
- How long will the work take?

  Be **realistic**. Don't propose 10 years worth of experiments in an Application in which you ask for 5 years of support.

    A realistic, carefully planned budget is a good way to check that your project is not overly ambitious.
- How much will the project **cost** (**Budget**) and why (**Budget Justification**)?
    - —Even if you are submitting a modular budget, it is important for you to create a detailed budget for yourself.
    - —Some universities require you to submit such a budget to the grants office even if you are submitting a modular budget.

—Writing a Budget Justification—or at least envisioning one—is a good way to make sure that you are asking for a reasonable budget that is commensurate with the project you plan to carry out.

- Where will the work be carried out (project site)?
- What facilities will the work require?

  —Assure the Reviewers that you have access to such facilities to the extent required by the project described in the Grant Application.

  —If you will depend on shared or borrowed equipment, document this. **Provide detailed letters** of commitment or support for unique facilities and/or shared equipment.

- Is the environment conducive to carrying out your project expediently?

  —Do you have access to the space required to carry out the project?

  —Do you have adequate access to the services required to carry out the project?

  —Are all the services required to carry out the project within easy reach of your laboratory and other ancillary resources?

- What are the expected results?

  For each set of experiments proposed in your Application, have you considered what the possible outcomes might be and how to proceed in each case? You should **explain in the proposal** how you will proceed if you find "X"—and how you will proceed if you find "Y" instead.

- What are your contingency plans in case you hit a "snag?"

  Have you proposed **alternative methods** for resolving your Specific Aims? Providing alternative methods is a bit akin to having an insurance policy!

- What is the cost/benefit ratio for the project?

  —How will the project benefit your institution?

  —How will the project benefit the granting institution?

  —How will the project benefit society?

  For example, what is the health-relatedness of the project?

  —For corporation grants: How will the project make money for, or add to the stature of, the corporation?

- What other funds are available to support your project?

  —Describe possible cost-sharing by your institution
    - Cost-sharing refers to the value of third-party in-kind contributions and the portion of the costs of a federally assisted project or program **not** borne by the Federal Government.
    - Cost-sharing may be required by law, regulation, or administrative decision of an NIH Institute or Center.
    - Costs used to satisfy matching or cost-sharing requirements are subject to the same policies governing other costs under the approved budget.

  —Describe possible financial resources available for the project from other funding agencies/sources (public or private)—but explain/show **CLEARLY** that there is no overlap.

- If applying to an agency other than NIH, have you determined whether the agency requires a **pre-Application**?

Before you begin to create the final draft of your Application

- Arrange for **wise, experienced** colleagues to read the **pre-final draft** of your proposal
- **Consider seriously ALL** the comments made by these colleagues— but **incorporate only those** suggestions with which you agree

RECAP FOR PART IV: PLANNING THE RESEARCH PLAN

Before you write the Research Plan:

- Discuss your project with established, experienced colleagues to be sure your idea is good and can be carried out successfully by you and your staff.
- Consult the funding agency to determine whether your project has high relevance priority (i.e., is of great **current** interest to the agency).
- Check the NIH Web site to get a sense of the current funding rate for Applications in your area of expertise (i.e., in your **potential** NIH funding component).
- Outline your project.
- Analyze your "track record." Then plan and organize pilot experiments and preliminary experimental results accordingly.
- Research how much time and what personnel, equipment, supplies, etc., will be required to do the project. (Be reasonable about your budget and schedule.)
  Create a budget for yourself—and for your grants office—even if you plan to submit a Modular Grant Application.
- Get pre-submission advice from staff of the potential funding agency. Some agencies will help you develop your proposal if you contact the agency sufficiently early.
- Plan to **have Readers/Colleagues critique your Application.**
  - —Make appointments with at least 2 or 3 people well in advance and ask them how much time they want to read your proposal.
  - —Commit to getting a good, **close-to-final** draft of your Grant Application to them by a **specific date** that is in keeping with the amount of time the Readers ask for.
  - —Allow the amount of time the Readers ask for—generally plan for **at least** 2 to 4 weeks for them to read your Application.
  - —Allow **at least** 2 to 4 weeks—after you get your Application back from the Readers—for you to implement their suggestions (which might perhaps involve doing additional experiments!)
- Read—and meticulously outline—the agency instructions for completing the Application.
- Try to read one or more Applications (in your area of research if possible) that have been funded by the potential funding agency.
- If available, read Summary Statements or Reviewers' reports from the potential funding agency in response to other Grant Applications.

- Gather all the information you will need to prepare the Application.
- Plan the Research Plan:
  —Be sure your project idea is **innovative**.
  —Have a clear **rationale** and obvious **significance**.
  —Be sure the proposal is **focused, well-thought-out, and timely**.
  —Address a **specific problem** or set of related problems that can be solved by a logical sequence of experiments.
  —If appropriate for your project, demonstrate **clinical relevance**—especially if the potential funding agency is committed to solving problems related to health.
  —Provide a **context** (Research Design) within which you present the Methods to be used.
  —Describe experiments that are feasible and designed to answer **specific** questions.
  —Suggest and explain **alternative approaches**. (Providing alternative approaches to resolve your Specific Aims is a very important part of a good Grant Application.)

PART V

WRITING THE RESEARCH PLAN

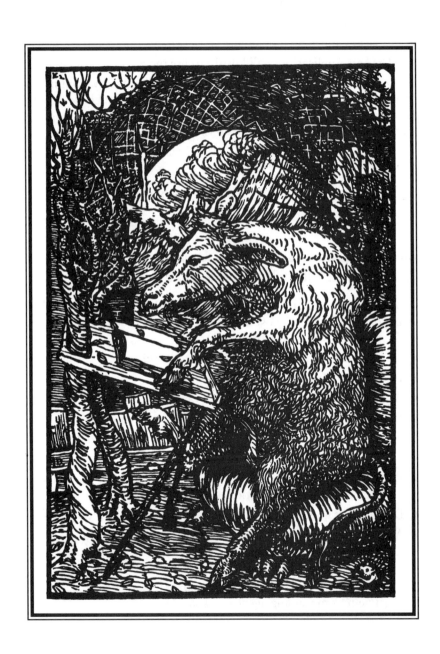

INTRODUCTION

If you want to get funded, it is imperative to write a superb (competitive) Grant Application. When the available grant funds decrease, the competition for these funds will increase and it then becomes even more important to write a superior Grant Application. "A superior Application is one that

- "states a project purpose clearly"
- "documents its need compellingly"
- "describes its uniqueness or appropriateness convincingly"
- "sets forth its methods competently"
- "discusses anticipated outcomes conservatively but confidently"
- "The best Applications will [also] capture the Reviewer's imagination."

The quoted text above is taken from a brochure distributed by Capitol Publications and is reprinted with permission of Capitol Publications. Note that I have changed the text only by changing the original paragraph form into a bulleted list. Also note that Capitol Publications was acquired by Aspen Publishers in 1998.

> Aspen Publishers, Inc.
> 7201 McKinney Circle
> Frederick, MD 21704
> Orders: 800-638-8437; Customer Care: 800-234-1660
>
> **www.aspenpub.com**

THE WAY YOU WRITE YOUR GRANT APPLICATION

You should be aware that the way you write your Grant Application tells the Reviewer a lot about you—both as a scientist and as a person.

- Do you show originality of thought?
- Do you plan ahead—and do so with ingenuity?
- Do you think logically and clearly?
- Are you up to date in all matters relevant to your project?
- Do you have good analytical skills?
- How meticulous are you? How much care do you give to detail?
- Do you recognize limitations and potential pitfalls?
- Do you think about alternative procedures in case your proposed project does not go according to expectation?
- Do you have good managerial skills? For example, how do you handle a budget?
- Are your interpersonal skills good enough to allow you to
    - —maintain a stable work group?
    - —get help from colleagues?
    - —get help from other department personnel?
    - —get help from funding agency personnel?

Begin to write your grant proposal EARLY

A bit of NIH history:

The 10/88 revision of the PHS 398 Instructions stated:

> "PHS estimates that it will take from 10 to 15 hours to complete this Application. This includes time for reviewing the instructions, gathering needed information, and completing and reviewing the form."

The 9/91 revision stated:

> "The PHS estimates that it will take approximately 50 hours to complete this Application for a regular research project grant. This estimate does not include time for development of the scientific plan. Items such as human subjects are cleared and accounted for separately, and are therefore also not part of the time estimate for completing this form."

The statement in the above paragraph appears again in the 4/98 revision of the PHS 398, but the estimate given for completing the Application was 40 hours!!!

Over the years, I have heard occasional stories of proposals that were written in one week—just before the deadline—and were funded. I have also—on one or two occasions—prepared small **non-government** Grant Applications in a few days and been funded. However, in my experience—and that of many of my colleagues—it usually takes an appreciably longer time—several weeks to several months—to prepare a GOOD NIH (or other government agency) Grant Application. And, it is important to understand that the aforementioned time estimates do not include the many months that may be required to accumulate the preliminary data on which the proposal is based!

Moreover, it is also important to plan to set aside time

- to have others ("pre-reviewers") read the proposal (at least 2 weeks; 1 month is better!)
- for you to consider—and act on—relevant suggestions made by these "pre-reviewers"/"readers" (at least 2 weeks; 1 month is better!)
- for the grants office at your institution to check—at the very least—the administrative aspects of the proposal (usually between 5 days and 2 weeks). **Check with your Office of Grants and Contracts when you begin to work** on a proposal to determine
  —when the office wants to see your Application
  —whether they expect to see the complete Application or just certain sections of the Application

It is important to keep in mind that, although there are undoubtedly exceptions, in general, a hastily prepared Application tends to be a poorly prepared Application.

As a first step, it is imperative to check the NIH (or other funding agency) Web site to determine

- the submission deadline for your Application
- whether the due date is the mailing date or the receipt date!

A missed deadline may cost you at least 4 months of time at NIH and as much as a year at funding agencies that only have one deadline per year!

Once you know the deadline, plan ahead for the time required to do each of the steps listed below. Set deadlines for yourself for finishing each stage of the process—and stick to the deadlines you set.

- *Read and follow the agency instructions **meticulously***
- Think through and plan the project
- Obtain and compile the relevant preliminary data
  The objective is to convince the Reviewers that the project is:
  —realistic and viable
  —capable of yielding the desired data
  —do-able by you and your staff
  —do-able in your laboratory
  —worth doing
- Prepare appropriate
  —tables
  —figures/diagrams
  —photographs
- Work through the various stages of filling out/writing the Application:
  —Outline the Research Plan
    Use an Outline Processing program if possible.

NOTE: An Outline Processing program is a type of software program that facilitates creation of an outline. There is an Outline Processor within Microsoft Word™ and Word Perfect™. There is also a good Outline Processing program called "Inspiration" published by Inspiration Software.

>   Inspiration Software, Inc.
>   7412 SW Beaverton-Hillsdale Highway, Suite 102
>   Portland, OR 97225-2167
>   Tel: 800-877-4292 Ext. 134
>   Fax: 503-297-4676
>
>   **http://www.inspiration.com/awards.html**

The company will send you a free demo CD that you can try for 30 days. The outline you make in "Inspiration" can readily be exported to Microsoft Word™ and other word processing programs. **Please be honest and considerate: If you like the program and plan to use it, you should buy it! Don't cheat the company!!!**

- Write the first draft
  —Learn to overcome "writer's block"
    If you can't think of a first sentence, start with the second sentence!!!
  —Keep to the specified page limits
  —Stay within the recommended margins
  —Put information only where it belongs
    • Do NOT put "Background" information into "Specific Aims"
      but
    • **Do repeat—or summarize—"Specific Aims"** in the "Research Design and Methods" section, etc.
- Revise your own first draft into a readily comprehensible second draft to send to your "pre-reviewers"
- Have others ("pre-reviewers") read your proposal

Have a good second draft of the proposal ready to send to 2 or more readers/ colleagues/consultants for their appraisal at least 8 to 10 weeks before the Grant Application is due at your institution's grants administration office. (The grants administration office often needs to have your Application—sometimes only the administrative parts—1 to 2 weeks before the grant proposal is due at NIH.) The suggested 10-week period gives

—the readers a month to read and critique your Application

—you a month to implement their suggestions and finalize the Application

—your grants administration office at least 2 weeks to review the Application

- Revise the second draft using the **relevant** "pre-reviewers'" comments
- Polish the final draft
- Fill in the various form pages

    —Be sure to leave enough time to do this **well**.

    —Ask some of your more senior colleagues how much time this might take. It is likely to take a lot more time than you anticipate!

    —Allow yourself **extra time** if this is your first Application to the agency in question.

- *Use a checklist*

    —Use the printed administrative checklist that NIH requires as the last page of the Application to see that you have attended to all administrative matters.

    —Use the general checklist provided in Appendix I of this book:

    - before you begin writing; i.e., when you are planning the proposal
    - before you finish the second draft
    - before you finish the final draft of the Application

- get all necessary letters of collaboration

    such letters should

    —indicate the Collaborator's willingness to participate in the project

    —specify what specific role the Collaborator will have in the project

- If you are requesting assignment to a particular Study Section or awarding component, *include*—with the Grant Application—*a cover letter* about your request.

> **NOTE:** Be aware that obtaining the information to enable you to suggest—wisely—a particular Study Section or awarding component may require a significant amount of research and thoughtfulness—and hence a significant amount of time.

Check the NIH Web site to:

- get a sense of the types of Applications that are reviewed by the various Study Sections
- find out who are the current sitting members of these Study Sections
- be aware of the dates on which these Reviewers are scheduled to finish their term of service on the Study Section
- find out what type of research these Reviewers are doing

    —Check Medline

    —Check the CRISP database

- get a sense of the sorts of projects that have been funded recently by those awarding components that you consider appropriate to review an Application about the type of research you are proposing
- get administrative Approval; i.e., obtain signatures of required relevant officials at your institution
- assemble the Application. Place all items in the order requested by the funding agency
- photocopy the Application

  Make enough copies for:

  —the funding agency
    (The funding agency generally specifies the required number of copies.)
  —your department
  —your institutional administrative offices
  —Colleagues and Collaborators
  —your own files
- **mail the Application in time** for it to arrive at the funding agency when the agency wants it!!!

OUTLINING THE RESEARCH PLAN

Make an outline for each section of the proposal

In the long run you will probably save much more time at the writing and editing stages of proposal preparation if you take the time to **make a good outline at the start.**

Many good writers spend their total project time as follows:

  —60% to make and revise an outline
  —10% to write the first draft
  —30% to revise the document one or more times to obtain a **good** final draft

There are several ways to make an outline. You can use:

- Index cards
  —Have one "topic phrase" per index card.
  —Color code the corners or use different color index cards to help keep track of related topics/subjects.
  —Work on a large flat surface and rearrange all the cards until you have the topics in **optimal logical order.**
- 3M Post-it® notes
  —Have one "topic phrase" per Post-it® note.
  —Color code the corners or use different color Post-it® notes to help keep track of related topics/subjects.
  —Work on a large flat surface—or on a wall—and rearrange all the Post-it® notes until you have the topics in optimal logical order.

> **NOTE:** Word processors are very useful programs *but are NOT a substitute for making an outline.* Make an outline using your word processor, and then write from the outline. Or use an Outline Processor.

- An Outline Processor on your computer
    - —An **Outline Processor** is software that facilitates creation of an outline.
    - —There is an **Outline Processor** within Microsoft Word™ and within Word Perfect™.
    - —There is also a **good** Outline Processing program called "**Inspiration**" published by Inspiration Software, Inc. in Portland Oregon (see page 136 above).
- Your outline should fit *logically* into the obligatory outline given in the NIH (or other agency) instructions.
- Your outline should include, in good logical order, everything you plan to include in the Application.
- Consider: *It is much easier to see and check the logical flow of ideas in an outline than in multiple pages of text.*
- Consider: *Outlines are much easier to revise than text.*
- Check the outline for
    - —adequacy of detail
    - —logical progression of ideas
    - —parallel construction
- *Do NOT begin to write prose until you are 99.99% happy/satisfied with your outline.*

GETTING READY TO WRITE

Plan to *refer to the literature* thoughtfully and thoroughly but selectively

Know when to look at original papers and when it's okay to consult a review article. If in doubt, go to the original paper rather than a review article.

Plan to include well-designed and carefully-labeled tables and figures with clearly-written legends.

- Clever Readers will often peruse your figures before they read any of your text! Thus, Readers should be able to understand tables and figures without referring to the text.
- *Before* you write your proposal, prepare

    figures

    tables

    photographs (plates)

    - —Use tables and figures as a guide to organize your material (sequence).
    - —**Be sure all tables and figures are referred to in the text.**
    - —Be sure tables and figures are **labeled** with an **informative title** and have a **clear legend** in a type size that conforms to NIH (or other agency) specifications.
    - —For graphs, coordinates should be clearly labeled. The Reader should be able to understand the essence of a table or figure without referring to the text.
    - —Be sure tables and figures are interpreted/discussed in the text.
    - —Be sure the units, abbreviations, and other terminology, as well as the findings depicted in the legends to figures and tables, agree with the corresponding discussion in the text.
    - —Don't put too much information into one figure! Figures should be easy to understand.

—Be sure that all figure legends, coordinate labels, and other text on figures and photos that have been reduced on a computer or photocopy machine remain legible; that is, have not become too small to read **easily**.

WRITING THE FIRST DRAFT

Refer to the advice given below and in Appendix II before writing and revising the first draft of your proposal.

- *Follow the outline.*

  If you have made a well-thought-out and thorough outline, it should be easy for you to write the first draft of your Application. Those who truly understand and practice the "art" of outlining, often have little work to do when they are ready to convert the outline to prose. If you have made a superb outline, you will have only to delete the indents and add some connecting words or phrases to flush out the text and produce a **clear, concise, perfectly organized** document.

- Try to write each **section** of your Application at one sitting.

  —If the section is long, try to write each sub-section at one sitting.
  —If you must take a break, when you get back to the writing, re-read what you wrote before you proceed to the next part of your draft. If you neglect to do this, you are likely to introduce changes in tense or style into the text.

- Unless otherwise noted in the instructions of the agency to which you are applying, it is now generally acceptable to use the first person when writing the research plan.

  Note, however, that for an NIH Application the first person is *not* permitted in the *Description (Abstract)* of the proposal.

- Don't worry about "niceties" in the first draft; just let the sentences flow.

  While writing the first draft, do not allow yourself to be interrupted to look up details. Keep a pad at your side, and jot down the things that you need to check, find, or look up later.

- *Write to express, not to impress!!!*

  —Overt attempts to impress the Reviewers will tend to depress/"turn off" these busy people rather than impress them.
  —Avoid putting self-laudatory statements into Grant Applications.
   Self-praise tends to have a negative affect on Reviewers and can be a cause for unnecessary mirth (at your expense) during the Study Section meeting!

- Never assume that the Reviewers will know what you mean.

  —Your Reviewer is NOT a "mind-reader."
  —Even if your Reviewer is in your field, s/he is not in your lab—or likely to know what happens there.
  —Write **CLEARLY**—as though you are explaining something to a bright person in a different field.
  —Never use "lab-jargon" in a Grant Application.
  —Do NOT use abbreviations that you have not yet defined.
  —Do not use non-standard abbreviations!

- Don't be afraid to repeat words.

> **NOTE:** In contrast to what many people were taught about **creative writing** in grade school—in **expository writing,** it is important to "call a spade a spade" every time you refer to that thing/entity. Do **NOT** take the risk of confusing the Reader or Reviewer by varying the word you use to refer to some specific thing/item.

- Convince your Reviewers that your project has a high likelihood of succeeding by providing
  —a solid, well thought out approach to achieve your Specific Aims
  —a reasonable amount of good pilot data
  —sound plans for evaluating your progress

REVISING (SELF-EDITING) THE FIRST DRAFT

When you revise the first draft, think about:

      Accuracy

      Clarity

      Consistency

      Brevity

      Emphasis/impact

      Style

      Tone

      Presentation

Each of these subjects is discussed briefly below and also in Appendix II.

Be accurate

- Provide correct information to maintain your credibility.
- Convey correctly the information you provide.
- Use words correctly.
- Don't call something a fact unless it *is* a fact.
  According to the dictionary, a fact is something that "has been objectively verified/is known with certainty."
  It is generally a wise policy to avoid usage such as:
  —The fact is, …
  —In fact, …
  —As a matter of fact, …
  —The fact of the matter is, …
  The above phrases/expressions waste valuable space and rarely add anything useful to your text!
- **Don't use superlatives** unless you are certain that they apply.
  You are less likely to be challenged if you write,
     "Method X is **a good way** to purify substance Y."
  than if you write,
     "Method X is **the best way** to purify substance Y."

Be clear

The Reviewer should be able to

- Understand easily what you wrote
- Perceive easily how you got from point A to point B

    Keep in mind that the Reviewer may be less familiar with your project than you are. What seems perfectly clear to you may be confusing to a Reader who is not as involved with the project as you are. This is well illustrated in the *New Yorker* cartoon on page 87.

    Having colleagues read and critique your Application can be very useful for catching
    —unwarranted assumptions
    —unclear exposition

To achieve clarity:

- Use a logical sequence of presentation
- If you discuss 3 topics, give similar information (if available and appropriate)—in the same sequence—about each topic

    e.g., Method 1 should go with Specific Aim 1, Method 2 should go with Specific Aim 2, and so forth.

- Avoid uncommon/unfamiliar vocabulary

    Never send your reader to the dictionary

    —Just because someone knows a lot about science does not mean that s/he has a large general vocabulary.
    —Many scientists now come from abroad and are not native English speakers

- Don't use jargon!

    Terminology limited to a given field may be unfamiliar—and irritating—to a Reviewer who is not in that specific field.

- Try to avoid using the words "former" and "latter"

    Using "former" and "latter" slows the Reader down. Some Reviewers are likely to have to re-read the previous text to determine what was "former" and what was "latter."

- Use acronyms and abbreviations sparingly and only if they are in fairly common usage and are defined at the first occurrence

    —Reviewers may be forced to read more slowly and may, therefore, be annoyed by
      • acronyms and abbreviations defined many—or even just several—pages earlier
      • use of **multiple** unfamiliar acronyms and abbreviations

> **NOTE:** If you do use more than 2 or 3 acronyms and/or abbreviations, you can help the Reviewer by inserting an **un-numbered** page in the Application with an alphabetical listing of the acronyms and abbreviations and an explanation of what they stand for. **Mark this page "For the convenience of the Reviewers" and insert it at the beginning of the Research Plan.**

- Be sure sentences and paragraphs in your Application are not too long
    —Sentences of 17 to 23 words tend to make for easy reading. Longer sentences are more difficult for fast reading.

—Avoid more than 1 or 2 subordinate clauses in a sentence.

—Paragraphing should be done around topics.

However, if your text has excessively long paragraphs, consider splitting these long paragraphs into 2—or more—shorter paragraphs to avoid overwhelming the Reader with a large solid block of text that provides no relief (in the form of white space) for the reader.

■ Start paragraphs with clear, informative *topic sentences*

—The topic sentence tells the Reader what you are going to discuss in that paragraph.

—*Note:* When long paragraphs are broken into two or more paragraphs simply to avoid presenting the Reader with a large block of uninterrupted print, the continuation paragraphs may not need topic sentences.

■ Don't disappoint the Reader

Be aware that a heading, a subheading, or a topic sentence is essentially a "promise" to the Reader about what s/he will find in the text that follows. Thus, in the paragraph below, taken from an actual grant proposal, the writer has broken his promise to the Reader. The subheading promises a discussion of "Alternative Approaches," but none is forthcoming in the brief paragraph that followed!

> "*Alternative Approaches:* All the approaches planned for years 1–5 of the proposed project are very low-cost strategies. Each will be carefully evaluated to gauge its effectiveness and those which prove most successful will be repeated, and where possible expanded."

■ Avoid ambiguity

Think about possible gaps/misunderstandings between what you *intend* to convey and what the Reader may *perceive*.

Consider:

—misplaced modifiers

—uncommitted pronouns

—words or phrases that can be interpreted in more than one way

—overly complex sentences

See Appendix II.

■ Avoid irrelevant information

Irrelevant information is information that is irrelevant in a given context.

—Irrelevant information wastes valuable space that could be better used to present pertinent information.

—Irrelevant information may confuse the Reviewer/Reader.

—Irrelevant information may annoy the Reviewer/Reader.

—Don't "pour out" all you know just to impress the Reviewer/Reader.

—Think about what the Reviewer/Reader needs/wants to know in relation to *this* section of *this* proposal about *this* subject/project.

To avoid putting information in the wrong section of a proposal, think about the following:

• If it's future tense, it probably doesn't belong in the Background Section or Progress Report.

• If it's past tense, it probably doesn't belong in the Methods Section.

Irrelevant information is often a weak point in proposals.

> Because they are afraid that they are not saying or doing enough, novice Grant Application writers are sometimes prone to buttress their proposals with information that is not relevant to their project. But irrelevant information tends to confuse rather than impress Reviewers. Limit your proposal to the relevant, strong points about your project. If your Application is complete and you have responded to everything in the instructions, Reviewers will be thankful for having to read less rather than more!

Be consistent

Consistency helps the Reader understand the proposal; it is important to be consistent in all aspects and all parts of the proposal.

- In the outline form

  Are your headings at a given level of the outline at equivalent levels of importance?

  > I, II, III—Should all be major topics presented in a logical order

  > A, B, C—Should be of equivalent levels of importance and all relate to the major topic defined by the Roman numeral topic under which the A, B, C topics appear

  > 1, 2, 3—Should be of equivalent levels of importance and all relate to the major sub-topic defined by the capitol letter topic under which the 1, 2, 3 topics appear

- Although it is sometimes difficult, you must try to maintain a good outline within the confines of the one imposed by the NIH (or other agency) instructions.
  An Outline Processor can help immensely.

- Text should agree with the information in figures and figure legends (including the units you use).

- Terminology and abbreviations should be **defined at first use** and should be consistent throughout the whole Application.

  —Do not use different words (or different acronyms) for the same thing just for literary reasons. Use of different terms for the same thing may create ambiguities—which can slow the Reader down. Keep in mind that this is a Grant Application (expository writing)—not a work of fiction.

  —Also keep in mind that Reviewers may not have time to read a whole proposal at one sitting. Consistent terminology makes it easier for reviewers to pick up where they stopped reading earlier.

- Tenses should be appropriate and uniform throughout a document, or at least throughout a section of the document.

- Subjects and verbs should agree (singular or plural):

  —The ***group*** of scholars ***is*** getting an award.
  —The ***scholars are*** getting an award.
  —Be aware that the word "data" is plural; hence:
    The data are...

NOTE: Grammar Checkers (sometimes included in word processing programs) are useful for detecting, for example, when the subject and verb do not agree—and can also help detect numerous other grammatical errors.

- Appropriate sections of the proposal should agree with each other in form (order of presentation; parallel construction) and content:
  —Body of proposal with Description (Abstract)
  —Specific Aims with Methods
  —Methods with Budget (if you have to submit a detailed budget)
  —Budget requests with Facilities Available
  > If you ask for a microscope in the Budget and then say under Resources that your department has 3 microscopes, you had better have a very good justification for why you need another microscope.
- Separate clearly for the Reviewer/Reader what you say you
  —have done (Progress Report)
  —are doing now (time between writing proposal and, you hope, getting funded)
  —propose to do in the project period for which you are requesting funding
  —want to do (or should do) in the future but are *not* planning to do in the project period for which you are requesting funding. That is, if you want to discuss future projects (e.g., to discuss long-range goals or establish significance), be very explicit about designating what might be a direction for a subsequent renewal project period but is not a current Specific Aim.

Be brief (concise but complete)

In the case of a competitive renewal Application, the Reviewers may be provided with a copy of your previous Grant Application. However, the instructions specify that the present Application must be complete by itself. Within that context, keep the following maxims in mind:

- In expository writing, the Reader wants the **maximum** information in the **minimum** number of words.

- *Avoid information that is irrelevant in the context of the proposal*
  —Don't discuss things just to show how much you know.
  > Limit your discussion to information that relates to your project.
  —Don't overwhelm the Reviewer with a "shopping list" of facts or findings devoid of any effort on your part to summarize, compare, contrast, evaluate, and provide the Reviewer/reader with context.
  > Beware of this tendency especially, for example, in the Background and Significance section—and even more so in the Research Design and Methods section.
  —Don't put information in an inappropriate part of the proposal. For example, the 2 excerpts below were found in the **Progress Report** of an actual proposal.
  > *Excerpt 1:* "X-cell cultures, on the other hand, are characterized by.... These cells are presumed to derive from..., based on a number of criteria such as.... Substance Y, however, is not a useful marker in cultures because...."
  —The above excerpt would be more appropriate in the Background section.
  > *Excerpt 2:* "The...was next used to determine if.... We purified the...by separating the samples on an SDS gel and transferring the fractions to.... The...was then stained with..., and the band of...was cut out. This strip was then de-stained and reacted with.... Following an x-hour incubation, the...was eluted from the strip using a...buffer. This was then used on...."

  —The above excerpt would be more appropriate in the Research Design and Methods section.
- Do NOT provide information in your proposal
  —that is not likely to be useful to the Reviewer
  —that detracts from your image as a scientist or a person

Some foundation Applications require a free-form biographical sketch. When you write this part of the Application, be aware that the agency is NOT testing your ability to do creative literary writing.

  —The agency is trying to assess whether you are a good scientist/researcher and a productive, innovative worker/thinker.

  —Think about what the agency wants to know about you in the **context of the proposal** and the **mission of the agency**.

  —Steer clear of personal details, especially those that do not show you in the best light.

   For example, the statement, "I was an awkward child" (which someone wrote in a Grant Application!), may well suggest to the Reviewer that the writer grew into an awkward adult. Awkward adults do not tend to do well in a laboratory situation!

Avoid unnecessary words and redundancy

Unnecessary words and redundancy

- waste your space (page limitations)
- waste the Reviewer's precious time
- may irritate the Reviewer
- may confuse the Reviewer

  (Why is the writer telling me this?—telling me this again?)

Also, consider that sentence redundancy may give the Reviewer the idea that you are an insecure person. Whatever you plan to write: **say it once and say it right**. One exception to this suggestion is redundancy for the purpose of emphasis. For example, **when there are *no* page limits**, it is often useful to formulate expository reports (including oral presentations) so that you:

1. Tell the Readers (listeners)—in outline form—what you are going to tell them.

2. Tell them—in appropriate detail—what you want to tell them.

3. Tell them briefly (summarize) what you just told them.
   See Appendix II.

Think about emphasis and impact

Don't begin a paragraph with unimportant words. In a compound sentence, put the important phrase first.

  For example:

   If you want to stress that the work was done *in the previous project period*, write:

   In the previous project period, three approaches were developed to solve...

If you want to stress that *three approaches were developed,* write:

> *Three approaches were developed* in the previous project period to solve...

Think about style

- Use simple (but not simple-minded/simplistic) words.
- Use short, direct sentences (about 17 to 23 words is a reasonable length), but avoid a choppy first-grader sound by judicious use of transition words (although, however, nevertheless, etc.).
- Use short paragraphs that begin with *informative topic sentences.*
- Avoid modifiers that do not add to the critical essence of what you want to say:
  This *cleverly conceived* experiment...
- Avoid an undue amount of self-praise. Let your data speak for you!
  —Our *fantastic unique* method for...
  —Our laboratory is the *best known in the world* for...
  —We have *by far the largest* collection of... in the country.
- Replace "opinion" modifiers with quantitative modifiers.
  —Not: *most* or *many*
  —But: 68%–70%
- Don't overstate your case.
  Avoid superlatives unless you are very sure "it" really is *best, most,* etc.
- **Try not to split infinitives,** unless splitting the infinitive avoids ambiguity or improves the flow of the sentence.
  Consider the difference in meaning in the sentences below:
  (a) She will try *to **more than** justify* the cost of the computer.
  (b) She will try *to justify* **more than** the cost of the computer.
  (c) She will try **more than** *to justify* the cost of the computer.
  The 3 sentences above do not have identical meanings. To achieve clarity (get the correct meaning), the modifier words "more than" must be located in the correct position with respect to the word (or words) they are intended to modify, in this case, "justify." The intention is to convey that the "she" is going to justify the cost of the computer extremely thoroughly. In this context, (a) is the sentence with the appropriate meaning.
  See Appendix II.
- **Know when to avoid highly technical language**
  —Don't write: "Nosocomial infection."
     Write: "Hospital-acquired infection."
  —Don't write "Iatrogenic condition."
     Write: "Physician-induced condition."
  —Remember that **some of your Reviewers may not be MDs!**

Avoidance of unnecessary, "heavy" medical jargon is especially important if you are a physician-researcher proposing a disease-oriented project that involves a large number of basic science experiments. Such a proposal is highly likely to have one MD Reviewer and at least one PhD Reviewer. Sending the PhD Reviewer on frequent trips to a medical dictionary wastes her/his time!

On the other hand, failure to use the proper terminology in a given field may be perceived by some Reviewers (such as your MD Reviewer) as a lack of familiarity with the subject. There is a fine line here, and **a PI must make an educated judgment** about such issues. Assessments of likely Study Section assignments and familiarity with the work of the members of those Study Sections (Review Groups) can sometimes help you to decide how much or how little technical terminology and field-specific jargon to use. This is an area in which experienced proposal-writers may be able to advise you.

Think about tone

Attitude, mood, and tone can be "contagious."
Avoid words that have a negative tone, such as "unfortunately."

Be positive

Don't write: I/We won't be able to finish this project by the end of the first year.

Write: I/We expect to be able to finish this project by March of the second year.
  or

     I/We expect to finish this project by March of the second year.
  or

     I/We plan to finish this project by March of the second year.

Think about presentation

Some scientists seem to think that if they have a superb project idea, they do not have to worry about the presentation. This shows a naïve view of human psychology. Although an attractive presentation will **NOT** fool any Reviewer into mistaking a poor proposal as a good proposal, a well-formatted, easy-to-read proposal can certainly affect the attitude of the Reviewer as s/he reads your proposal. It is especially important to think about this and to realize that when the Reviewer pulls **YOUR** Application out of the box, s/he may already have read numerous other proposals—or may have 100 more Applications waiting to be reviewed/read after yours.

- Adhere strictly to the page limitations.
- If you are strapped for space, consider that 12 letters per horizontal inch type allows more text on a page than 10 letters per inch, but don't antagonize your Reviewer by using smaller than 10- or 12-point type (to circumvent the page limitations!).
- Do NOT use fancy fonts that are hard to read.
- Choose a type style and size that result in a neat and easy-to-read document.
- If you are submitting a proposal on paper, use good "letter-quality" print (black ink, white paper) for all drafts that will be read by others.

If the agency to which you are applying specifies acceptable type styles and type-size limitations for proposal preparation, follow these instructions meticulously. If possible, use a font size that is larger than the smallest size the agency will allow. Many of your Reviewers are likely to wear reading glasses and may be reviewing your proposals late at night when these busy people are tired.

- Face page
  Determine whether type density specifications for the Face page are different than for the rest of the Application
- Rest of the Application:
  —Type must be clear and readily legible
  —Type must be a standard easy-to-read size. Usually, 10- to 12-point font

The article below is reproduced with permission of IMV, Ltd, Greenbelt, MD, Publishers SCI/GRANTS News.

Perspective

Neatness and Grammar Count

A colleague who provides grant consultation and assistance to not-for-profit organizations tells of a prospective Applicant who called to ask if it is advisable to type Applications, rather than printing them neatly by hand. When the same consultant returned a proposal draft to another Applicant with the suggestion that the grammar and syntax be improved, the Applicant dismissed the criticism, saying that the granting agency would be able to decipher the Application.

Representatives of granting agencies, grant reviewers, grant consultants, and repeatedly successful Grant Applicants are nearly unanimous in urging careful attention to the form and structure of a grant proposal. Despite that advice, granting agencies are deluged with Applications that look more like poorly done undergraduate exercises than the work of serious professionals.

It is hard to fathom the apparently cavalier attitude with which many Grant Applicants approach the preparation of a proposal. The charitable assumption—that they know better and are capable of better—is probably correct in a great many cases. It is probably true that, given more time and less stressful circumstances, they would prepare a neat, well-ordered document. It is probably also true that grant seekers who submit poorly done proposals console themselves with the thought that the merits of the request outweigh any esthetic considerations.

That view is correct, to a degree, but largely in a negative sense. A poorly justified proposal is not likely to be funded, no matter how well written and visually attractive it may be. The danger is that a worthy proposal may not receive due consideration if it is poorly prepared. In order to discern the merit of an Application, a reviewer must first read the Application with as little bias as possible. Faced with smudged type, scrambled pages, and sentences that defy translation, a reviewer may be hard pressed to read a proposal, and may be incapable of reading it with any degree of objectivity.

A gem is a gem, whether it be wrapped in velvet or burlap. One who is searching for a gem, however, is more likely to look in a velvet pouch than in a burlap sack. A reviewer is more likely to expect an outstanding idea in an outstanding package than in one that is carelessly prepared. Fair or not, the quality of a presentation is sometimes as important as the quality of the idea that it presents. Billions of dollars in advertising turn on that very concept.

In very rare cases, an obvious lack of sophistication may actually work to the advantage of a Grant Applicant. There are those few agencies that seek to aid organizations with little or no sophistication, and submitting a polished package to such an agency would be a mistake. Since agencies with that type of philosophy almost always make their preferences very clear, there is little danger that a grant seeker will inadvertently approach them with too much polish.

For the vast majority of granting institutions, a proposal cannot be too well done. Proper proposal preparation never guarantees success, but its absence often guarantees failure.

SCI/GRANTS News, Vol. II, No. 6, June 1990

—**Horizontal spacing** (constant-spacing or proportional-spacing type): Unless you are otherwise instructed, do NOT have more than 15 characters per horizontal inch (cpi)

—**Vertical spacing**: Unless you are otherwise instructed, do NOT have more than 6 lines of type per vertical inch

—Figures, charts, tables, figure legends, and footnotes may be in smaller type but must be clear and **readily legible**. In making this judgment, think about the size font that you might like to read at 1 AM if you were tired and had to use reading glasses.

If you are submitting an Application on paper, note the readability of the type and size of the font you choose:

- This is Times 12 point. It is a serifed font and is easy to read, but it is fairly spread out and takes up a lot of space. Apparently, many people find it easier to read a serifed font.
- This is Times 10. OK for most readers.
- This is Times 9. This is too small.
- *This is Zapf Chancery 14*. This is too ornate for use in a Grant Application.
- This is Helvetica 10.
- This is Helvetica 12. This is a condensed, nonserifed font. It takes up a lot less space than Times 12 point.

It is very difficult to read a page of small text that has no visual relief; i.e., at least some white space. For dense text it is helpful to skip a line between paragraphs. If you do this, do not indent the beginnings of paragraphs. However, because of page limits at some agencies, it is generally better NOT to skip lines between paragraphs in Grant Applications to such agencies. Instead, start paragraphs by indenting 5 spaces and avoid having long paragraphs by breaking them into shorter paragraphs.

Consider placing tables and figures so as to relieve the look of densely packed text and let text flow around the tables and figures. But be sure the tables and figures are placed as close as possible to the text in which the tables and figures are discussed.

If it is acceptable to the funding agency (call the agency to ask!!!)—and if it seems appropriate—consider presenting your proposal in a 2-column-per-page format. A few Reviewers have told me that they find this format actually saves space and is easier and faster to read and digest. The "ease of reading" issue is probably more true of people who are very fast readers. Interestingly, you will find that you often use fewer pages for the same number of words with 2-column-per-page format. Do a comparison test with a few pages of text and see for yourself.

If you are submitting to NIH:

- Do **NOT** use a 2-column-per-page format without first checking with your SRA.
- If you get permission to use a 2-column-per-page format, try to fit tables and figures into one of the columns—but, if necessary for clarity, have the tables and figures go across the whole page even though the text does not.
- If you are submitting to NIH for the first time and are not sure which Study Section will review your Application, do **NOT** use a 2-column-per-page format!

Although many people prefer the neat look of text justified at both margins, I have heard several Reviewers say that they find text with a ragged right margin easier to read—especially because Reviewers are frequently interrupted. **The pattern recognition of the irregular margin in ragged-right text helps Readers—especially very fast Readers—to keep their place.**

Further suggestions for editing your first draft

It is important to realize that, unless you are a very good and experienced writer—and have made an extensive outline before writing your first draft—you should NOT give anyone—except perhaps a parent, a spouse, or an offspring—a first draft to read. First drafts of manuscripts are often somewhat tedious and unattractive and you would be ill advised to show such an early draft of your work to any colleague or mentor.

It is **your** responsibility to **edit your own first draft** of your Grant Application (or research paper). Fortunately, modern technology has provided some very useful aids (see below) to help you edit your own first draft. Be sure you make optimal use of these aids. However, you will, in the final analysis, still need to proof-read your own "masterpiece" before subjecting others to it. You will also need to impose on kindly colleagues to read your Application to help assure that what you have written is comprehensible to others and that it is the best that it can be. Listed below are some resources for creating a good second draft of your Grant Application that is unlikely to embarrass you in the hands of the people who I refer to as "Pre-Reviewers."

Use computer aids to help you improve the first draft

- Outline Processors

  Outline Processors are extremely valuable for making outlines and **getting your thoughts organized into a good logical flow** of ideas/concepts

  —There are **Outline Processors** within both MS Word™ and Word Perfect™.

  —There is a very good outline processor program called "Inspiration." You can get a 30-day trial CD of this software from the company: Inspiration Software (800-877-4292).

- "Search mode" in word processors to find overused words

  If you do not check carefully, you may find that you have used some form of the same root word many times in a few pages, e.g., interest, interested, interesting. If you put the root word (interest) into the "Search mode" of your word processor and search your text you will find all forms of the word. This puts you in a good position to delete—or change—at least some of these iterations if you find it appropriate to do so.

- Spell checkers

  Spell checkers are now generally integrated into word-processing programs. Some of these programs allow you to request that the program automatically alerts you to the presence of misspelled words **as you type**. But spell checkers cannot help you if you do not use them or if you ignore the auto-alerts. It pays to do a "Spell check" on the pre-final version of every document you produce that will be read/seen by others!

  Spell checkers generally also alert you to adjacent duplicate words; e.g., if you have written "I later went to **the the** lab."

NOTE: But be aware that **spell checkers do not "catch" words that are correctly spelled but incorrectly used,** such as "there" instead of "their" (or vice versa) or "Principle Investigator" instead of "Principal Investigator." Likewise, the spell checker will not catch "typos" that result in correct English words that you did not intend. For example, if you meant to write, "We dissected one eye from each fruit **fly,**" but accidentally typed, "We dissected one eye from each fruit **fry,**" the program will not catch the error. Thus, even after you spell check your proposal or other document, **you must do a "human" proofreading** of the document to be sure that all word usage is correct.

- Stylistics and grammar checkers
  Word-processing programs can generally check for the following types of incorrect or poor usage:
  —Sentences that are too long
  —Paragraphs that are too long
  —Passive versus active verb constructions
  —Adjacent identical duplicate words
  —Vague phrases
  —Incorrect punctuation
  —Missing spaces
       e.g., words/sentences that are run together
  —Too many spaces between words/sentences
  —Overused words
  Although such errors may not seem very important, they are easy to find with the help of a grammar checker. Correcting these errors will make your proposal easier for the Reviewer to read.

Your grant proposal should be thorough but as concise as possible; do not repeat, but rather refer to, material in other sections. For example, if you have already described a procedure or an experiment, write "See section Y, page X" rather than repeating text content.

When you are finished preparing your best possible first draft, print out a clean copy and read through it **twice.** If you can afford the time, it is good to put the proposal away for a few days before you read it for the second time. The second reading is likely to be more fruitful if you have taken a break from working on the document and come to it with a "fresh" frame of mind.

More editing

The first time you read your completed first draft of your Application, check again for each of the items listed below:

- Lack of logical flow
- Bad grammar (especially the kind that causes ambiguity)
  Did you use the grammar checker?
- Jargon
  Get rid of it!
- Insufficient references
  Among other things, be especially sure that you have acknowledged the work of scientists who may be on your Study Section and have published papers relevant to the subject of your Application. **People do not take kindly to having their work overlooked!**

- Circular sentences

    Be careful to avoid errors like the following: You write, "The important conclusion from these findings is…." But instead of giving a conclusion, you repeat the findings!

- Sentences and paragraphs that are too long

    A grammar checker can generally help detect sentences and paragraphs that are too long.

- A messy presentation

    If your grant Application has too many "typos"/spelling errors, misplaced modifiers, and other evidence of careless writing, the Reviewer is likely to extrapolate: Carelessness in writing indicates carelessness in experimentation! People who are thought to do sloppy experiments, are not likely to get funded!

The second time you read your proposal ask yourself:

- Is my proposal well organized?

    The organization is much more likely to be good if you made a good outline before you began to write complete sentences.

- Is my proposal convincing?

    —Do I have sufficient preliminary results/data to convince the Reviewers that I can do the work and that I'm on the "right track"?

    —Is my proposal authoritative and persuasive without being arrogant?

    —Do I have sufficient references to support my approach to the problem?

- Did I adequately examine, analyze, and interpret preliminary results and the other information presented in the Application, rather than just list the information?

- Did I add my own thoughts and insights about information obtained from the published literature?

- Did I give sufficient credit to the work of others?

- Is the proposal easy to read?

- Was I careful to eliminate ambiguities from my Application?

    Be sure that you are writing for the Reviewer/Reader, rather than just for yourself. There may be information in your Application that is obvious to you but may not be obvious to the Reviewer! Try to imagine reading your Application as though you were not very familiar with the subject matter. A senior professor who attended one of my workshops remarked to me, **"I never notice my ambiguous statements because every time I read my own proposal, I know exactly what I mean."**

- Is the proposal up to date?

    Have you checked **recently** for new developments in your field that may have occurred since you began work on the proposal—which may have been several months ago?

- Is the bibliography up to date?

    If anything significant has been published in the field of your Grant Application up to a week before you generate the final draft of the Application, it behooves you to mention the subject matter and reference the publication.

NOTE: Always check the literature again just before you are ready to print the last draft of your Application!

GETTING HELP AFTER YOU HAVE A GOOD SECOND DRAFT

Preparing a draft for the pre-reviewers

When you have edited your first draft in accordance with each of the above criteria, print out and check a single-spaced version of your Application—or at least the Research Plan—with margins designated by NIH (or other funding agency) to be sure that you are within the required page limits. Then, if you wish, you can print out a second draft—with a different format—for your pre-reviewers.

Before you send a draft of your Application to your pre-reviewers, ask them about their preferences:

- Transmit electronically
- Send a draft on paper
- Ask about their preference for typeface size and margin size. If they do not express a preference, it is a good idea to prepare and print the document you plan to send to the pre-reviewers using

  —a standard easy-to-read font

  —type size of 12 or 14 points

  —**double-spacing to allow easy insertion of comments**

  —**wide margins** (2 inches) to make it easy for the readers to insert suggested changes

Alternatively,

- suggest to the readers that they insert circled numbers within the manuscript and use these numbers to make relevant comments or changes on separate sheets of paper
- arrange to send the Research Plan via e-mail. This allows the pre-reviewers to edit the text directly on the computer or print it out in a form they prefer.

  In Microsoft Word, the **"Track Changes"** feature (located in the "Tools" Menu) allows you to highlight changes and insert comments. Then you can accept or reject changes and compare document drafts in a convenient manner on-screen. This is a very useful editing feature.

Getting help from others when you have a good second draft

The best stage at which to get help with your Application is when you have a clean, comprehensible draft —but one that is not yet at the point at which you will feel resentful about making suggested changes.

When you have a good second draft, which you would not be embarrassed to show to colleagues, arrange to have **at least 3 people** review your Grant Application:

1. Someone who understands your specific research—to check for **accuracy**.

2. Someone who understands science and research but does **NOT** know about your specific research—to check for **clarity**.

   If your institution has an in-house "Study Section," take advantage of this generous service.

3. Someone who is a **good** editor—to help you polish the proposal.

   —If your institution has an in-house editorial service, take advantage of this service.

—Sometimes one of the "content" readers may have a sufficiently good command of the English language to act as the editor. If this is the case, you may be able to make do with 2 pre-reviewers, but this puts an additional burden on one of the 2 pre-reviewers because that person will have to spend more time working on your Application.

—Having your proposal read by a professional editor is a great advantage. Do NOT have an editor read the proposal until you are quite sure that you will NOT change anything other than items suggested by the editor.

—In addition to getting help from the aforementioned individuals, you may be able to get help from your institutional grants office (Office for Sponsored Research) and sometimes even from your potential funding agency. For example, some program officers at NIH may be willing to read the Abstract or the Specific Aims of your Grant Application for form (if given sufficient time and warning)—but generally will not comment on the scientific content.

When you send your proposal to others for critique, send only those parts that are appropriate for the particular reader(s). For example, if your reader is an eminent scientist in your field with whom you have had only professional contact, send only the Research Plan. If your reader is a kindly mentor whom you have known for some time, you might consider also sending the budget and budget justification (if there is a budget)—or even the whole Application.

Before you submit the Application to your institutional grants office (Office for Grants and Contracts), find out whether the officials in the office want to see the whole Application or just the administrative portions (i.e., everything **except** the Research Plan).

Colleagues

Try to make an "I'll read your grant proposal, if you read mine" agreement with at least one or two **bright, responsible, conscientious colleagues who are intimately familiar with your field of research and who are successful grant getters.**

- Ask way ahead of time so the person can block out an appropriate amount of time in her/his schedule to read your proposal **thoughtfully.**

- Give your colleague(s) *at least* 2—and preferably 4—weeks to read your proposal.

  —Colleagues who are in your field of research can make valuable scientific suggestions, but someone who is not totally familiar with your specific area of research may be a **better judge of clarity** (and may, in some cases, better simulate the secondary Reviewer).

  —A colleague who is a successful proposal writer (preferably with multiple successes) and has had experience as a Reviewer can have valuable comments even if he/she knows little about your field.

  —Someone with good editorial skills can help with the final polishing of the proposal and greatly improve its readability/comprehensibility.

To optimize the chance for your Application to succeed, you should plan to have your grant proposal read by each of the aforementioned types of "critics."

Your choice of readers is extremely important. To make the pre-review process a worthwhile endeavor, **choose readers who**

—**are knowledgeable/savvy**

—have an eye for detail
—are conscientious
—are candid with you
—**are willing to spend the necessary time to read and critique your Application with care**

It is to your advantage to try to find readers who have the necessary attributes and with whom you already have a long-term working relationship. Someone who has the relevant **experience and also really cares about you and your career** will generally spend more time and pay more attention to the particulars of your proposal than someone you know only casually. A colleague who reads your proposal in an hour and tells you "it's fine" has probably not helped you very much. As a consultant, I spend at least 30 hours to critique an R01 Application! *Assure your readers at the start that you invite harsh criticism and are not afraid of "a lot of red ink."*

The value of having your proposal read by **several readers** is well illustrated by my experience with the manuscript for my 1995 book about proposal-writing. I sent copies of the main part of the book to the 5 readers named in the "Acknowledgments" section of that book. Each of them made extremely valuable and cogent suggestions for improving the text. Two of the readers each sent me more than 100 numbered comments and suggestions for changes and improvements. Interestingly, there were very few suggestions or corrections that overlapped, that is, were made by more than one reader. This confirmed for me that different people bring very different expertise, criteria, and perspectives to what they read. The totality of their comments made my book a much better book than it otherwise might have been. Thus, I suggest that it will generally benefit your proposal to have—within reason—more, rather than fewer, pre-readers.

If you are mailing your Grant Application to your pre-reviewers, always enclose **for each pre-reviewer:**

- **A cover letter**

  —Thank the person in advance for taking her/his precious time to read your proposal.
  —Suggest an appropriately far off date for the return of your proposal (at least 2 weeks, but preferably one month after they receive your Application).
  —Specify when and how the person can best reach you in case s/he has questions. (Provide your correct mailing address, e-mail, and telephone and fax numbers.)

- **A self-addressed return envelope**

  Be sure the envelope is large enough—and has affixed to it the correct amount of postage to accommodate the original proposal plus any extra sheets the reader may wish to enclose. As a rule of thumb: for return of your Application by regular first class mail, put twice the amount of postage on the return envelope as you put on the outgoing envelope. The U.S. Postal Service 2-day priority mailers are often a convenient way to send manuscripts. In either of the aforementioned, it is imperative that the pre-reviewer retains a photocopy of your Application with her/his comments on the slight chance that the item is lost in the mail. Otherwise, express mail or registered mail or a courier service should be used so the package can be traced if lost. But even then, it's the better part of wisdom to suggest to the pre-reviewer that s/he makes and retains a copy of her/his comments. As a courtesy, offer to pay for the photocopying if there is a charge involved.

Funding agency staff members

Applicants can get various degrees of pre-submission advice from their potential funding agency. Some foundations will actually work with you to prepare your proposal.

As mentioned earlier, at NIH Applicants can sometimes get some pre-submission advice regarding the general approach taken in preparing an Application, and a staff member may occasionally discuss with you the appropriateness of certain components of your Application. But for the most part, agency pre-review will be only with respect to form and adequacy of the presentation—not for scientific content. If you want to try to get help from agency staff members, the Grant Application must be sent to the agency several months before the required submission date!!! (Call to ask when and where to send the proposal.)

Do NOT expect agency personnel to
- *make suggestions about material (scientific) content*
- *give "estimates" on fundability*
- *do routine editing*

Office for sponsored research at your institution

At many institutions, personnel in the Office for Sponsored Research/Office for Grants and Contracts will want to check the administrative parts of your Application before you submit the Application to the agency. **This is a valuable service.** *Give them ample time to do the best possible job for you.* Some institutions have people in the Office for Sponsored Research/Office for Grants and Contracts who can help with more than the administrative details. **If such help is available, take advantage of it.**

In the more than 15 years that I have been giving workshops about proposal writing, I have conferred with personnel at many university Offices for Sponsored Research/Office for Grants and Contracts. To date, I do not recall even one such office in which the personnel did not tell me how difficult it is to get the faculty to submit their Applications to the office in a timely fashion! The story is almost invariably some variation of "we ask for 2 weeks and we are lucky if we get the proposals an hour before they have to be mailed." The officers tell me that they cannot adequately check the Applications when several arrive in their office for processing at the last minute. **Your institution is paying for these individuals to help you.** You are cheating yourself out of this service if you do not get your Application to them **at the time THEY ask to see it!**

Consultants as pre-reviewers

A good consultant can help you organize your ideas, write, rewrite, critique, and/or generally improve the presentation of your idea in your Application. Consultants are generally unlikely to help you with your research idea. Therefore, before you spend money on a consultant, be sure that
- the science is sound
- your project idea is good and feasible
  Check with knowledgeable colleagues/mentors
- the intended granting agency is interested in—and enthusiastic about—the idea

Do NOT change the draft you gave to the pre-reviewers while they are reading that draft
- If you generate a new draft of your proposal and change it substantially, it will be difficult for you to locate changes suggested by the pre-reviewers!
- The time during which others are critiquing your proposal is a good time for you to get some distance from the proposal.

- If you have given yourself the time to "distance" yourself from the proposal, you are likely to approach it with a fresh view when you read it again and—in some sense—YOU essentially become an additional pre-reviewer.

REVISING THE SECOND DRAFT AFTER IT COMES BACK FROM THE READERS/ PRE-REVIEWERS

Do NOT revise the second draft until you have the copies back from **ALL** the readers/ pre-reviewers. A conscientious reading of a grant proposal is a lot of work.

- **You owe your readers the courtesy of** *considering* **their suggestions** *seriously.*
- However, you are *NOT* obliged to *use* all their suggestions!
- YOU are responsible for the proposal.
- YOU should feel comfortable with the proposal that you submit.
- YOU must decide which of the readers' suggestions are useful and appropriate.
- Incorporate only those of the readers' suggestions that you consider pertinent.

    But be open-minded in your assessments. Sometimes another person's comment may wound your ego. Re-read the comment in question a few hours or—preferably—a day or two later. When your ego has recovered, you may realize that the reader made a good point. Remember that **the objective is to get funded**.

While reading the pre-reviewers' edits, you may find that their comments suggest other changes to you that you had not thought of before. This process tends to work better if you have put the proposal aside for a while. Leave your mind open to the possibility of making such changes.

When you have finished this revision process, you should have a pre-final draft of your proposal.

> **NOTE:** You should now **do one final edit of your Application.** Consider this your last opportunity to make changes. Be sure you are satisfied with your proposal before you do the final polishing and checking.
>
> **See Appendices I-D, II, and III.**

The final copy of the proposal should look neat. Spelling and grammar should be correct. Poor grammar makes extra work for the Reviewers and, if they are of the "old school," may sour them about the Applicant. More importantly, some grammatical errors can lead to unfortunate misunderstandings about your science!

Certain spelling and grammatical errors—or a large number of such mistakes—may provide comic relief during the long and sometimes tedious Study Section meetings. Be sure your proposal is not the origin of such humor. An occasional minor error is not a calamity, and a neatly "whited-out" correction is usually perfectly acceptable. But a carelessly written—or sloppy-looking—Grant Application may give the Reviewers the idea that this is a **reflection of how you do your science**. If a Reviewer thinks that an Applicant could not be bothered putting out a decent final product, the Reviewer is likely to get a bad impression of the PI and start her/his review of your grant proposal with a negative attitude.

If you have checked all the items mentioned in this section and everything appears to be in good order in the pre-final draft of your Application, it is time to print the final draft of the Application and make the necessary copies for submission.

RECAP FOR PART V: WRITING THE RESEARCH PLAN

The way you write your Grant Application tells the Reviewer a lot about you.

To be competitive, do the necessary background work and write a superb grant Application.

Begin to write your grant proposal early. It may take several weeks to several months to prepare a **good** Application—not counting the time it takes to accumulate preliminary data or the time to have others read the proposal.

Prepare before you write:
- Collect ample pertinent preliminary data
- Read and follow instructions meticulously
- Use a good **checklist** when you plan the proposal
- Set deadlines for yourself for finishing the various stages of the project

Writing the Research Plan:
- **Make a good and extensive outline**
- Compile and analyze relevant data
- Prepare clearly labeled tables, figures, and photographs with clear legends
- Write the first draft
  - —Write to express, not to impress
  - —Provide alternative approaches for the project
  - —Don't put information in inappropriate parts of the proposal
  - —Avoid ambiguity and irrelevant information
  - —Be quantitative and specific
  - —Be consistent (tenses, nomenclature—including abbreviations; check that figure legends agree with descriptions in the text)
  - —Be complete but concise (avoid redundancy and unnecessary words)
  - —Use simple (but not simple-minded or simplistic) words
  - —Use short, direct sentences
  - —Use short paragraphs that begin with **informative topic sentences**
  - —Avoid pompous language and self-praise (let your data speak for you)
  - —Be positive
  - —Stay within the recommended margins
  - —Strictly adhere to the page limits
  - —Strictly adhere to the instructions about type size
- Revise the first draft to generate a good second draft
  - —Consider
    - Accuracy
    - Clarity
    - Consistency
    - Brevity
    - Emphasis and impact
    - Style

       Tone

       Presentation

—Use computer aids to help you improve the first draft

       Spelling checker

       Grammar checker

       Search mode to find over-used words

—Use a good checklist to make sure you have followed all the instructions and that everything has been completed to the best of your ability

- Print out a good second draft
- Have at least 2 or 3 pre-reviewers (colleagues and/or consultants) critique the second draft. At least one of these pre-reviewers should be someone with a good command of English grammar.
- Revise the second draft using the **relevant** comments of the pre-reviewers
- Generate a pre-final draft
- When you are sure that all has been completed to the best of your ability, print out a final draft

■ PART VI ■

SUBMITTING AND TRACKING THE GRANT APPLICATION

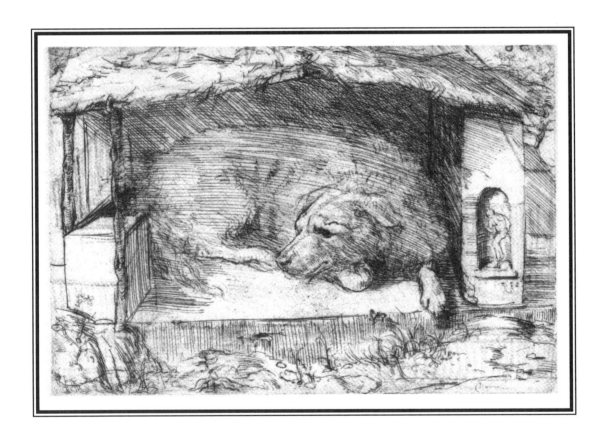

Now that you have finished filling out most of the administrative forms of the Application and have finished writing the Research Plan, you are ready to prepare the Application for submission.

POLISHING AND CHECKING THE PRE-FINAL DRAFT OF THE GRANT APPLICATION

If your total budget is such that you have to submit an itemized budget:
- Have you rechecked the budget calculations?
- Have you checked that budget totals are entered on the Face page?
- Is the budget adequately justified?

Other things to check:
- Have you signed the Application (If you are submitting on paper, you should sign *before* you make the requisite number of copies)?
- Has the responsible institutional official signed the Application (If you are submitting on paper, have the official sign *before* you make the requisite number of copies)?
- Is your name (last name first!) filled in on the top right corner of each page?
- Are the pages all numbered consecutively and correctly?

  NIH does not permit page numbers with suffixes (e.g., pages 5A, 5B, 6a, etc.); some other agencies permit and even request such numbering. Check the instructions.
- Do you have a **Table of Contents**?

  —Are the page numbers entered in the Table of Contents *in accordance with the page numbers of the **final** draft* on the text pages?

  —Have you listed the Appendix items in the Table of Contents?
- Have you compared the **Project Description (Abstract)** with the final version of the Application to be sure it is appropriate and parallel in content to your Research Plan?

  Write the Project Description (Abstract) **after** you have printed out the final draft of your Research Plan.
- Do you have a reasonable, realistic **tentative timetable** for your project at the end of the Research Design and Methods section?
- Do you have a **Biographical Sketch for each professional person** you have listed under

  —"Personnel?" and "Consultants/Collaborators"?

  —Have you stayed within the permissible page limits for the Biographical Sketch?

  —Did you follow all other instructions about what the agency wants in the Biographical Sketch?

  —Did you check to be sure that all the Biographical Sketches are in the **same format**?
- Do you have a **letter of collaboration** from each "Consultant" and "outside Collaborator"?

  —Have you placed the letters in the appropriate section of the Research Plan?

  —Have you checked that these letters give substantive and specific information about the role the Consultants/Collaborators will have in the project?

- Do you have the necessary documentation if you have Consortium or Contractual Arrangements?
- Have you completed the necessary forms concerning
  —Other Support?
  —Resources?
    If you are submitting a budget, be sure that "Facilities" and "Equipment" listed under "Resources" are not at odds with items you have requested in the budget.
  —Personal Data Form
    Self-explanatory. Follow the instructions.
  —Checklist pages
    Self-explanatory. Follow the instructions.
    The NIH Checklist must be
    - filled in
    - placed at the end of the Application (if you are submitting on paper)
    - given a page number
- Have the dates of the various institutional agreements and assurances been filled in on the Face page?
- Have the indirect costs been calculated on the Checklist pages and filled in on the Face page?
- Is the Appendix complete and in order?
  Is each Appendix item labeled correctly?
  —Name of PI
  —Title of Grant Application
  —Number of Appendix item
  —Title of Appendix item
  Have you collated the Appendix items into the required number of Appendix sets?

  Have you included a list of Appendix items as a cover sheet for each copy of the Appendix?

  Have you included a list of Appendix items in the Table of Contents for the Grant Application?
- Have you checked the formatting, including margins, of each page of the Application?
- Have you checked that no page limits have been exceeded in the final formatted draft?

> **NOTE:** Applications with as little as half page over the page limit have been returned to PIs without review!

- Have you made a final check of all items in your Application to be sure you have included everything listed on the NIH checklist?
- Have you made a final check of all items against the checklist in Appendix I in this book or some other checklist that is at least as detailed as the NIH checklist?

PREPARING THE APPLICATION FOR SUBMISSION

- Print out a final draft (unless you are submitting electronically!).
- If you are **not** submitting electronically, make the appropriate number of photocopies of the Application and the Appendix.

  Aside from the photocopies of the Application and the photocopies of the Appendix required by NIH, you will need extra copies of the Application and the Appendix for

  —your own files

  —professional colleagues listed on your Application may want to have copies of all or parts of your Application for their records:
    - Co-investigators
    - Collaborators
    - Consultants listed on the Application

  —the Office of Grants and Contracts at your institution

  —other administrative offices in your own department/institution

- Use paper clips or rubber bands to fasten pages together.

  Do not staple or bind the Application unless the instructions specifically suggest that you do this.

- To keep copies neat

  —put each copy into a separate folder

     or

  —cut off the top third or half of manila envelopes and use the lower part to keep the pages of each copy of your Application together

     or

  —use tension-binder clips

     Do not use regular paper clips—especially small ones! Small paper clips tend to slip off multiple sheets of paper that are handled frequently. Do not allow your Application to arrive at the funding agency as a set of loose sheets that are not in the correct page order!!!

- Label items: "Original Application," "Original Appendix," etc.
- Consider providing a cover letter requesting/suggesting up to 3 specific Study Sections that would be appropriate to review your Application—and the reason you are making the request—and attach it to the front of the **original copy** of the Application. You may also suggest a potential funding component in this letter. Unless there is some good reason not to do so, NIH is obliged to honor your request.

> **NOTE:** If you make such a request/suggestion, be sure you have thoroughly researched who is on these Study Sections and what sorts of projects have been funded by which agencies in the recent past.

- If the Application is in response to an RFA (Request for Application), read carefully and follow all available instructions.

- Postcards submitted with Applications are no longer returned by NIH. Instead, "snapout" mailers are returned to PIs after Study Section assignments are made. Moreover, PIs can now access the NIH Commons to check on the status of pending Applications.

The NIH Commons opened in September 2003 for registration by all NIH grantee institutions. In January 2004, I was informed that there was a pilot deployment at NIH whereby Applicants can submit competitive Applications electronically. This pilot deployment is slated for expansion, such that by the end of 2004 all institutions should be able to submit Applications electronically.

By the end of 2003 about 700 grantee institutions had registered and some 10,000 investigators had Commons accounts. The predominant use to date is the so-called "status" interface whereby PIs can check on

- the status of pending Applications
- upcoming deadlines for renewals
- access to summary statements and priority scores several days after Study Session meetings rather than the 4–6 weeks that were previously the norm when Summary Statements were sent via U.S. mail

The NIH Commons has a full-time eRA liaison to the extramural community:
David Wright
Tel: 301-435-1792
E-mail: david.wright@nih.gov

If you are dealing with an agency OTHER than NIH, it might still be wise to include, with your Grant Application, a self-addressed, *stamped* postcard that someone at the agency can easily fill out and drop in the mail to confirm receipt of your Application. Attach the postcard to the original copy of your proposal. The postcard can read simply:

Grant Application: (Fill in your grant proposal title) by (Fill in your name) was received at (Name of agency)_____

By (Name of person)_____

E-mail address _____

Telephone # _____

On (date) _____

Thank you.

MAILING THE APPLICATION

Perhaps by the time this book is in print, Grant Applications to NIH will be transmitted by electronic means. Until then, all Applications and other deliveries to the Center for Scientific Review must come either via courier delivery or via the United States Postal Service (USPS). **NOTE:** Applications delivered by individuals to the Center for Scientific Review are **NOT** accepted—so do **NOT** plan to fly to Bethesda to deliver your Application!

Mail the *original* + *5* **copies** (= 6 complete sets) **of the Application** plus *5 complete sets of the Appendix.*

NOTE that the number of Application sets required is one more than the number of Appendix sets required!

Some NIH proposals (e.g., those with expedited review processes) may require submission of a different number of copies of the proposal. **Always READ THE INSTRUCTIONS!** If in doubt, call the Program Officer at the relevant Institute.

- If you are submitting by mail, use a box from bond paper or something similar to pack the Application so that it arrives at NIH (or other funding institution) in good condition.
- Use the following address:
  Center for Scientific Review
  National Institutes of Health
  Suite 1040
  6701 Rockledge Drive, MSC 7710
  Bethesda, MD 20892-7710

NOTE: If you use Express Mail or courier service, use zip code 20817 and telephone # 301-435-0715.

NOTE: NIH does NOT accept C.O.D. packages!!!

- Use the proper amount of postage.
  Weigh the package. **Do NOT guess!**
- Mail the Application in ample time **to get to NIH on time.**

  For Grant Applications processed through the NIH Center for Scientific Review, Applications must be *received* by the published Application receipt dates. However, an Application received after the deadline may be acceptable if it carries a legible proof-of-mailing date assigned by the carrier and the proof-of-mailing date is not later than one week **prior** to the deadline date.
- Get a legible proof-of-mailing receipt from the Post Office or commercial mail carrier.

  On arrival at NIH, each Application is stamped with the arrival date in large letters. **It is important that your Application arrive on time.** If you cannot mail the Application early enough to use regular mail, use U.S. Postal Service Express Mail or a private express delivery service such as Federal Express.

TRACKING THE APPLICATION

Follow the travels of your Application after you send it to the granting agency—in this case, NIH:

- Did you receive your proposal ID number, and Study Section and Institute assignments from NIH within about 6 weeks after you submitted your

Application? This ID number will likely arrive sooner once electronic grants administration is fully implemented.

If your Application is assigned to a Study Section or funding component that you consider inappropriate, you should immediately

—contact the Referral Office (301-594-7250) to discuss the possibility of reassignment

—follow up with a written request to the Referral Office

As with suggestions for Study Section assignments submitted with the original proposal, requests for reassignment will be considered carefully, but **the final decision rests with NIH.**

■ Know when your Study Section meets.

This information is available online at

http://www.csr.nih.gov/Committees/meetings/ssmeet1.asp

It's good to keep the dates in mind in case you have generated some pertinent additional data to send to the Study Section (see below).

> **BE AWARE: You must get permission from the SRA before sending additional materials to the Study Section!**

■ Know the members of the Study Section.

—As soon as you get your assignment, go to

http://era.nih.gov/roster/index.cfm

and

http://www.csr.nih.gov/Committees/rosterindex.asp

to determine who is on the Study Section to which your Application was assigned, and the name—and contact information—of the SRA.

—As soon as you get your assignment, it's a good idea to call the SRA to find out whether there is anyone on the Study Section who is not listed on the NIH Web site list of Study Section members.

—If there is someone on the Study Section whom you consider to have a conflict of interest with respect to your project, **alert the SRA** not to send your proposal to that person for review.

It is *your responsibility* to contact the Center for Scientific Review (CSR) Referral Office if you do not receive, within 6 weeks of submitting the Application the:

■ Study Section assignment
■ Scientific Review Administrator's
  —Name
  —Address
  —Telephone number
■ Number assigned to your Grant Application.

In the months between submission of your Application and the Study Section meeting, you may have new findings in your laboratory that might improve the quality of your proposal—and perhaps lead to a better review. It is to your advantage to inform the Study Section about new developments such as:

- New exciting data
- An additional paper you had submitted has been accepted for publication
- You got a promotion
- Something else occurred that might strengthen your Application

If you have new information in support of your Application, contact the SRA of your assigned Study Section and ask for permission to send supplementary materials (new data, reprints, etc.). If permission is granted, ask the SRA:

- how many copies to send (unless you are submitting electronically)
- to please forward the additional information to the Reviewers

  —Do not send data just to impress the Reviewers that you are working hard.
  —Use good judgment about what sort of information is important for the review process.
  —Do not send data that you would not have put into the original Grant Application.
  —Do not abuse the option to send additional data.
  —Do not send too much material.
    Try to keep it to 3 to 5 pages.
  —Understand that even if you do get permission to send additional material, the Reviewers have the option **not** to consider it!

In fairness to the Scientific Review Administrator, the staff, and the members of the Study Section, the optimal time to send such additional material **is at least 6 weeks before the Study Section meeting.** However, if an experiment that will help the status of your grant proposal materializes a week before the meeting, call the SRA. *If you get permission,* send the materials by Express Mail; there is no harm in trying. But keep in mind that sending new information at "the last minute" is a common "abuse" and tends to irritate Reviewers. Use good judgment!

If you do send material close to the time of the Study Section meeting, it is especially important to ask the SRA how many copies s/he would like to have—and send that number of copies—so that this busy person will not have to deal with the task of making photocopies. Some SRAs send additional materials only to the primary Reviewers/Readers. Some may send them to all the Study Section members. It is possible that some may not distribute them at all!!!

Unless you are submitting the materials electronically, enclose a self-addressed, *stamped* postcard (with an appropriate message on the blank side that can be easily filled in) with the materials you send so that you can get acknowledgment that the materials were received by the SRA in a timely fashion.

If you get permission and send additional materials to the Scientific Review Administrator, it is a good idea to also send a copy of the materials and the cover letter to the Institute program staff person who is responsible for your Application.

You will usually be notified of the status of your Application within 2 weeks after the end of the Study Section meeting. This notification will include the priority score and percentile ranking (if the Application was scored) for your Application and will provide the name of the Program Official from the potential funding component who is responsible for your Application.

Prompt access to your priority score and percentile ranking can give you an appreciable head start on revising an Application that is not likely to be funded.

Do not call the SRA for information about priority scores. The SRA needs time to recover from the Study Section meeting, averaging scores, calculating percentiles, and preparing the Summary Statements. The SRA has to prepare some 60 to 100 or more of these reports within the month after the meeting. In the past, the SRA had to synthesize these Summary Statements from the 2 or 3 written reports of the primary Reviewers, notations of the Readers (Discussants), and what she/he remembers of (or took notes about) the discussion during the meeting that follows the oral reading of the Reviewers' reports. It was no easy task! This burden was immensely decreased as of the February 1995 Study Section meetings, by the adoption of a "Streamlined Review" procedure (often still referred to as "triage") and associated modifications in the form of the summary statements for CSR-wide use for all Investigator-initiated research grants (R01) and certain other grant Applications reviewed by CSR. Under the "Streamlined Review" process, Reviewers are expected to identify the Applications that are likely to score in the bottom 50% of Applications being reviewed at that Study Section meeting. These latter Applications get a full written review by at least 2 Reviewers, but are not discussed at the Study Section meeting, do not get a numerical rating (and, hence, no priority score), and get a somewhat modified Summary Statement that consists primarily of the individual Reviewers' reports (critiques). (See Reif-Lehrer, L., article about changes at NIH, *Journal of the National Grantseekers Institute*, Vol. 2, No. 1, 1995 and Reif-Lehrer, L., "Science Community Gives Mixed, Review To 'Triage,'" *The Scientist*, Vol. 8, No. 23, November 28, 1994, pages 1, 8–9.)

> An Application can be "streamlined out" only if the decision to do so is **unanimous**. Before the Study Section meeting, an Application can only be "streamlined out" if both primary Reviewers agree to the appropriateness of this action. Moreover, any Reviewer on the Study Section can recall an Application, which has been "streamlined out" by the primary Reviewers, for full review by the full Study Section. Thus, **the decision to "streamline out" an Application must be unanimous.**

Applications which are not "streamlined out" ("triaged") are referred to as the "scored" Applications. The Reviewer's comments for each "scored" Application are read at the Study Section meeting and the Application is discussed by the whole group in session. The Reviewers are expected to modify their written critiques during the review of the Application at the Study Section meeting—for example, by removing a criticism that was deemed to be invalid during the group discussion. Under this revised review system, the Summary Statement consists of the revised individual critiques of the 2 or 3 primary Reviewers. SRAs are expected to edit critiques only "lightly"—to eliminate bad grammar and unnecessarily hurtful comments—but are no longer required to integrate the Reviewers' reports into a single cohesive piece of prose. Summaries of the Study Section discussion (including budget recommendations, if the Application has a detailed budget) are also included, under the heading of "Resume," for Applications that underwent full review by the Study Section. Summary Statements for scored Applications also have a "Description of Project." Summary Statements for Applications that were "streamlined out," consist of the individual critiques of the 2 or 3 primary Reviewers plus an explanation of the "Streamlined Review Process."

> **NOTE:** *Do not call the assigned Program Official on the day after the Study Section meeting to ask about the outcome of the review of your Application!* Wait at least until after you receive your priority score before making contact with the SRA or your Program Officer.

You should receive your Summary Statement 4 to 6 weeks after the Study Section meeting (sooner, if your proposal was "streamlined out"). Mark your calendar, and call the SRA if you have not received your Summary Statement by the expected time. **NOTE that this time frame will be much shorter when electronic grant proposal processing is implemented.**

After you receive your priority score, you may contact the SRA or the Program Official assigned to your Application if you need

- more details about the review
- information about the likelihood of funding

Such information can be useful for planning ahead. For example, you may need to

- start revising the proposal
- develop a totally new project
- plan a career move if the grant is not likely to be funded and your institution cannot support you!

RECAP FOR PART VI: SUBMITTING AND TRACKING THE GRANT APPLICATION

Prepare the Application for submission:

- Polish the pre-final draft (Use a good checklist.)
- Generate a final draft
- Incorporate the final draft of the Research Plan into the whole Application
- Assemble the rest of the Application packet
- If the Application is in response to an RFA (Request for Application), make this clearly apparent
- Sign and date the Application

> **NOTE:** Watch for changes that will occur once electronic grants administration is fully implemented.

Get administrative approval for the Application from your institution's office for grants and contracts

- Photocopy the Application
  Make the correct number of copies for the funding agency plus extra copies for yourself, for Collaborators, for the Office for Grants and Contracts, and for other administrative offices at your own institution.
- Organize the pages of the copies
  —Fasten the pages together—but do not staple or bind!

—Label copies ("Original Application," "Original Appendix," etc.)
- Provide a cover letter (optional)
    —Suggest up to 3 Study Sections for Application review
    —Suggest an appropriate funding component
    —Give cogent reasons for your requested choices
    —Paper-clip the cover letter to the front of the original copy of the Application (use a jumbo size paper clip that will not easily get dislodged!)

When you mail the Application:
- Pack the Application neatly and well
- Use the correct mailing address
- If using Express Mail or courier service to NIH, use the alternate zip code designated for this type of service
- Mail your Application in time to be **received** by the agency deadline
- If using U.S. Post Office or a commercial delivery service, get a legible proof-of-mailing receipt

Follow ("Track") the travels of your Application

In the case of an NIH Application:
- Did you get the Application ID number and Study Section assignment within 6 weeks after submitting Application?

    Contact CSR if you do not receive this information within 6 weeks after submitting the Application (sooner once electronic grants administration is fully implemented).

- Did you ascertain when your Study Section meets?
- Did you look up the membership of your assigned Study Section?
- If you get new pertinent results after submitting your Application, consider sending the additional information to the Study Section—provided that you first get permission from the SRA.
- Did you get your priority score and percentile ranking (if the Application was scored) within 2 weeks after the end of the Study Section meeting?
- Did you receive your Summary Statement 4 to 6 weeks after the Study Section meeting? (Sooner than 4 to 6 weeks once electronic grants administration is fully implemented.) If not, call the SRA.

PART VII

SUMMARY STATEMENTS, REBUTTALS, AND REVISIONS

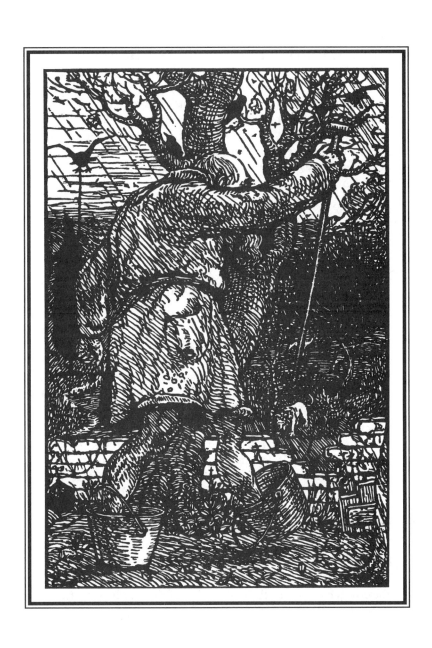

SOME HINTS ABOUT THE SUMMARY STATEMENT

The Summary Statement (sometimes still referred to as the "Pink Sheets," although it has not been printed on pink paper for several decades) will probably soon be sent electronically rather than on paper.

Before 1994, the Summary Statement was an integration of the reports of the primary Reviewers and the comments of the Readers/Discussants. The Summary Statements were put together by the SRA after the Study Section meeting, which placed a rather large workload on the SRAs. Since 1994, the Summary Statement has consisted of the individual Reviewers' reports (lightly edited by the SRA of the Study Section to eliminate bad grammatical errors and offensive comments) plus a summary of the discussion about the Application that took place during the Study Section meeting.

Most Summary Statements have some positive and some negative things to say about the proposal under review. It is a common—and human—response for PIs who find criticism of their proposal in the Summary Statement to respond with negative feelings or comments about the Reviewers. These comments seem to range from an exasperated, "The Reviewers did not understand this at all" to some exclamation implying that the Reviewers are just short of retarded. It is wise to keep such thoughts to oneself for a day or two and then to re-read the Summary Statement in a more dispassionate frame of mind. Although occasional mishaps may occur, it is important to know that Reviewers

- are chosen with care
- are bright people
- have extensive experience writing proposals
- have usually read many proposals—even if they are new Study Section members

Do not let your wounded ego get in the way of carefully considering the Reviewers' comments. The following story, which was told by a physician-writer who spoke at a writing workshop I attended, may help to make the point:

> The writer gave his editor a book manuscript. The editor gave it back saying it needed more work. This scenario happened multiple times. Finally, the writer got annoyed and said to the editor, "If you're so smart, why don't *you* rewrite the book." The editor responded, "I'm not a writer and I can't write, but I read a lot of manuscripts and this one stinks." The writer rewrote the manuscript several more times. When it was finally published, it became a best seller!

There is an "art" to *reading **between** the lines* of the Summary Statement. Learn to interpret the Summary Statement and to use this advice from the Reviewers to help you write a better Grant Application. If you are a novice Grant Application writer, it may be useful to have an experienced and successful PI read your Summary Statement. In any event, as you read your Summary Statement, you should consider the following possibilities before deciding what action to take in response to the critique:

- Comments that represent the proposal inaccurately often result from unclear writing by the Principal Investigator.
- Criticisms about protocols, techniques, or data analysis often indicate that the Principal Investigator didn't do enough homework.
- If the critique questions the ability of the Principal Investigator to carry out the proposed work, an appropriate Collaborator may be in order.

- If the critique questions the choice of problem, it may mean that
  —the significance was poorly explained, in which case you should consider rewriting the proposal

  or

  —the problem per se lacks merit, in which case you should consider finding a new problem
- If the Summary Statement is not sufficiently explicit about what the Study Section did and did not like about your proposal, you can sometimes get additional information by contacting the SRA of your Study Section and/or a member of the Institute program staff.

At NIH, the worst priority score is 500; the best score is 100. The **"payline"** is the priority score for the Grant Application with the highest/worst priority score that was funded from the group of proposals reviewed **at that review cycle** or the percentile equivalent to that score in that review round. If your priority score was just beyond (slightly higher than) the "payline," your Summary Statement may be quite positive and may provide relatively little information for you to use in writing a revised Application. The Institute program staff member responsible for your Application, who is likely to have been present during the Study Section review of your Application, may be able to provide some insight into what the Reviewers did and did not like about your project and may be able to make suggestions about rewriting your proposal if you plan to submit a revised Application.

It is important to understand, however, that a major reason why some grants do not get funded is that the ideas, although perhaps good, are not quite good enough to compete in the funding climate of the time at which the Application was reviewed. Applicants sometimes find it difficult to comprehend that the priority score for a second or third revision has not markedly improved and does not get funded because the proposal is based on

- a less-than-very good idea
- a very good idea that is being—or has been—investigated by too many other researchers
- a very good idea but one in which the funding agency is not interested at that time—or at all!

> **NOTE:** You can feel confident that an extremely well-written proposal based on a superb idea—but one that is NOT within the mandate of the agency to which it has been submitted—will **NOT** be funded!

On the other hand, if, after checking with knowledgeable colleagues, you are convinced that your project idea is good **and** matches the current mandate of the agency to which you are applying, you should be tenacious about reapplying. To reinforce this point, I call your attention to 5 Applications reviewed by CSR (then called Division of Research Grants, DR) in 1992: Four were A6 Applications (6th revision; i.e., the 7th Application submitted under the same title by the same PI). Two of these were funded. The fifth was an A7 Application (7th revision; i.e., the 8th Application submitted under the same title by the same PI) that was also funded! Keep in mind, however, that since that time, NIH has instituted the so-called "Three strikes and you're out" rule. Thus, one may now re-submit an Application with the same title only 3 times (i.e., the original Application and 2 revisions).

Do NOT "play games" with NIH. You will only waste your own precious time and the precious time of the Reviewers.

- If you have issues with the Reviewers' comments, you may rebut them politely—but do not ever "argue" with a Reviewer!!!
- Do NOT resubmit an Application if you have not responded to ALL the Reviewers' comments and made relevant substantive changes to the Research Plan.
- Do not submit the same unchanged Application with a new/different name.

  "A rose by any other name would smell as sweet"—and a bad proposal is just as bad no matter what you call it! Remember that Reviewers are generally neither dumb nor gullible!

REBUTTALS

When you receive your Summary Statement, you may not agree with what the SRA and Reviewers have written. "The Reviewers totally misunderstood …" is a common response from unsuccessful proposal writers! It is important to consider that the fault is very likely to be a problem with your writing. If "they" misunderstood, perhaps you did not explain the project clearly enough! However, if after recovering from the initial pain and disappointment of not getting funded, you still think that the review was flawed, you may consider writing a rebuttal. But you should understand that unless your priority score was close to the funding level, or your proposal was really grievously misjudged, the rebuttal process may just cost you time that you could spend more fruitfully by revising and improving your Application.

If you want to write a rebuttal, contact an appropriate staff member at the assigned Institute or other funding component for information about procedures to seek redress of your concerns. Detailed information about communicating concerns regarding the review of an Application is available from the NIH Grants Information Office.

If you decide to write a letter of rebuttal, be sure that it is constructive and written in a positive tone.

- Do not *complain* to the granting agency.
- Do not berate the Institute staff about what is in the Summary Statement—no matter how "right" YOU think you are.
  —The Institute staff does not initiate the critique.
  —The Institute staff is only the intermediary between the Study Section and the Principal Investigator.
  —The Institute staff generally does not communicate with the Study Section about an Application once the Study Section meeting is over.
  —The Institute staff consists of professionals. They are also human beings; it is important to treat them with courtesy and respect.
- Be aware that intrusion of sarcasm, righteous indignation, and/or "sour grapes" statements in a letter of rebuttal helps no one, least of all you!

Under NO circumstances should you attempt to contact individual Study Section members. Never put a Study Section member in a compromising position either by

- trying to influence him/her personally prior to the Study Section meeting

or

- asking questions about the deliberations of the Study Section after the meeting

WHAT TO DO IF YOUR APPLICATION IS NOT FUNDED

It is painful to deal with rejection. Thus, it is common for Grant Application writers to respond with some negative reaction to Summary Statements bearing bad news about the outcome of their efforts. Many proposal-writers find—after their disappointment subsides and they reread the Summary Statement—that the Reviewers were not as far off the mark as had initially appeared. It is also important to realize that a major reason for NOT getting funded is that there was **not enough money** to fund all the good Applications. This knowledge does not help your particular situation and may do little to salve your wounded ego, but it may help you realize that—after giving yourself a few days to recover from the disappointment—it's time to begin to plan realistically what you need to do next. For many grant seekers, this next step is to

- prepare a revised and improved proposal that is responsive to the Reviewers' comments

  or

- plan a new proposal, possibly to a different funding agency

SUBMITTING A REVISED APPLICATION

You should revise the proposal and try again if you

- are fairly sure that your proposed project is within the mandate of the agency to which you submitted the Application
- have funds to tide you over for another grant cycle
- have new data to present that supports your Application more substantively than the preliminary data you submitted with the original Application

It has become more the rule than the exception to have to revise at least once—and even twice (check the funding statistics on the NIH Web site).

If you perceive that you have a chance of getting funded, be persistent. But know when it is appropriate to persist and when it is time to stop.

Be aware that priority scores for revised Applications generally do not improve by more than 50 points. So if your priority score is more than 50 points away from the "payline," you should seriously consider

- making **major** changes to your proposal
- preparing **a totally new proposal** about some other project
- reworking your project idea for submission to **another appropriate funding agency**

A revised NIH Application requires a 3-page **Introduction** (see below) and must be responsive to every point in the critique of the Summary Statement. In writing the Introduction section, please consider the advice given earlier for writing rebuttals. The way you respond to constructive criticism, the manner in which you deal with criticism that you consider invalid, and the general tone of your response are all important factors in the way Reviewers will view your revised proposal. It is a courtesy to overworked Reviewers to thank them for praise they bestow on your proposal and to be open-minded about criticism. If you disagree with comments in the Summary Statement, it is a good idea to leave such comments for last and then state your counter-opinion firmly but politely and, whenever appropriate, back up your arguments with sound data and references to published work. Insults or other negative comments to or about the Reviewers rarely, if ever, produce a positive effect and serve only to sour the Reviewers and other Study Section members about you and your Application. Likewise, flattery, in the form of excessive compliments to the Reviewers, is more likely to turn the Reviewers "off" rather than win them over. Be neutral and make it clear that you have **carefully** considered the comments in the Summary Statement.

> **NOTE:** To make the Reviewers' job as easy as possible, **summarize in the Introduction** the **changes that you have made** in the proposal—do not repeat them. If your revisions are so extensive that you cannot mark them in the manner requested in the PHS 398 Instructions, clearly indicate this in the Introduction.

If you prepare a *revised Application*, you may wish to get help from the Institute program staff member responsible for your Application.

Also see:

http://www.niaid.nih.gov/ncn/grants/basics/basics_d3.htm

http://grants.nih.gov/grants/guide/notice-files/NOT-OD-03-041.html

http://www.nlm.nih.gov/ep/FAQRevise.html

- Be sure the revised Application has substantive improvements.

  "A revised Application will be returned if substantial revisions are not clearly apparent."
- Be sure the revised Application is responsive to all questions and criticisms raised in the Summary Statement.

  Being responsive means acknowledging and responding to—not necessarily agreeing with—all the comments in the Summary Statement.
- Indicate all substantive changes you have made in the revised Application.
  - —"Highlight these changes within the text of the Research Plan by appropriate bracketing, indenting, or changing of typography." *Do not underline or use shading!*
  - —Discuss these changes in the Introduction part of the Research Plan. Note that this "Introduction" has a page limit.
- "Incorporate into the Progress Report/Preliminary Studies of the revised Application any **[pertinent]** work done since the prior version was submitted."
- Make note of, and be responsive to, the deadline for submission of revised Applications.

If you submit a revised Application, remember that the composition of the Study Section changes with time. Thus, although a resubmitted Grant Application is generally returned to the same Study Section that reviewed the initial Application, the Reviewers who reviewed your initial Application may have rotated off the panel. If this is the case, your Application will be reviewed by different Reviewers who may find a whole set of different faults with the proposal!

RECAP FOR PART VII: SUMMARY STATEMENTS, REBUTTALS, AND REVISIONS

Some hints about the Summary Statement ("Pink Sheets"):

- Summary Statements combine

  —the primary Reviewers' reports

  —the Readers' comments

  —a summary of the Study Section members' discussion about the proposal

- Ask an experienced, successful grantee to read and "interpret" your Summary Statement.

- Before blaming the Reviewers for negative comments about your proposal, ask yourself:

  —Was my choice of problem good—or does the problem per se lack merit?

  —Was the significance of my project adequately and clearly explained?

  —Did the project match the mandate of the funding agency?

  —Was my writing sufficiently clear or did unclear writing mislead the Reviewers?

  —Did I do enough homework?

  —Should I have enlisted the help of a Collaborator?

- If the Summary Statement is not sufficiently explicit, contact the SRA or Institute program staff. **Never try to contact individual Study Section members!**

If you think your Application was grievously misjudged, write a letter of rebuttal:

- Contact a staff member at the assigned Institute or grants information office about procedures.

- Do not complain or berate the granting agency.

- Do not be sarcastic.

What to do if your Application is not funded:

- If your priority score is more than 50 points away from the "payline," seriously consider:

  —preparing a totally new proposal

  —reworking the old proposal for submission to another funding agency

- If your priority score is less than 50 points away from the "payline," and if you have funds to tide you over for another grant cycle or two, submit a **revised** Application at least once—and even twice.

If you prepare a *revised Application:*

- Get help from the Institute program staff.

- Write an Introduction (note page maximum):

  —Summarize the changes you have made in the proposal.

  —Be responsive to the critique in the Summary Statement but do NOT "argue" with Reviewers.

  —Back up your statements/comments with sound data and references to published work.

  —Do not indulge in "sour grapes" rhetoric.

  —Do not excessively compliment/flatter Reviewers.

  —Do not "ARGUE" with Reviewers!

- Indicate changes in the body of the proposal by bracketing, indenting, or changing typography. *Do not use underlining or shading.*

- Incorporate into the Progress Report/Preliminary Studies, pertinent work done since the prior version of Application was submitted.
- Do **NOT** submit a revised Application **unless** you have made *substantive* changes.
- Be sure that you submit your revised Application in time for the deadline for submission of revised Applications.

Success rates and other data about Grant Applications to NIH can be accessed via the NIH Web site

http://grants2.nih.gov/grants/award/success.htm

Although the data are not always up to date, they may give you some idea of recent trends in funding.

PART VIII

Some Final Words

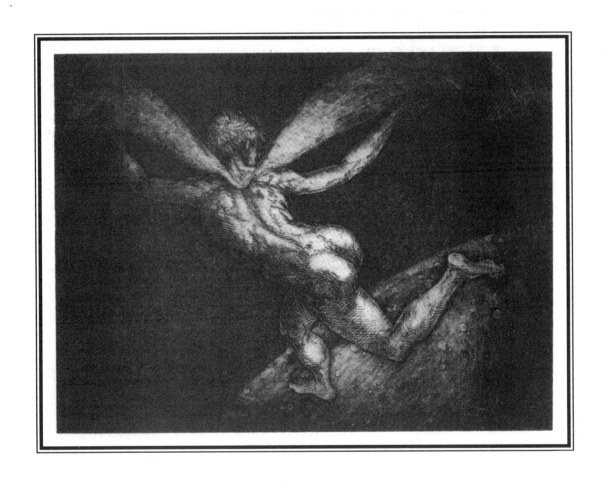

DON'T GET DISCOURAGED: WRITING A GOOD GRANT PROPOSAL IS A READILY LEARNABLE SKILL

Writing a grant proposal, like many other things in life, is not as daunting as it first appears. If you have a good idea, start early, and "put one foot in front of the other"—and follow the instructions—you will get the job done little by little. You are likely to submit a good proposal that stands a reasonable chance of being funded if you

- apply to an appropriate funding agency that is interested in the subject of your proposal
- do your homework thoroughly
- get help and advice from **wisely chosen** colleagues
- follow the advice given in this book about how to write the proposal

> **NOTE:** If you don't get funded by NIH or some other government agency, try private foundations and/or business and industry.

BE PERSISTENT

Revise, Revise, Revise! If you want to get funding, you must be persistent

In the last decades of the 20th century, it was not unusual for 25% or more of the Study Section workload to consist of reviewing revised Applications! And it is NOT at all unusual for investigators to revise more than once before getting funded. Likewise, during that time, new Research Project Grants (RPGs) accounted for about the same percentage of the research project dollars as competing continuations (Renewals). During that period, success rates for Renewals were about twice as high as for new RPGs. You may find it both useful and enlightening to check some statistics—about Revised (Amended) Applications—on the NIH Web site.

The Robert Wood Johnson Foundation states in its guidelines for Grant Applicants:

> "Unsuccessful Applicants should approach the foundation again, and, if necessary, again. *Most grantmakers regard tenacity as a virtue, and we are certainly among them.*"

You should think of tenacity as a prerequisite for doing research. If you really intend to do what you want to do, you must keep trying to get financial support for your project until you succeed in getting funding.

> **NOTE:** As Connie Weaver wrote in a 1990 edition of the Purdue University Research manual, *"The One Truth: If you don't submit a grant [proposal], you won't get a grant."*

THE GRASS IS ALWAYS GREENER . . .

If you think life is tough in the sciences, talk to people in other fields, especially in the arts and humanities. Scientists have the advantage of getting referees' comments when they submit papers to journals, and Reviewers' reports and Summary Statements when they submit Grant Applications. The comments of such readers in your own or related fields can be extremely useful for helping you improve your papers and grant proposals. **Be grateful for this type of help.**

Literary writers often get rejection slips without any feedback! A professor of creative writing at a large university in Boston told me that she submitted a book manuscript to over 100 publishers before it was finally published by a fairly prestigious university press. **Persistence can pay in the long run.**

On the other hand, banging your head against a stone wall is painful and may not always be fruitful. An important thing to learn from experience and from colleagues is when to be persistent and when to change direction.

AD HOC REVIEWING: A CHANCE TO SEE PEER REVIEW FROM THE INSIDE

If you get a chance to be an ad hoc reviewer on a Study Section (i.e., on a one-time basis), do it! Watching the peer review system work, from the inside—and observing and experiencing the enormous task of the Reviewers—will not only be enlightening but is almost guaranteed to improve the way you write your own Grant Applications. When you get to the appropriate stage of your career, you should consider it an obligation to serve on a Study Section. Others have reviewed your proposals. You should feel obliged—at the right stage of your life—to review the proposals of younger scientists.

Good Luck!

RECAP FOR PART VIII: SOME FINAL WORDS

- Don't get discouraged
- Be persistent
  —Writing a good grant proposal is a readily learnable skill.
  —REVISE, revise, revise!
  —If you don't get funded by NIH try
    - other government agencies
    - private foundations
    - business and industry
- "If you don't submit a Grant [Application], you won't get a grant."
- Try to be an ad hoc reviewer on a Study Section so you can see the review process first-hand.

GENERAL CHECKLIST FOR AN APPLICATION

This checklist was adapted from a list I received from a Federal agency that funds proposals in the social sciences. It was a list of reasons why some proposals at that agency are not funded. I have reworded the reasons into positive statements and made some minor changes and additions to the list.

A.   ARE THE RESEARCH GOALS APPROPRIATE AND CLEAR?

A1. Is the topic/purpose of the Application:
   a. Feasible in your environment and in the requested time?
   b Appropriate for support by the granting agency? If in doubt, call or write the agency to ask.
   c. For an RFP (Request for Proposal): Is the topic responsive to the scope of the announcement?

A2. Are the purposes of the study clear and sufficiently detailed? Are the hypotheses explicit?

A3. Are the research goals worthy of support?

A4. Have the collected data been analyzed appropriately and fully?

A5. Where pertinent, have you included specific end points, Applications, or products in the research goals?

B.   IS THE STUDY DESIGN GOOD?

B1. Have you determined that the research proposed has **not** been done by others? Don't waste your time! Perhaps the study design was tried and judged inadequate by others (insofar as it is possible to assess this statement). Don't reinvent the wheel!

B2. Is there sufficient attention given to related research by others? Have you cited their work?

B3. Is the study design carefully related to the purposes of the project?

B4. Will the study design provide the data needed to achieve the aims of the project? Will the study yield enough data (cases) to support the analysis?

B5. Is there evidence of a coherent direction in the study rather than parts just thrown together?

B6. Is the proposal well-coordinated and clearly related to a central focus?

B7. Is the sampling design appropriate? Have you justified the sample size?

B8. Are the data unbiased? Is there recognition of the problems of bias and ways to correct the bias?

B9. Is the methodology sufficiently detailed?

B10. Have you spelled out:
   a. the major dependent and independent variables?
   b. how the data will be obtained and analyzed?
   c. how the data will be interpreted?

d. whether the data contain enough information to support the proposed analysis?

B11. If appropriate, have you built into the study design a means and time frame for evaluating progress toward fulfilling the aims of the project?

C. ARE STAFF, TIME, AND BUDGET APPROPRIATE?

C1. Are specific tasks clearly related to personnel, time, and budget?

C2. Is there sufficient time commitment by the Principal Investigators? (Avoid small allocations of time among a large number of Investigators.)

C3. Are the scientific disciplines of the research team (including Consultants) appropriate for the topics to be investigated?

D. IS THE OVERALL PRESENTATION GOOD?

D1. Have you spelled out a specific plan of research rather than expected the Reviewers to trust in your past reputation?

D2. Have you accounted for the possibility that the Reviewers have not read about your past research? That is, is the proposal complete without the Reviewer having to refer to additional materials?

D3. Is there a balanced presentation in the proposal?

a. Does the proposal focus on particular data sets and techniques of analysis without obscuring the overall research goal?

b. Does the proposal relate each specific focus to the overall goal?

c. Have you started with a problem or topic and looked for data sets that address the issues rather than started with a data set and looked for a research problem that might be appropriate for that data set?

E. ADMINISTRATIVE DETAIL

E1. Is the Budget realistic for the work proposed?

E2. Is the Budget Justification sufficiently detailed to allow Reviewers to relate each phase and level of the project to the budget?

E3. Have you provided letters that outline willingness to participate and extent of commitment for all Consultants, Collaborators, and Subcontractors?

E4. Have you

a. filled out and obtained signatures for the cover page? If you wait until the last minute, the appropriate official may be out of town.

b. entered the appropriate page numbers in the Table of Contents?

c. made sure the Abstract reflects the contents of the Application?

d. provided the necessary information and forms concerning

    i. human studies (including gender and minority inclusion)?

    ii. humane treatment of vertebrate animals?

    iii. Other assurances (inventions and patents, debarment and suspension, drug-free workplace, lobbying, delinquent Federal debt, misconduct in science, civil rights, handicapped individuals, sex discrimination, age discrimination, recombinant DNA)?

    iv. personal data on ethnic origin, etc.? (optional)

    v. other grant support?

    vi. resources and environment (facilities and equipment)? Include support services and description of work ambiance (who is available for collaboration and exchange of ideas?)

    vii. checklist (2 required pages for NIH Applications)? Have you numbered them as the last 2 pages of the Application?

e. mailed the Application in time **to be received by the deadline?**

f. provided a stamped, self-addressed postcard or/and an e-mail address (to receive acknowledgment of Application receipt)?

g. marked your calendar at 2 weeks after submission to be sure you have received a postcard or an e-mail acknowledging receipt of your Application by the agency?

h. marked your calendar at 6 weeks after submission to be sure you have received your review board assignment?

NOTE: Some of the above items will change as NIH (and perhaps other agencies) move toward electronic grants administration. Keep up to date!!!

STRATEGIES FOR GOOD WRITTEN AND ORAL PRESENTATIONS

A. STRATEGIES FOR GOOD EXPOSITORY WRITING

Strategies for getting started

Write for the Reader

- Always write for the Reader rather than for yourself, the writer.
- Ask yourself, "What does the Reader need and/or want to know about this subject?"

Consider the evaluation criteria

- Think about the criteria for the evaluation of the grant proposal (or research paper or other document).
- What are the Reviewers (Readers) being asked to assess?
- Thinking about the evaluation criteria will help to clarify the objectives for you.
    - —The more measurable the objectives, the easier the evaluation.
      Think about the difference between having to grade a multiple-choice test compared to one that consists of a set of essay questions.

Make an outline

- An outline is like a road map or blueprint, a plan of "*what* you will write" (the ideas).

  The text is "*how* you write it;" i.e., the words and sentences that express the ideas.
- Begin to write only after you have made a good outline.
    - —An outline will save you much time in the long run and will help you avoid a lot of frustration.
    - —Working on the outline often helps to put into focus what additional information you may need to gather for the project.
- Many good writers spend their project time as follows:

50%–60%	making an outline
10%–20%	writing
About 30%	revising

***Do not begin to write until you are* 99.99% satisfied with your outline.**
To help you make an outline, write down the answers to the following questions for **each** pertinent section of the grant proposal:

- What should the scope of this section of the grant proposal be?
- How should I introduce the subject of this section of the grant proposal? (The first paragraph of the particular section.)
- What are the main ideas (main topics) to be included in this section of the grant proposal?

If you are writing a proposal, use a checklist to be sure you have included all the information required by the funding agency to which you plan to apply.
Consider:

- What is the best logical sequence for your main ideas/topics?
- If subheadings would help the Reader, use the main topics to create subheadings.
- The main topics should also be used to generate good informative **topic sentences** for each paragraph.

—**In Grant Applications, the first sentence of EACH paragraph should generally be the TOPIC sentence.**

—Tell the Reader in the **first** sentence of **each paragraph**—or at least each major paragraph—what you are going to discuss in that paragraph.

—Be aware that Readers who skim may never get beyond the **topic sentence.**

—Many efficient/fast Readers decide whether or not to read the rest of a paragraph on the basis of what they read in your **topic sentence.**

- What information should go into each paragraph to support the main idea in the paragraph?

    —These will be **subtopics** for the outline.

    —What is the **best logical sequence** for these subtopics within the paragraph?

    —Which of the pieces of information requires particular emphasis?

- What illustrations, diagrams, and/or photos, if any, should you provide in each paragraph or section?

    Where in the text should each illustration, diagram, or photo be placed for optimal clarity and effectiveness?

    Figures should be placed as close as possible to the text that describes them.

- What is an effective closing paragraph for this section of the grant proposal?

    —A conclusion?

    —A summary?

    —A recommendation?

    —A plan for future directions?

- Which of the topics and subtopics that you wrote down are essential and relevant, and which ones can be omitted, i.e., are not important for this section of the grant proposal?

In the **first outline**, do not force a structure (i.e., I, II, III, A, B, C, etc.) *if you find it hard to do.*

- Just get the main and supporting ideas in the form of key words and phrases (not whole sentences) onto

    —index cards

    —Post-it® notes

    —an outline processor, such as "Inspiration" (Inspiration Software, Inc, Portland, OR) or the one within the Microsoft Word™ program

- After you have all the ideas written down, organize them so that they have good logical flow. An outline processor can help make this task faster and easier!

- Then flesh out the outline so that it includes everything you want to have in the document.

- Add formal structure (I, II, III; A, B, C; 1, 2, 3; etc.) at the end, if at all.

- Be sure to check whether the various outline levels are of equivalent importance to other items at the same level.

Write a first draft

- Use your outline as a **guide** when you write the first draft.

- Do not interrupt the flow of writing the first draft by stopping to check spelling, references, or other details.

- Keep a list of items you need/want to check; attend to the list **after** you finish writing the first draft.
- Use easy, short, familiar words, short sentences, and short **paragraphs that start with topic sentences.**
  —Note that in expository texts, such as grant proposals, the topic sentence should always be the first sentence of the paragraph.
  —However, when long paragraphs are divided into several shorter paragraphs just to provide "white space" for ease of reading, the subordinate paragraphs may not require topic sentences.
- In a complex sentence, put the most important phrase first (emphasis).
- Use subheadings to help the Reader easily and quickly find specific information.
- Use easy-to-read formatting—with an appropriate amount of white space—but stay within the designated page limits.
- Write the way you speak, that is, in a direct, not overly formal manner—but DO NOT USE jargon or slang.

Revise the first draft
- Be sure everything you wrote is
  —accurate
  —clear
  —concise
- Use a checklist to locate and correct common writing problems.
- Give the Reader a choice about how much to read by providing:
  —Table of contents
  —Subject line/summary
  —Subheadings
  —Topic sentences that tell what the paragraphs are about
  —Appropriate format
- **Don't let your ego get in the way.** The less of your document the Reader has to read to get the information he/she wants, the better the job you've done!

Strategies for achieving clarity and brevity in your writing

Don't make the Reader do extra work
Readers of expository prose generally want the maximum information in the minimum number of words.
- Don't use long or complex sentences that have to be read more than once to be understood.
- Tell the Reader **"up front"** what you will discuss in that paragraph.
  —Start each paragraph with a good topic sentence.
  —A good topic sentence provides the Reader with a context into which s/he can fit details that you give subsequently.
  —The object of **expository** writing is to **expose**; the Reviewer should never have to guess what you mean.
  —Remember that busy efficient people, who have time only to skim, use the first (topic) sentence of each paragraph to decide whether or not to read the rest of that paragraph!

- Avoid using words that the Reviewer–Reader may not understand. Never send your Reviewer–Reader to the dictionary.

  —Be aware that a brilliant scientist does not necessarily have an extensive literary vocabulary.

  —Be sensitive. Many scientists now come from other countries and may speak only rudimentary English.

- Avoid jargon.

  Think about a computer specialist talking to a cardiac surgeon! They might not understand each other at all if they spoke in the jargon of their own fields.

- Avoid use of the "*former* and *latter*" construction.

  The tired Reader may have to re-read what came before to see what was *former* and what was *latter*. If the Reader is not careful or has a poor memory, unfortunate misunderstandings may occur.

  —**Consider:**

  "Please take care of my son and my cat while I'm away. Let the former stay out all night. Be sure the latter is in by 11 P.M.

  —**Instead of:**

  "Please take care of my son and my cat while I'm away. Be sure the former is in by 11 P.M.; let the latter stay out all night."

Avoid ambiguity caused by misplaced modifiers or other "reference" problems

Not:
On Tuesday, a volumetric flask was brought to the glassware washing room by a technician with a broken neck.
Who had the broken neck, the volumetric flask or the technician?

But:
On Tuesday, a volumetric flask with a broken neck was brought to the glassware washing room by a technician.

After spilling the drink, the photomicrographs were ruined.
How did the photomicrographs manage to spill the drink?

After the drink was spilled on them, the photomicrographs were ruined.

The spectrophotometer should be turned off before leaving the laboratory.
Does the spectrophotometer really leave the laboratory?

The spectrophotometer should be turned off before you leave the laboratory.

A fasting urine specimen should be collected.
Have you ever heard of a urine specimen fasting?

A urine specimen should be collected after the patient has fasted for x hours.

Avoid ambiguity caused by uncommitted pronouns

Not:
It has been shown that ...
Who showed ... ?

But:
Hooper and Cooper (1984) showed that
...

Not:	**But:**
It is well known that ...	A survey done by Smith and Jones at ABC University has indicated that 57% of faculty members at the university know that ...
By whom?	
We noted that most of the rabbits were sick and all the rats had bald spots. This finding ...	Taken together, the findings that most of the rabbits were sick and all the rats had bald spots indicated that ...
Which finding—or both taken together?	

Avoid ambiguity caused by complex sentences

- Use short, direct, unambiguous sentences.
- Avoid long convoluted sentences such as:

    Looking back on it, it is curious that nobody was heard to ask why, since vitamin A has long been known to be very insoluble in aqueous media in general, scientists did not set about looking for a likely carrier protein that might be responsible for transporting vitamin A to its target tissues. (Adapted from a sentence by Russell Baker, *New York Times*, February 1, 1986, page 27.)

    This sentence is acceptable in a piece of creative writing **but not in a grant proposal.**

Avoid words and phrases that can be interpreted in more than one way

- **Vague modifiers**

    Replace vague modifiers that state opinions with quantitative information

    > **Not:** "*most*" or "*many*"
    > **But:** 68%–70%

    > **Not:** This experiment requires *enormous* numbers of test tubes ...
    > **But:** This experiment requires **133** test tubes ...

    What is enormous to you may not seem enormous to someone else!!!

- **Vague reference to time or place**

    Specify time and place rather than using words like "*recently*" or "*here.*"

    —What will the word *recently*, in an article you publish in 1995, mean to someone who reads the article in 2005?

    —What will the word *here*, in an article you wrote in Boston, mean to someone who reads the reprint in China?

- **Words or phrases that can be interpreted in more than one way**

    —The phrase "lightly anesthetized animals ..." was used by a PI to indicate that he was treating the animals with great care but the phrase was apparently interpreted by a Reviewer as implying that the animals were subjected to pain because they were only lightly anesthetized.

    —The word "tree" may bring a palm tree to mind for someone who grew up in Hawaii but will perhaps bring a fir tree to mind for someone from Maine.

    —"If you leave the door with the venetian blind open, the alarm will go off."
    Does this mean:

    > If you leave the door (the one that has a venetian blind on it) open, the alarm will go off?

    or

If you leave the door closed—but leave the venetian blind open—the alarm will go off?

- Here are some amusing examples from *The Lexicon of Intentionally Ambiguous Recommendations (Acronym: LIAR)*, by Prof. Robert Thornton, Economics Department, Lehigh University, Bethlehem, PA 18015. Published by Meadowbrook, Inc., Deephaven, MN 55391; Distributed by Simon and Schuster, New York, NY; copyright 1988. ISBN 0-88166-111-2.

  To recommend a lazy friend:

  "In my opinion, you will be very fortunate to get this person to work for you."

  To describe a totally inept person:

  "I most enthusiastically recommend this candidate with no qualifications whatsoever."

  To describe a "difficult" ex-employee:

  "I am pleased to say that this person is a former colleague of mine."

  To describe a job Applicant who is not worth further consideration:

  "I urge you to waste no time in making this candidate an offer of employment."

Avoid sentences that don't provide substantive information (e.g., circular sentences)

- "X-related complications will be treated according to general institutional guidelines for X-related complications."
- "In these experiments, we found that sterility is very important. Thus, we concluded that sterility is an important factor in these experiments."

Be brief

Use short, simple words

Not:	But:
Contemplate	Think
Endeavor	Try
Equitable	Equal, Fair
Facilitate	Help
Is indicative of	Indicates
Magnitude	Size
Require	Need
Terminate	End
The Reader	You
Utilize	Use

Eliminate unnecessary words/phrases

- Extra words waste the Reviewer's time—and your space. Save space for more important information. Remember the page limitations.
- When you edit your proposal, ask yourself—*for each word*: Is this word really necessary? Does it add anything to the meaning of the sentence?

Not:	But:
Arrived at the conclusion	Concluded
As a matter of fact	Actually
At the present time	Now
At this point in time	Now
Data given in the 3d column are	Data in the 3d column are
Do a study of the effects of x on y	Study the effects of x on y
Due to the fact that	Because
Every single night	Every night
For the purpose of	For, To
Give assistance to	Assist, Help
Have a preference for	Prefer
If you should have any questions feel free to contact me at XXX	If you have questions, call XXX
In a number of cases	Some, Several
In addition to	Also
In all probability	Probably
In excess of	More than
In order to	To
In the amount of $x	For $x
In the course of	While, During (Note: *while* and *since* generally refer to time)
In the event that	If
In the majority of instances	Usually (most of)
In the nature of	Like (similar to)
In the near future	Soon
In the neighborhood of	About
In the not too distant future	Soon
In the vicinity of	Near
In view of	Because
In view of the fact that (Don't use the word *fact* unless it refers to a fact)	Because
It is imperative that	Be sure that
It is interesting to note that	Note that, Note:
It is of interest to note that	Note that, Note:
It is possible that the cause of	The cause may be
It would thus appear that	Apparently
Last but not least	Finally, Lastly
Make decisions	Decide
Make decisions about	Decide on; Decide about
May result in damage	May damage
Must necessarily	Must
Needless to say	Then why bother to say it?
On a few occasions	Occasionally
On the assumption that	Assuming that
On the other hand	Or
Prior to	Before
Serve to make approximations	Approximate

Not:	**But:**
Subsequent to	After, Following
Take action	Act
Take into consideration	Consider
The instruments which are located in	The instruments in
The process of extracting the	Extracting the
With regard to	Regarding
With the exception of	Except
Reports were lengthy this year because the page limitations were eliminated from the instructions.	Reports were long this year because there were no page limits.
Please find enclosed, herewith, my new paper that was published in January of this year.	Here is my January 20XX paper.
At the present time we are experiencing precipitation.	It's raining.
One of the members of the group said ...	A group member said ...
There is a new method that helps ...	A new method helps ...
He said the reason the grant was late was because ...	He said the grant was late because ...
It was suggested by the Reviewers that the Principal Investigators include an Appendix to amplify the background section.	The Reviewers suggested the Principal Investigators include an Appendix to amplify the background section.
The reason I am worried is because I think she is writing a very poor grant proposal.	I am worried because I think she is writing a very poor grant proposal.
The Progress Report was in need of additional data.	The Progress Report needed more data.
It is imperative that you fill out the personal data sheet.	You must fill out the personal data sheet.

Avoid redundancy

Don't say the same thing in three different ways out of insecurity. Say it once, and say it right.

In the expressions below, you only need one of the words; for example, "each" or "every" (Not both!). Decide which is the better word in the context in which it is to be used.

- Each and every
- First and foremost
- In this day and age (Consider using "Now" instead.)
- One and only

Avoid obvious, trite phrases

You can often *omit:*

- Needless to say (Then why bother to say it?)
- In summary
- In the last analysis
- In actual fact (How can a fact not be actual? Is it really a fact?)

- The fact of the matter is (Is it really a fact?)
- It is apparent that
- In my opinion (If you say something, it is usually understood to be your opinion. If you must make clear that something is your opinion, use the shorter expression, "I think.")

Consider omitting **unnecessary transition words** and phrases such as "In conclusion, ..."

- But *keep* transition words that tell the Reader that you are "changing direction." For example:

  —In contrast, ...
  —Nevertheless, ...

I think, I feel, I believe:

- If your field is psychology it **may** be appropriate to say, "I feel."
- If your field is religion, it **may** be appropriate to say, "I believe."
- If your field is science, or you are engaged in a research aspect of your profession, it is generally more appropriate to say, "I think."

Use active voice rather than passive voice when appropriate

- Passive voice contains some form of the verb "to be" before the main verb. Therefore, the passive voice form may have extra words.
- Active voice is more direct, more clear; it tells you up front who (or what) did (or does, or will do) the action of the verb. The passive voice is often used to evade this issue and does not give this information.
- To turn a passive voice sentence to an active voice sentence, answer the question—up front—"Who (or what) is doing the action of the verb?"

Passive/passive:

It *was suggested* that the laboratory reports *be revised*. (9 words)

>   Who did the suggesting?
>   Who will do the revising?

Note that one can provide the desired information in passive voice, but it makes for an awkward sound:

> It *was suggested* by John that the laboratory reports *be revised by Joe*.

Active/passive:

John *suggested* that the laboratory reports *be revised*. (8 words)

> Who will do the revising?

Active/active:

John *suggested* that Joe *revise* the laboratory reports. (8 words)

> Note that providing the desired information may make the sentence longer but clearer:

>> The head of the department suggested that the post-doc revise the laboratory reports. (14 words)

When trying to decide on the best form to use, the priorities should be:

>   —accuracy first
>   —clarity second
>   —brevity third

Note that passive voice occurs in all tenses:

Past tense:

Passive voice:	The solutions were mixed.
	The solutions were mixed by John.
Active voice:	John mixed the solutions.

Present tense:

Passive voice:	The solutions are being mixed.
Active voice:	John is mixing the solutions.

Future tense:

Passive voice:	The solutions will be mixed.
Active voice:	John will mix the solutions.

Avoid turning verbs into nouns

Not:

Utilization of marine plant species for food *production* will bring about a *reduction* in food costs and *creation* of cheaper sources of calories. (23 words)

But:

Utilizing (Using) marine plant species to *produce* food will *reduce* food costs and *create* cheaper sources of calories. (17 words)

Avoid unnecessary "ing" words

Not:

They were meeting to ...
He will be going to ...

But:

They met to ...
He will go to ...

Be aware of style

Try to EXPRESS rather than IMPRESS

- Use simple (but not simple-minded or simplistic) words.
- Use short, direct sentences (about 17 to 23 words is a reasonable length), but avoid a choppy first-grader sound by judicious use of transition words (Although, However, Nevertheless, etc.).
- Use short paragraphs that begin with *informative topic sentences*.
- Be quantitative.
- Replace "opinion" modifiers with quantitative modifiers.
  - **Not:** *the majority of*
  - **But:** 88%–90%
- Avoid phrases or modifiers that *may* not add to the critical essence of what you want to say:
  - **Not:** Let us concentrate first on the X molecule, which is very large and, therefore, it ...
  - **But:** The X molecule is very large; therefore, it ...
  - **Not:** This interesting observation suggested to us that we should perhaps carefully examine X, which revealed that ...
  - **But:** Careful examination of X revealed that ...

      Let your data and presentation speak for you:

Not: This *cleverly conceived* experiment ...

But: This experiment . . . (and then provide a table or figure that makes the reader immediately aware of how cleverly conceived the experiment is—without having to point it out to the Reader.)

- ■ Avoid an undue amount of self-praise:
    - —Our *tremendously unique* method for ...
    - —Our laboratory is the **best known in the world** for ...
    - —We have the *largest collection* of ... in the country.
- ■ Avoid pompous language

Not:	But:
Unless all parties to the plan interface imminently, the project will be rendered inoperative. (Negative tone)	Unless everyone cooperates now, the project won't work. OR If everyone cooperates, the project will be successful. (Positive tone)

Think about who will read what you wrote

Not:	But:
Nosocomial infection	Hospital-acquired infection
Iatrogenic condition	Physician-induced condition

Keep in mind that one of your Reviewers may not be an M.D.! Avoiding unnecessary "heavy" medical jargon is especially important if you are a physician researcher proposing a project that involves a lot of basic science. Such a proposal is likely to have at least one Ph.D. Reviewer. Sending this Reviewer on frequent trips to a medical dictionary wastes her/his time! On the other hand, you don't want your M.D. Reviewer to wonder how you got through medical school without learning appropriate medical terminology. Take a reasonable "best-compromise" approach.

Be consistent with respect to:

- ■ Form/format
- ■ Pronoun versus the noun to which it refers
- ■ Singular versus plural
- ■ Subject versus object
- ■ Tense

Use parallel construction

Not:	But:
His job consisted of *organization* of new projects, *researching* current projects, to *write* progress reports, and *being available to help* the junior staff.	His job consisted of *organizing* new projects, *researching* current projects, *writing* progress reports, and *helping* the junior staff.
We couldn't decide between *rental,* leasing, and buying a new spectrophotometer.	We couldn't decide between *renting,* leasing, and buying a new spectrophotometer.

Avoid short, choppy sentences

Use, but don't overuse, transition words.

Not: Good expository writing is difficult. It is an important skill to master. It requires much time and effort. It is worth it. Writing is necessary for job advancement. It improves self-image. It provides satisfaction. Everyone should take a good course in business writing.

But: Good expository writing is difficult, but it is an important skill to master. Although it requires much time and effort, it is worth it. Writing is necessary for job advancement. It also improves self-image and provides satisfaction. Everyone should take a good course in business writing.

Avoid excessive multiple modifiers

- The attractive, upgraded, computerized, large, heavy, expensive, recently purchased, spectrophotometer ...
- The computer-based integrated decision support environment ...

Avoid jargon "ize" and "wise" words

Acceptable:	Not acceptable:
The car has been winterized.	The plan has been operationalized.
Clockwise (in the manner of)	Budgetwise (meaning: with respect to the budget)

Try not to split infinitives

Not: Be sure *to quickly go* ...

But: Be sure *to go quickly* ...

However, splitting the infinitive sometimes avoids ambiguity or makes for a better flow. Consider the difference in meaning in the following sentences:

- She will try *to more than justify* the cost of the computer.
- She will try *to justify more than* the cost of the computer.
- She will try *more than to justify* the cost of the computer.

    Note that the 3 sentences above do not have identical meanings! Position the modifying words "more than" so as to achieve clarity (i.e., to convey the correct meaning).

Don't overstate your case

- Avoid superlatives: Use "best," "most," etc., only if you are *sure* the superlative is correct:

    Not: One of the best ways to purify ... is ... (There can be **only ONE** *best* way!)

    But: ... is the best way to purify ...

- Avoid useless modifiers:

    "I repeat this experiment every *single* month." (Are there double months— or married months?)

Think about emphasis

Emphasis is important in the context of the psychology of the Reader.

- In a sentence, start with the clause you want to stress:

    —*In the previous project period*, three approaches were developed to solve ...

    —*Three approaches were developed* in the previous project period to solve ...

    —*Three approaches* to solve ... were developed in the previous project period.

- **Don't begin a paragraph with unimportant words:**

  Not: *First let us consider that* rain helps plants grow.

  But: Rain helps plants grow. Let us consider the significance of this in relation to …

Be aware of tone

- Remember that attitude, mood, and tone are sometimes "contagious."
- Be positive.

  Not: I won't be able to finish this project by the end of the first year.

  But: I will be able to finish this project by March of the second year.

- **Avoid words that may upset the Reader.**

  —Words that are inherently negative, such as: *intolerable, misguided, unfair, wrong, unfortunately*

  —Words that have negative connotations

Positive or neutral connotation	Negative connotation
Methodical, Meticulous	Fanatical, Nit-picking
Economical, Frugal	Cheap, Chintzy
Uninformed	Ignorant
Firm	Inflexible
Forceful, Persevering	Overbearing, Dogged
Colorful	Gaudy
Problem	Disaster

NOTE that, in addition to the overt connotations, the words you choose to use may also have more subtle psychological impact. For example, if something is a "problem," people generally assume that one can find a solution. But if something is a "disaster," there may be a sense that the problem can't be fixed—that one needs to start from "square one."

- **Use neutral words to avoid sexual bias.**

  The English language is **inherently masculine**. Don't make it more so.

  The use of "s/he" or the plural "they" instead of "he or she" are now generally considered polite and acceptable.

Say	Instead of
Business executive or manager	Businessman or Businesswoman
Chair, Chairperson, or moderator	Chairman
Member of the clergy	Clergyman
Firefighter	Fireman
Supervisor	Foreman
Police officer	Policeman
Flight attendant	Stewardess or Steward
Human race, humanity, humankind	Mankind
Synthetic	Man-made
Utility hole	Man-hole

See *Guide to Nonsexist Language*, which can be purchased from:
    Project on the Status and Education of Women
    Association of American Colleges
    1818 R Street, NW
    Washington, DC 20009

> **NOTE:** Keep in mind, however, that the **main purpose** of your proposal is to **communicate what you propose to do** to the Reviewer, so don't go "overboard" about trying to make up for the shortcomings of the English language.

- **Understand where you stand with respect to the Reader.**
    This issue is important in interaction, correspondence, and collaboration with people from other countries or cultures and at other authority levels. Be aware of the issues listed below.
    —**Cultural differences**

United Kingdom	**United States**
Tendency to be more formal especially when dealing with older people	Tendency to be quite informal unless dealing with older people or people from other cultures

Dear Sir:
    Having been privileged to receive your esteemed patronage in the past, we think you will be interested to know that ...
	Dear Bill:
	    Because you've been so generous with funding for our project in the past, we thought you'd like to know that ...

    —**Authority**
        —If *you* have the authority, say: "*I suggest ...*"
        —If you are addressing "the boss," say: "*I would like to suggest ...*"

Grammar Hotline
If you have a question on English language usage, call the National Grammar Hotline. In Massachusetts the hotline is located at Northeastern University. Tel: (617) 373-4540 or

http://www.tcc.edu/students/resources/writcent/GH/hotlinol.htm

Scroll down to get to a list, organized alphabetically by states, of where the Grammar Hotlines are located.

Grammar Hotline Directory
A Publication of Tidewater Community College
    The **Grammar Hotline Directory** lists telephone services that provide **free answers to short questions about writing,** including syntax, diction, grammar, punctuation, and spelling.
- Most of these services are staffed by faculty members, graduate students, editors, and former teachers.

- **Days and times of operation are subject to change** according to teaching schedules.
- Many hotlines reduce or suspend service during college breaks and summer sessions.
- Unless otherwise noted, the Hotlines do **NOT** accept collect calls.
- Unless otherwise noted, the Hotlines will **NOT** return long distance calls.
- Some hotlines offer Fax or e-mail service as indicated in their listings.
- All information in the directory is provided by the services listed.

For further information you may contact:

Tidewater Community College
Writing Center
1700 College Crescent
Virginia Beach, VA 23453
Tel: 757-822-7183
Fax: 757-427-0327
e-mail: writcent@tcc.edu

A **free directory (published annually)** of Grammar Hotlines in other areas of the **U.S.** is available. To order the directory, send a self-addressed, **stamped,** 7×10 or 9×12 inch clasp envelope with $1.25 postage to:

Grammar Hotline Directory
Tidewater Community College Writing Center
1700 College Crescent
Virginia Beach, VA 23453
Tel: 757-822-7170 (Hotline)
e-mail: writcent@tcc.edu

B.   STRATEGIES FOR GOOD ORAL PRESENTATIONS

Your **reputation as a scientist** depends a great deal on talks/seminars you give at your institution, as well as at other institutions and at professional meetings. The **quality of the science** is the most important factor. However, the **quality of your presentation** cannot help but make an impression. Therefore, it is important to **learn to give a good talk.**

There is also a small possibility that you may get site-visited when you submit a grant Application. Should this occur, it is important that you be able to present your project clearly to the site visit committee and convince the members that you have a good project and will be able to carry it out well.

In this Appendix, you will find some strategies for giving a good talk. Like proposal writing, **public speaking is a learnable skill**. As with many other learnable skills, it takes knowledge of the **principles** and a certain amount of **practice** to become good at it.

Not **all** the advice given below pertains to **all** kinds of talks. For example, a 10-minute talk requires some strategies that are different from those that are required for a one-hour talk. Likewise, a formal talk at a professional meeting where the physical setup has been organized for the occasion by experienced personnel requires less attention to details about equipment than does a talk you will give in a place where the host (and sometimes the speaker) must arrange things specifically for your talk.

Giving a lecture to a class of young students and giving a workshop to a group of adults require somewhat different but related skills. Before you agree to give a talk, be sure that

- you have something significant to say about the subject
- you can speak about the subject with authority and conviction

It is important to understand that your excitement—or boredom—about a subject tends to be highly contagious to the audience.

General considerations for presenting a good talk

- Make **frequent eye contact** with the audience.

    It makes a bad impression if you read your talk and only rarely look at the audience.
- Practice good voice projection.

    The mind of even the most interested listener is likely to wander if the person cannot hear you.
- Develop—and learn to convey—an air of confidence (even if you are nervous inside).

    If you are nervous, there is a tendency for the audience to

    —wonder why you are not more sure of yourself
    —also feel a bit ill-at-ease/edgy
- Avoid having the audience be distracted from what you say by what you do or what you wear:

    —Don't fiddle with things (the microphone cord, your papers, your fingers, etc.); don't scratch your head, etc.
    —Avoid **excessive** pacing or gesticulation.
    —Be aware of appropriate dress and general appearance; the audience is likely to get distracted by
    - unusual clothes
    - inappropriately low-cut necklines
    - stains on your tie or other visible parts of your clothing
    - a green Mohawk hairdo
    - a button missing in an awkward place

Combat nervousness

- Know your subject matter extremely well.
- Be well-prepared.

    If necessary, practice your talk ahead of time. Some people can do a practice run alone in the seminar room; others do better if they have a small live audience. Get a few colleagues to listen to you rehearse and tell them to ask questions.
- **Get used to giving talks by offering to give them rather than avoiding them.**
- The following is true for many people:

    —the more talks you give the easier it becomes and the less nervous you get when you have to give a talk
    —age and experience tend to eliminate the anxious feelings about public speaking

- Deep breathing and appropriate exercise, prior to the talk, help some speakers calm down.
- The **longer** the talk, the **longer** the time you should plan to spend to research the topic, make slides, practice the talk, etc.
- The **shorter** the talk, the **longer** the time you should plan to spend to prepare for the presentation per se.
  —There is no time to be casual in a 10-minute talk.
  —To give a good very brief presentation, you need to memorize —or almost memorize—the talk.
- Practice giving the talk, preferably in front of one or more experienced colleagues.
  —Ask colleagues to critique both the **content** and the **presentation**.
  —Practice good tone and good timing; don't drone and don't race.

Aim to communicate

- Be aware that people come to your talk with different perspectives/expectations.
- Consider that different words mean different things to different people.
- Think about connotation versus denotation of words.
- Understand that for communication to occur, what you intended to say must match what the audience perceives you to have said.

How many people will be in the audience and how large is the room?

- Be sure the print size on your slides is appropriate.
- Determine whether you will need a microphone. If yes, arrange to
  —have one ready at the site
  —bring one
- Determine whether a flip-chart will be visible at the back of the room, or whether you will need an overhead projector.

Call ahead to ensure that/determine whether the host institution will provide all the equipment you need for your talk

Many presenters and Institutions are now equipped for PowerPoint presentations, but some institutions still use slide projectors. Call ahead to determine what sort of equipment will be available to you for your talk. Think about:

- Projector (extra projector or lamp housing or at least an extra bulb)
- Does the projector project from behind the screen (from a projection booth/room) **or** onto the front of the screen?
  This will make a difference with respect to how you position your slides in the slide tray!!!
- Remote control for the projector
- Screen (what size?)
- Flip-chart/overhead projector (appropriate pens, plastic film on which to write)
- Blackboard, chalk, and erasers or whiteboard, pens, and moist towels
- Pointer (extra batteries; some laser pointers require a lot of energy)
- Microphone
- Lectern or podium
- Glass and drinking water within easy reach of the speaker's table

- If possible, ask about/get a sense of the physical facility.

  Be aware that at large hotel-based meetings, you may occasionally have to do the best you can with some difficult circumstances, such as simultaneous talks in adjacent rooms separated from the room in which you are speaking by a non-sound-proof movable wall!

Plan your talk based on the needs of the audience—not just your needs!

- Focus on what the audience needs and wants to know about the subject—in addition to what YOU want to tell the audience.
- Have some understanding of the audience's level of expertise in your subject:
  —Never talk down to the audience.
  —Never talk above the audience's level of understanding of the subject.
- Provide an appropriate **introduction** to your subject commensurate with the audience's level of understanding of the subject. When you are invited to speak, ask the host for guidance about the level of knowledge of the audience!
- Don't use jargon that the audience may not understand.
- Don't take leaps of logic when you talk. You know your subject intimately; the audience may not!
- Aim to **keep the audience with you** throughout your talk.

Make an outline for your talk

- Keep it simple:
  —Stick to one or two main points
  —Educate—don't overwhelm—the audience
  —Don't try to impress the audience in any overt manner: Let the quality of the content and the quality of the presentation impress the audience.
- Have good **logical** progression.
- Provide appropriate details.
- Prepare good, appropriate visuals: A picture is worth a thousand words.
- Give credit to the work of others.

Plan what you will say

- For each point in the outline
- For each visual (slide or overhead) you show

Prepare a thoughtful attractive handout/lecture outline

- Bring more than enough copies for the people in the audience—or, if appropriate, send the outline to the host ahead of time and ask her/him to have photocopies made on-site.

  Providing the audience with a good outline of what you plan to say allows people to pay attention to your talk rather than be distracted by taking notes.
- Include a bibliography in case someone wants additional details/information.
- Make the preparation time and the extent of detail in the handout commensurate with
  —the level of understanding of the audience
  —the occasion for the talk

Things to do/check before the talk

- If you are sponsoring the talk, check on refreshments and any other items that will be needed.
- If you are the speaker, get to the room early.
- Check to see that everything you need is available.
- Check to see that everything works properly—BEFORE—any audience members arrive.
- Have a **brief** typed (easy-to-read print) script about yourself ready to provide to the host if s/he asks how you wish to be introduced.
- Be prepared to introduce yourself if asked to do so.
- If you are using slides, put your slides in the projector tray, and review *every* slide to be sure it is right side up and frontward.

  It is good to arrange and review your slides at your home institution and, if possible, once again at the seminar site before the audience arrives in the room.
- If you plan to do a PowerPoint presentation, be sure that
  —the host institution is equipped to do PowerPoint presentations
  —your images are in the correct order
  —the color schemes are easy to view and read
  —type size is appropriate for the size of the lecture room
- **Before the audience arrives**, determine
  —the location of the switches for the overhead lights
  —who will turn the switches on and off
  —whether there is a microphone
  —how the microphone works/how to control the volume
  —the optimal microphone volume
    You may need to re-adjust the volume again before the start of your talk once the room is full.
- Distribute the lecture outlines for your talk:
  —leave one on each desk or seat in the room
  OR
  —leave a pile of the outlines in a place where each person can pick one up as s/he enters the room
- Things to think about before and during the talk
  —Talk **to** the audience—not at them—and be sensitive to their reactions.
  —Good speakers are able to adjust their delivery, if necessary, in response to subtle signals from the audience:
    • facial expressions
    • body language
    • interactions between people in the audience
      For example, if you notice that someone looks puzzled, you can say (**without directly addressing the person in question**—which might make her/him feel embarrassed), "Perhaps I could explain that in another way ..."
- Don't read your talk.
  —It's okay to use notes, but make frequent eye contact with the audience.
  —It's even better to use your slides or overheads—rather than notes—to remind you of what you want to say next.
  —**Don't "memorize" your talk unless you are a professional actor.**

- If you memorize your talk, you are likely to give a somewhat stilted delivery.
- During my first few weeks at college, I met two classmates—who were roommates—who seemed to know not only everyone's name but all sorts of information about them. I later discovered that each evening these two women went back to their room and made an index card for each person they had met that day. At bedtime, they would quiz each other about the information on the cards until they remembered everything they had learned about each person. Using the information as soon as possible helped to reinforce the information in their memory.
- If you want to remember the name of someone to whom you are introduced, it is useful to say, "Hi Cathy Young; I'm pleased to meet you," rather than just saying, "Hi, I'm pleased to meet you."
- Check out various nmemonic devices on Web sites such as

  http://www.utexas.edu/student/utlc/makinggrade/mnemonic.html

- Be positive. Negative attitudes are contagious.
- To keep the talk at a human level and keep the audience involved, interject humor and illustrative stories **when appropriate**.
- **NEVER** insult your audience.
  —Don't put the audience into the position of having to show their ignorance:
    - Don't ask, "How many of you **don't** know ...?"
    - Instead, say: "Some people do not seem to be aware that ..."
  —Don't call on people or embarrass them in any other way.
  —Don't use words that people in the audience may not understand. If you must use words/technical terms that are likely to be unfamiliar to people, define them.
  —Don't tell jokes that may hurt people's feelings; e.g., ethnic jokes—even if you are sure that no member of that group is in the audience!
  —Restate highly technical material into simpler language.
  —Don't sound pompous or arrogant.
- Try to make your audience feel sufficiently comfortable to ask questions.
  —No matter how ridiculous a question may seem to you, answer the question as though it is an interesting question.
  —Try to remember that, "The only stupid questions are the ones people don't ask."
  —If you embarrass someone who asks a question you may inhibit others from speaking and, thus, are less likely to have a lively discussion about your talk.

When the talk begins
- Thank the host for her/his introduction.
- If the host has not given sufficient background information about you and your work, introduce yourself further—and fill in the gaps—before you begin your talk. The audience usually wants to know about your authority to talk to them on the subject in question.
- Try to establish rapport with the audience as soon as possible.
- Tell the audience whether you prefer
  —to be interrupted if people have questions
  or
  —people to hold questions and comments until the end of the talk

- **Tell the audience—at the start of your talk—what your presentation is about.**
  Have this information on a slide, an overhead, a flip-chart, or a blackboard.
- Present the main part of your talk.
- Be sure that you point to specific things on your slides, and let the pointer rest on the part of the slide you are discussing **long enough** for everyone to concentrate on that piece of information.
- Try to help the audience make connections between what you are telling them and information they probably already know.
  People remember things better when they can make such associations; help them by discussing the connections between your recent findings and the background work in the field.
- Tell the audience outright and clearly when you are about to make a transition from one topic to another.
- If and when appropriate, try to involve the audience rather than just lecturing at them.
- Periodically, give a brief summary of what you have said up to that point, "So at this point we knew (know) that ..." These periodic summaries
  —reinforce what you have already told the audience
  —help those who got derailed (mind wandered, fell asleep, etc.) to get back on track
- End your talk with
  —a strong positive **closing statement** (perhaps the direction your work will take in the future or some possible long-range benefit of your work to society)
  and
  —a **summary:** Tell the audience what you have told them and what the "take-home" message is. Have this information on a slide or write it on a flip-chart, board, or overhead.
- Stay on schedule. This includes leaving an adequate amount of time for questions!
- Take questions and comments from the audience and, if appropriate, ask for feedback.
  —If your host does not help you choose who gets to ask questions, then it is your job to do so in a fair, orderly manner.
  —Don't let one person monopolize the discussion.
  —Don't get into arguments with the audience. The objective is to discuss and enlighten, not to "win."
  —Don't be afraid to say, "I don't know."
  —If appropriate, offer to find out the answer to an unresolved question and call the person who asked the question when you have the answer.
  —If appropriate, offer to remain after the talk and answer additional questions on a one-to-one basis.
- Have business cards and appropriate reprints with you for people who may want to contact you or read about your work in more detail.

APPENDIX III

INFORMATION ABOUT NIH

> **NOTE:** Although the **Public Health Service (PHS) has been discontinued as an entity,** the agencies that comprised the PHS continue to exist as part of the Department of Health and Human Services (DHHS).

THE DEPARTMENT OF HEALTH AND HUMAN SERVICES (DHHS) IS A DEPARTMENT OF THE EXECUTIVE BRANCH OF THE U.S. GOVERNMENT

Agencies that comprise DHHS:

- Administration for Children and Families (ACF)
- Administration on Aging (AoA)
- Agency for Healthcare Research and Quality (AHRQ)
- Agency for Toxic Substances and Disease Registry (ATSDR)
- Centers for Disease Control and Prevention (CDC)
- Centers for Medicare & Medicaid Services (CMS)
- Food and Drug Administration (FDA)
- Health Resources and Services Administration (HRSA)
- Indian Health Service (IHS)
- **National Institutes of Health (NIH)**
- Program Support Center (PSC)
- Substance Abuse and Mental Health Services Administration (SAMHSA)

Thus, NIH is an agency of the Department of Health and Human Services (DHHS). Despite the demise of PHS as an entity, the grant Application forms continue to be designated as PHS 398 and 2590. A summary of 2003 enhancements to these forms is given at

http://grants.nih.gov/grants/guide/notice-files/NOT-OD-03-062.html

THE MISSION OF NIH

http://www.nih.gov/about/NIHoverview.html

Begun in 1887 with an appropriation of about $300, the NIH is now one of the world's foremost medical research centers, and the Federal focal point for medical research in the U.S. In 2002, the appropriation was nearly $23.4 billion. NIH is part of the U.S. Department of Health and Human Services (DHHS) and is comprised of 27 separate components, mainly Institutes and Centers. Based in Bethesda, Maryland, NIH has more than 75 buildings on over 300 acres of land.

About 50,000 Principal Investigators—working in every state and in several foreign countries, from every specialty in medicine, every medical discipline, and at every major university and medical school—receive NIH extramural funding to explore unknown areas of medical science.

About 18,000 employees, including more than 4,000 with professional or research doctorate degrees, support and conduct the NIH extramural and intramural programs. NIH staff includes intramural scientists, physicians, dentists, veterinarians, nurses, and laboratory, administrative, and support personnel, plus a continually changing array of research scientists in training.

The mission of NIH is to uncover new knowledge that will help prevent, detect, diagnose, and treat disease and disability, from the rarest genetic disorder to the common cold, and lead to better health for everyone. To fulfill its mission, NIH:

- conducts research in its own laboratories
- supports the research of non-Federal scientists in universities, medical schools, hospitals, and research institutions throughout the country and abroad
- helps train research investigators
- fosters communication of medical information

SOME SPECIFIC INFORMATION ABOUT NIH

For information about **REVIEW PROCEDURES FOR SCIENTIFIC REVIEW GROUP MEETINGS,** see

http://www.csr.nih.gov/guidelines/proc.htm

NIH Medical & Behavioral Research Grant Policies, Guidelines & Funding Opportunities
The NIH "Grants – Office of Extramural Research (OER) Home Page" is at

http://grants2.nih.gov/grants/oer.htm

and **provides access** to NIH Medical and Behavioral Research Grant Policies, Guidelines and Funding Opportunities organized into categories such as those listed below:

About OER
- Introduction to Extramural Research
- NIH Outreach Activities
- New Investigator/Grantee
- General Information
- Staff Directories
- OER Offices and Org Charts

NIH Guide for Grants and Contracts
- NIH Funding Announcements
- RFAs, PAs, and Notices
- Most Recent Weekly Index
- LISTSERV – Weekly e-mail
- Search the NIH Guide
- Description of the NIH Guide
- Grant & Application Submission Information

Research Training
- News
- Extramural Training Programs

- Intramural Research and Training Opportunities
- Job Links
- Career Resources
- Forms and Applications
- Training Q&A and FAQs

Grant Topics
- Funding Opportunities
- Grants Policy and Guidance
- Grants Compliance and Oversight
- Award Data
- CRISP Database
- Intellectual Property Policy
- iEdison: Invention Reporting
- ERA: Electronic Research Administration
- Forms and Applications
- Human Subjects
- Lab Animal Welfare (OLAW)
- Peer Review Policy and Issues
- Small Business Funding Opportunities (SBIR/STTR)
- NIH Roadmap Initiatives

Related Topics
- Bioethics
- Sites of Interest

News
- Current News Flashes
- News Archives
- Search News Archives

Frequently Requested Links:
a. PHS 398 and 2590 Applications/Forms
b. Receipt Dates & Submission Information
c. NIH Grants Policy Statement
d. Funding Program Guidelines
e. Career Development Award (K) Kiosk
f. Certificates of Confidentiality Kiosk
g. Human Subjects Research Enhancement Awards (HSREA)
h. Modular Research Grants
i. NIH Data Sharing Information

j. Study Section Information
k. Award Trends – Ranking Tables

To contact the **National Institutes of Health (NIH)**:
GRANTSINFO
Tel: 301-435-0714
TTY: 301-451-5936 (For hearing impaired)
e-mail: grantsinfo@nih.gov

Main NIH mailing address:
National Institutes of Health
9000 Rockville Pike
Bethesda, Maryland 20892

e-mail: NIHInfo@OD.NIH.GOV
Main telephone number: 301-496-4000
For toll-free NIH telephone numbers go to:
http://www.nih.gov/health/infoline.htm
To contact NIH on weekends, call 301-496-4000

Center for Scientific Review
National Institutes of Health
6701 Rockledge Drive, Room 1040 - MSC 7710
Bethesda, MD 20892-7710
For express/courier service, use: Bethesda, MD 20817
For information about grants e-mail to: grantsinfo@nih.gov

The NIH Roadmap

- **http://nihroadmap.nih.gov/**
  After becoming Director of NIH in May 2002, Elias A. Zerhouni, M.D. convened a series of meetings to chart a "roadmap" for medical research in the 21st century. The purpose of the "Roadmap" is to accelerate medical discovery to improve health. Familiarize yourself with the "NIH Roadmap." Some of the concepts are:
  —New Pathways to Discovery
  —Building Blocks, Biological Pathways, and Networks
  —Molecular Libraries and Imaging
  —Structural Biology
  —Bioinformatics and Computational Biology
  —Nanomedicine
  —Research Teams of the Future
  —High-Risk Research
  —Interdisciplinary Research
  —Public-Private Partnerships
  —Re-engineering the Clinical Research Enterprise
  —Re-engineering the Clinical Research Enterprise
- In September 2003, Dr. Ellie Ehrenfeld resigned as Director of the Center for Scientific Review. Dr. Brent Stanfield, CSR Deputy Director, became the Acting Director of CSR. For additional information, go to

http://www.csr.nih.gov

or

http://www.nih.gov/news/pr/sep2003/csr-22.htm

- ■ To get an idea of current funding for research related to various diseases go to

http://www.nih.gov/news/fundingresearchareas.htm

The easiest way to get information about—and from—NIH is via the NIH Web site

http://www.nih.gov

At this site you will find several helpful features:
- ■ **A search tool at the upper right where you can type in search terms**
- ■ A column with information about recent
  —Press Releases
  —Health Issues
  —Medical Research Issues
- ■ Portals to various features that can be accessed from the main NIH Web page:
  —Health information
    - • A–Z index of NIH health resources
    - • Clinical trials
    - • Health hotlines
    - • MEDLINEplus
    - • Drug information
  —Grants & funding opportunities
    - • Grants news
    - • Applications
    - • Grants policy
    - • NIH Guide
    - • Award data
    - • Research training
    - • Research contracts
    - • CRISP database
  —News & events
    - • Press releases
    - • Media center
    - • Calendars
    - • Radio & video
    - • Media contacts
  —Scientific resources
    - • Human Embryonic Stem Cell Registry
    - • Intramural research
    - • Special interest groups
    - • Library catalogs

- Journals
- Training
- Labs
- Scientific computing

—Institutes, Centers & Offices
- The individual organizations that make up the NIH

—About NIH
- Visitor information
- Jobs
- Science education
- Employee directory
- Public involvement
- Policy issues
- Organization & mission
- History
- Doing business with NIH
- Freedom of Information Act (FOIA)
- Director's Page

—Access to
- Q&A About NIH
- Career Opportunities
- Visitor Information
- Employee Information
- Information in Spanish
- Search the NIH Web site
- "Featured this week"
  - This feature changes each week; e.g., as I write this, the weekly feature is "NLM's Household Products Database."

NOTE: You may also be well served to look at "R01—NINDS Research Project Grant Guidelines" at

http://www.ninds.nih.gov/funding/nindsr01.htm

and see the NIH forms at

http://www.grants2.nih.gov/grants/funding/phs398/398_forms.pdf

WHERE TO GET INFORMATION ABOUT NIH AWARDS

Institute and Center Coordinators for NIH Awards are listed at

http://www1.od.nih.gov/ohrm/Awards/Award-Coords.htm

The funding components at NIH use a variety of award mechanisms to support extramural research. However, **not all the components support all the award mechanisms.** NIH periodically publishes a list of **activity codes** for the awards. The list indicates which funding components support which award mechanisms. It's a good idea to keep up-to-date by reading **every** issue of the *NIH Guide for Grants and Contracts.* You can ask to have the Table of Contents of each issue e-mailed to you:

> **NIH Guide LISTSERV:**
> **The *NIH Guide for Grants and Contracts* is the official publication for NIH medical and behavioral research Grant Policies, Guidelines and Funding Opportunities.**
>
> Each week (usually on Friday afternoon), the NIH transmits an e-mail with the Table of Contents (TOC) information for that week's issue of the *NIH Guide*, via the NIH LISTSERV. The TOC includes a link to the **Current NIH Guide Weekly Index** as well as links to each *NIH Guide* article published for that week.
>
> **To Subscribe** to the *NIH Guide* LISTSERV, **send an e-mail to listserv@list.nih.gov**
>
> with the following text in the message body (**not in the "Subject" line**):
>
> **subscribe NIHTOC-L** *your name*
> *(Example: subscribe NIHTOC-L Joe Smith)*
> Your e-mail address will be automatically obtained from the e-mail message and added to the LISTSERV.
>
> **To Unsubscribe** to the *NIH Guide* LISTSERV, **send an e-mail to listserv@list.nih.gov**
>
> with the following text in the message body (**not in the "Subject" line**):
> **unsubscribe NIHTOC-L** *your name*
> *(Example: unsubscribe NIHTOC-L Joe Smith)*
> Your e-mail address will be automatically obtained from the e-mail message and removed from the LISTSERV.
>
> More information on using the NIH LISTSERV can be obtained from the NIH LISTSERV FAQ page.

NIH tries to reach communities that are under-funded. For example, there are a number of grant opportunities targeted to minorities. Also, although NIH funds medical research or research training in every state in the U.S., about 23 states plus Puerto Rico have not been participating in research as fully as NIH would like. To help these regions increase their capacity for medical research, NIH launched a pilot Institutional Development Award (IDeA) program in 2001 to determine if institutions in these areas have the potential to do good medical research.

For further information about grant opportunities, go to

http://grants1.nih.gov/grants/oer.htm

and look under "Grant Topics."
Also check

http://nihroadmap.nih.gov

SOME SPECIFIC NIH CONTACT INFORMATION

NIH HOME PAGE
http://www.nih.gov

GRANTS PAGE
http://grants.nih.gov/grants/oer.htm

EXTRAMURAL RESEARCH
http://grants.nih.gov/grants/welcome.htm

NIH GUIDE TO GRANTS AND CONTRACTS
http://grants.nih.gov/grants/guide/index.html

CRISP (Computer Retrieval of Information on Scientific Projects)
http://crisp.cit.nih.gov

NIH INSTITUTES
http://www.nih.gov/icd

FORMS (including APPLICATIONS/INSTRUCTIONS)
http://grants.nih.gov/grants/forms.htm

Research Grants—use PHS 398
Fellowships (F31 and F32)—use PHS 416-1

STANDARD RECEIPT DATES
http://grants.nih.gov/grants/dates.htm

REFERRAL AND REVIEW
http://www.drg.nih.gov/refrev.htm

REVIEW PROCESS OVERVIEW
http://www.drg.nih.gov/REVIEW/peerrev.htm

NIH GRANTS POLICY STATEMENT
http://grants.nih.gov/grants/policy/nihgps_2003/index.htm

Special Opportunities
Research Training
http://grants.nih.gov/training/index.htm

Small Business
http://grants.nih.gov/grants/funding/sbir.htm

International:
Fogarty International Center (FIC)
http://www.nih.gov/fic

Policy
http://grants.nih.gov/grants/policy/nihgps_2003/NIHGPS_Part12.htm

PREPARING TO APPLY FOR A GRANT

Before you plan your Grant Application
Go to

http://www.niddk.nih.gov/fund/grants_process/grantwriting.htm

to read advice from one of the NIH institutes about "Writing a Grant Application" and to

http://www.niddk.nih.gov/fund/divisions/DEA/review_branch/revapps.htm

to read about what happens during the 9 months your Application is going through the NIH "pipeline."

TERMS USED BY NIH

For information about any of the topics listed below, go to

http://grants1.nih.gov/grants/funding/phs398/section_3.html

For a Glossary of NIH terms go to

http://www.grants2.nih.gov/grants/glossary.html#1 (see also page 228 in this book)

There is also an extensive Glossary of Funding and Policy Terms and Acronyms from NIAID at

http://www.niaid.nih.gov/ncn/glossary/default.htm#a

To find a specific term, click on the letter in the ALPHABET across the top or bottom of the screen that corresponds to the first letter of the term/expression that you want to look up. In the table that appears, the right-hand column defines the term or acronym in the left-hand column and also provides additional links.

Some definitions that may be useful:
- **AIDS Related** includes:
  —projects relating to the etiology, epidemiology, natural history, diagnosis, treatment, or prevention of AIDS
  —various sequelae specifically associated with AIDS
  —preparation and screening of anti-AIDS agents as well as vaccine development, including both pre-clinical and clinical studies
- **Note** that not all Applications examining various influences on T-lymphocytes or retroviruses will be appropriate for the **expedited** AIDS review process.
- Applications only **indirectly** related to AIDS will be evaluated by established Scientific Review Groups (SRGs)—commonly referred to as "Study Sections"— appropriate to the scientific discipline during regular NIH review cycles and should not be submitted in response to the expedited AIDS receipt dates.
- Applicants are urged to take note of the **yearly NIH Plan for HIV-Related Research**, and indicate how their Application addresses the NIH priorities set

forth in that Plan. The Plan can be found on the NIH Office of AIDS Research Home Page

http://www.nih.gov/od/oar/index.htm

Applicant organization types

Federal
A cabinet-level department or independent agency of the **Executive Branch** of the Federal Government or any component part of such a department or agency that may be assigned the responsibility for carrying out a grant-supported program.

State
Any agency or instrumentality of a state government of any of the United States or its territories.

Local
Any agency or instrumentality of a political subdivision of government below the state level.

Nonprofit
An institution, corporation, or other legal entity no part of whose net earnings may lawfully inure to the benefit of any private shareholder or individual.

For profit
An institution, corporation, or other legal entity, which is organized for the profit or benefit of its shareholders or other owners. A "for profit" organization is considered to be a small business if it is independently owned and operated, if it is not dominant in the field in which research is proposed, and if it employs no more than 500 persons. Also see definition (below) for Small Business Concern.

Small Business Concern
A small business concern is one that, at the time of award of Phase I and Phase II, meets ALL of the following criteria

1. Is independently owned and operated, is not dominant in the field of operation in which it is proposing, has its principal place of business located in the United States, and is organized for profit.

2. Is at least 51% owned, or in the case of a publicly owned business, at least 51% of its voting stock is owned by United States citizens or lawfully admitted permanent resident aliens.

3. Has, including its affiliates, a number of employees not exceeding 500, and meets the other regulatory requirements found in 13 CFR Part 121. Business concerns, other than investment companies licensed, or state development companies qualifying under the Small Business Investment Act of 1958, 15 U.S.C. 661, et seq., are affiliates of one another when either directly or indirectly, **(a)** one concern controls or has the power to control the other; or **(b)** a third-party/parties controls or has the power to control both. Control can be exercised through common ownership, common management, and contractual relationships. The term "affiliates" is defined in greater detail in 13 CFR 121.3-2(a). The term "number of employees" is defined in 13 CFR 121.3-2(t).

Business Concerns
Include, but are not limited to, any individual (sole proprietorship), partnership, corporation, joint venture, association,

or cooperative. Further information may be obtained by contacting the Small Business Administration Size District Office at **http//www.sba.gov/size/**.

Socially and Economically Disadvantaged Small Business Concern

A socially and economically disadvantaged small business concern is one that is at least 51% owned by (**a**) an Indian tribe or a native Hawaiian organization, or (**b**) one or more socially and economically disadvantaged individuals; AND whose management and daily business operations are controlled by one or more socially and economically disadvantaged individuals.

Women-Owned Small Business Concern

A small business concern that is at least 51% owned by a woman or women who also control and operate it. "Control" in this context means exercising the power to make policy decisions. "Operate" in this context means being actively involved in the day-to-day management.

SOME ADDITIONAL DEFINITIONS USED AT NIH

Child: NIH defines a child as an individual **under the age of 21 years**. It should be noted that the definition of child described above will pertain notwithstanding the FDA definition of a child as an individual from infancy to 16 years of age, and varying definitions employed by some states. Generally, state laws define what constitutes a "child," and such definitions dictate whether or not a person can legally consent to participate in a research study. However, state laws vary, and many do not address the age at which a child can consent to participate in research. Federal Regulations (45 CFR 46, subpart D, Sec.401-409) address DHHS protections for children who participate in research, and rely on state definitions of "child" for consent purposes. Consequently, the children included in this policy (persons under the age of 21) may differ in the age at which their own consent is required and sufficient to participate in research under state law. For example, some states consider a person age 18 to be an adult and, therefore, one who can provide consent without parental permission.

Clinical Research: NIH defines human clinical research as:

- Patient-oriented research. Research conducted with human subjects (or on material of human origin such as tissues, specimens and cognitive phenomena) for which an investigator (or colleague) directly interacts with human subjects. **Excluded from this definition** are *in vitro* studies that utilize human tissues that cannot be linked to a living individual. Patient-oriented research includes:
  —Mechanisms of human disease
  —Therapeutic interventions
  —Clinical trials
  —Development of new technologies
  —Epidemiologic and behavioral studies
  —Outcomes research and health services research. Note: Studies falling under Exemption 4 for human subjects' research are not considered clinical research by this definition.

Clinical Trial: For purposes of reviewing Applications submitted to the NIH, a clinical trial is operationally defined as a prospective biomedical or behavioral research study of human subjects that is designed to answer specific questions about biomedical or behavioral interventions (drugs, treatments, devices, or new ways of using known drugs, treatments, or devices).

Clinical trials are used to determine whether new biomedical or behavioral interventions are safe, efficacious and effective. **Clinical trials of experimental drug, treatment, device or behavioral intervention may proceed through 4 phases:**

Phase I clinical trials are done to test a new biomedical or behavioral intervention in a small group of people (e.g., 20–80) for the first time to evaluate safety (e.g., determine a safe dosage range, and identify side effects).

Phase II clinical trials are done to study the biomedical or behavioral intervention in a larger group of people (several hundred) to determine efficacy and to further evaluate its safety.

Phase III studies are done to study the efficacy of the biomedical or behavioral intervention in large groups of human subjects (from several hundred to several thousand) by comparing the intervention to other standard or experimental interventions, as well as to monitor adverse effects, and to collect information that will allow the intervention to be used safely.

Phase IV studies are done after the intervention has been marketed. These studies are designed to monitor effectiveness of the approved intervention in the general population and to collect information about any adverse effects associated with widespread use.

NIH-Defined Phase III Clinical Trial: For the purpose of the Guidelines an NIH-defined Phase III "clinical trial" is a broadly based **prospective** Phase III clinical investigation, usually involving several hundred or more human subjects, for the purpose of evaluating an experimental intervention in comparison with a standard or control intervention or comparing two or more existing treatments. Often the aim of such investigation is to provide evidence leading to a scientific basis for consideration of a change in health policy or standard of care. The definition includes pharmacologic, non-pharmacologic, and behavioral interventions given for disease prevention, prophylaxis, diagnosis, or therapy. Community trials and other population-based intervention trials are also included.

Co-Investigator: A co-investigator (collaborator) is an individual involved with the principal investigator in the scientific development or execution of the project. These individuals would typically devote a specific percent of effort to the project and would be identified as key personnel. The individual(s) may be employed by, or affiliated with, either the grantee organization or an organization participating in the project under a consortium or contractual agreement.

Commercialization: The process of developing markets and producing and delivering products for sale (whether by the originating party or by others). As used here, commercialization includes both government and private sector markets.

Consortium or Contractual Agreement: An agreement whereby a research project is carried out by the grantee and one or more other organizations that are separate legal entities. In this arrangement, the grantee contracts for the performance of a substantial and/or a significant portion of the activities to be conducted under the grant. These agreements typically involve a specific percent of effort from the consortium organization's Principal Investigator and a categorical breakdown of costs, such as personnel, supplies, and other allowable expenses, including Facilities and Administrative costs.

Consultant: An individual hired to give professional advice or services for a fee, normally not as an employee of the hiring party. In unusual situations, a person may be both a consultant and an employee of the same party, receiving compensation for some services as a consultant and for other work as a salaried employee. In order to prevent apparent or actual conflicts of interest, grantees and consultants must establish written guidelines indicating the conditions of payment of consulting fees. Consultants may also include firms that provide paid professional advice or services.

Consulting Fees: The fee paid by an institution to a salaried member of its faculty is allowable only in unusual cases and only if both of the following conditions exist:

- the consultation crosses departmental lines or involves a separate operation

or

- the work performed by the consultant is in addition to his or her regular workload

In all other cases, consulting fees paid to employees of recipient or cost-type contractor organizations in addition to salary may be charged to PHS grant-supported projects only in unusual situations and when **ALL** of the following 3 conditions exist:

- the policies of the recipient or contractor permit such consulting fee payments to its own employees regardless of whether Federal grant funds are received
- the consulting services are clearly outside the scope of the individual's salaried employment
- it would be inappropriate or not feasible to compensate the individual for these services through payment of additional salary

For additional clarification on the allowance and appropriateness of consulting fees, refer to the NIH Grants Policy Statement.

Cooperative Agreement: A support mechanism that will have substantial Federal scientific and/or programmatic involvement. Substantial programmatic involvement means that after award, scientific or program staff will assist, guide, coordinate, or participate in programmatic activities beyond the normal stewardship responsibility in the administration of grants. Proposed cooperative agreements will be published as policy announcements, program announcements, or requests for Applications.

Essentially Equivalent Work: This term is meant to identify "scientific overlap," which occurs when

(1) substantially the same research is proposed for funding in more than one proposal (contract proposal or Grant Application) submitted to the same Federal agency

OR

(2) substantially the same research is submitted to two or more different Federal agencies for review and funding consideration

OR

(3) a specific research objective and the research design for accomplishing that objective are the same or closely related in two or more proposals or awards, regardless of the funding source

Feasibility: The extent to which a study or project may be done practically and successfully.

Foreign Component: (1) The use of grant funds to support any element or segment of the project which is to be performed outside the U.S., either by the grantee or by a researcher employed by a foreign institution

or

(2) the use of grant funds for extensive foreign travel by grantee project staff for the purpose of data collection, surveying, sample collection, etc. Foreign travel for consultation is not considered a foreign component.

Full-Time Appointment: May be different in terms of actual months per year or days per week at the Applicant organization. The definition of a full-time appointment must be in accordance with the institutional policy and used consistently by the institution regardless of the source of support.

Gender: Refers to the classification of research subjects into either or both of two categories: women and men. In some cases, representation is unknown, because gender composition cannot be accurately determined (e.g., pooled blood samples or stored specimens without gender designation).

Grant: A financial assistance mechanism whereby money and/or direct assistance are provided to carry out approved activities.

Human Subjects: Human subject means a living individual about whom an investigator (whether professional or student) conducting research obtains

a. data through intervention or interaction with the individual

or

b. identifiable private information

The regulations governing the inclusion of human subjects in research extend to the use of human organs, tissues, and body fluids from individually identifiable human subjects as well as to graphic, written, or recorded information derived from individually identifiable human subjects.

Intervention includes both physical procedures by which data are gathered (for example, venipuncture) and manipulations of the subject or the subject's environment that are performed for research purposes. Interaction includes communication or interpersonal contact between investigator and subject.

Private information includes information about behavior that occurs in a context in which an individual can reasonably expect that no observation or recording is taking place, and information that has been provided for specific purposes by an individual and which the individual can reasonably expect will not be made public (for example, a medical record). Private information must be individually identifiable (i.e., the identity of the subject is or may readily be ascertained by the investigator or associated with the information) to constitute research involving human subjects.

The use of autopsy materials is governed by applicable state and local law and is not directly regulated by 45 CFR 46.

Innovation: Something new or improved, including research for
- development of new technologies
- refinement of existing technologies

or

- development of new Applications for existing technologies

For the purposes of PHS programs, an example of "innovation" would be new medical or biological products, for improved value, efficiency, or costs.

Institutional Base Salary: The annual compensation that the Applicant organization pays for an employee's appointment, whether that individual's time is spent on research, teaching, patient care, or other activities. Base salary excludes any income that an individual may be permitted to earn outside of duties to the Applicant organization. Base salary may not be increased as a result of replacing institutional salary funds with grant funds.

Some PHS grant recipients are currently subject to a legislatively imposed salary limitation. Any adjustment for salary limits will be made at time of award. Applicants are encouraged to contact their offices of sponsored programs or see the *NIH Guide for Grants and Contracts* for current guidance on salary requirements.

Key Personnel: Key personnel are defined as individuals who contribute to the scientific development or execution of the project in a substantive way, whether or not salaries are requested.

Principal Investigator, Program Director, or Project Director: The one individual designated by the Applicant organization to direct the project or program to be supported by the grant. The Principal Investigator is responsible and accountable to Applicant organization officials for the proper conduct of the project or program.

Program Income: Gross income earned by the Applicant organization that is directly generated by a supported activity or earned as a result of the award. The PHS Grants Policy Statement or NIH Grants Policy Statement contains a detailed explanation of program income, the ways in which it may be generated and accounted for, and the various options for its use and disposition.

Examples of program income include:
- Fees earned from services performed under the grant, such as those resulting from laboratory drug testing
- Rental or usage fees, such as those earned from fees charged for use of computer equipment purchased with grant funds
- Third party patient reimbursement for hospital or other medical services, such as insurance payments for patients when such reimbursement occurs because of the grant-supported activity
- Funds generated by the sale of commodities, such as tissue cultures, cell lines, or research animals
- Patent or copyright royalties

Prototype: A model of something to be further developed and includes designs, protocols, questionnaires, software and devices.

Research or Research and Development (R/R&D):   Any activity that is:
- A systematic, intensive study directed toward greater knowledge or understanding of the subject studied.

- A systematic study directed specifically toward applying new knowledge to meet a recognized need.
- A systematic Application of knowledge toward the production of useful materials, devices, and systems or methods, including design, development, and improvement of prototypes and new processes to meet specific requirements.

Research Institution: A United States research organization that is one of the following:

- A nonprofit college or university
- A nonprofit research institution, including nonprofit medical and surgical hospitals.

    A "nonprofit institution" is defined as an organization that is owned and operated exclusively for scientific or educational purposes, no part of the net earnings of which inures to the benefit of any private shareholder or individual.

- A contractor-operated, federally funded research and development center, as identified by the National Science Foundation in accordance with the Government-wide Federal Acquisition Regulation issued in accordance with section 35(c)(1) of the Office of Federal Procurement Policy Act (or any successor legislation thereto).

> **NOTE:** Laboratories staffed by Federal employees do not meet the definition of "research institution" for purposes of the STTR program.

Significant Difference: For purposes of NIH policy, a "significant difference" is a difference that is of clinical or public health importance, based on substantial scientific data. This definition differs from the commonly used "statistically significant difference," which refers to the event that, for a given set of data, the statistical test for a difference between the effects in two groups achieves statistical significance. Statistical significance depends upon the amount of information in the data set. With a very large amount of information, one could find a statistically significant, but clinically small difference that is of very little clinical importance. Conversely, with less information one could find a large difference of potential importance that is not statistically significant.

Socially and Economically Disadvantaged Individual: A member of any of the following groups: Black Americans; Hispanic Americans; Native Americans; Asian-Pacific Americans; Subcontinent Asian Americans; other groups designated from time to time by the SBA to be socially disadvantaged; or any other individual found to be socially and economically disadvantaged by the SBA pursuant to Section 8(a) of the Small Business Act, 15 U.S.C. 637(a).

Subcontract: Any agreement, other than one involving an employer–employee relationship, entered into by a Federal Government prime contractor calling for supplies or services required solely for the performance of the prime contract or another subcontract.

United States: The 50 states, territories and possessions of the U.S., Commonwealth of Puerto Rico, Trust Territory of the Pacific Islands, and District of Columbia.

Valid Analysis: The term "valid analysis" means an unbiased assessment. Such an assessment will, on average, yield the correct estimate of the difference in outcomes between two groups of subjects. Valid analysis can and should be conducted for both small and large studies. A valid analysis does not need to have a high statistical power for detecting a stated effect. The principal requirements for ensuring a valid analysis of the question of interest are:

Allocation of study participants of both sexes/genders and from different racial/ethnic groups to the intervention and control groups by an unbiased process such as randomization; unbiased evaluation of the outcome(s) of study participants; and use of unbiased statistical analyses and proper methods of inference to estimate and compare the intervention effects among the gender and racial/ethnic groups.

AN NIH GLOSSARY

Taken from NIH Grants Policy Statement (Revised 03/01):

http://grants2.nih.gov/grants/policy/nihgps_2001/part_i_1.htm

I have made some minor changes to the text taken from the above Web site. The glossary defines terms commonly used throughout the aforementioned policy statement. These definitions may be amplified and additional definitions may be found in other sections of this document and in source documents such as applicable statutes, grants administration regulations, and OMB Circulars.

The GLOSSARY (Definitions of some terms used by NIH)

Application: A request for financial support of a project/activity submitted to NIH on specified forms and in accordance with NIH instructions. (See "Application and Review Processes" for detailed information about the Application process, including an explanation of the types of Applications.)

Approved Budget: The financial expenditure plan for the grant-supported project or activity, including revisions approved by NIH as well as permissible revisions made by the grantee. The approved budget consists of Federal (grant) funds and, if required by the terms and conditions of the award, non-Federal participation in the form of matching or cost sharing. The approved budget specified in the Notice of Grant Award may be shown in detailed budget categories or as total costs without a categorical breakout. Expenditures charged to an approved budget that consists of both Federal and non-Federal shares are deemed to be borne by the grantee in the same proportion as the percentage of Federal/non-Federal participation in the overall budget.

Authorized Organizational Official: The individual, named by the Applicant organization, who is authorized to act for the Applicant and to assume the obligations imposed by the Federal laws, regulations, requirements, and conditions that apply to grant Applications or grant awards.

Award: The provision of funds by NIH, based on an approved Application and budget, to an organizational entity or an individual to carry out an activity or project.

Awarding Office: The NIH Institute or Center responsible for the award, administration, and monitoring of grant-supported activities.

Budget Period: The intervals of time (usually 12 months each) into which a project period is divided for budgetary and funding purposes.

Competitive Segment: The initial project period recommended for support (up to 5 years) or each extension of a project period resulting from a competing continuation award that establishes a new competitive segment for the project.

Consortium Agreement: A collaborative arrangement in support of a research project in which some portion of the programmatic activity is carried out through a formalized agreement between the grantee and one or more other organizations that are separate legal entities administratively independent of the grantee.

Contract Under a Grant: A written agreement between a grantee and a third party to acquire routine goods or services.

Consultant: An individual that provides professional advice or services on the basis of a written agreement for a fee. These individuals are not normally employees of the organization receiving the services. Consultants also include firms that provide professional advice or services.

Cooperative Agreement: A financial assistance mechanism used when substantial Federal programmatic involvement with the recipient during performance is anticipated by the NIH Institute or Center.

Co-Investigator: An individual involved with the Principal Investigator in the scientific development or execution of a project. The co-investigator may be employed by, or be affiliated with, the Applicant/grantee organization or another organization participating in the project under a consortium agreement. **A co-investigator** typically devotes a specified percentage of time to the project and **is considered "key personnel."** The designation of a co-investigator, if applicable, does not affect the principal investigator's roles and responsibilities as specified in this policy statement.

Cost Sharing: See "Matching or Cost Sharing."

Direct Costs: Costs that can be specifically identified with a particular project(s) or activity.

Domestic Organization: A public or private nonprofit institution (including Federal, state, and other agencies) or for-profit organization that is located in the United States or its territories, is subject to U.S. laws, and assumes legal and financial accountability for awarded funds and for the performance of the grant-supported activities.

Equipment: An article of tangible non-expendable personal property that has a useful life of more than 1 year and an acquisition cost per unit that equals or exceeds the lesser of the capitalization threshold established by the organization or $5,000.

Expanded Authorities: The operating authorities provided to grantees under certain research grant mechanisms that waive the requirement for NIH prior approval for specified actions.

Expiration Date: The date signifying the end of the current budget period, after which the grantee is not authorized to obligate grant funds regardless of the ending date of the project period or "completion date."

Facilities and Administrative Costs: Costs that are incurred by a grantee for common or joint objectives and that, therefore, cannot be identified specifically with a particular project or program. These costs were previously known as "indirect costs," and referred to at NIH as "F&A costs."

Federal Demonstration Partnership: A cooperative initiative among some Federal agencies, including NIH, select organizations that receive Federal funding for research, and certain professional associations. Its efforts include a variety of demonstration projects intended to simplify and standardize Federal requirements in order to increase research productivity and reduce administrative costs.

Federal Institution: A Cabinet-level department or independent agency of the executive branch of the Federal Government or any component organization of such a department or agency.

Fee: An amount in addition to actual, allowable costs incurred that is normally paid to a for-profit organization under a contractual arrangement. This increment above cost also is referred to as "profit."

Financial Assistance: Transfer by NIH of money or property to an eligible entity to support or stimulate a public purpose authorized by statute.

Foreign Component: Under a grant to a domestic organization, the performance of any significant element or segment of the project outside of the United States, either by the grantee or by a researcher employed by a foreign organization, with or without grant funds.

Foreign Organization: An organization located in a country other than the United States and its territories that is subject to the laws of that country, regardless of the citizenship of the proposed principal investigator.

For-Profit Organization: An organization, institution, corporation, or other legal entity that is organized or operated for the profit or financial benefit of its shareholders or other owners. Such organizations also are referred to as "commercial organizations."

Full-Time Appointment: The number of days per week and/or months per year representing full-time effort at the Applicant/grantee organization, as specified in organizational policy. The organization's policy must be applied consistently regardless of the source of support.

Grant: A financial assistance mechanism providing money, property, or both to an eligible entity to carry out an approved project or activity. **A grant is used whenever the NIH Institute or Center does NOT anticipate any substantial programmatic involvement with the recipient** during performance of the financially assisted activities.

Grant-Supported Project/Activities: Those programmatic activities specified or described in a grant Application or in a subsequent submission(s) that are approved by an NIH Institute or Center for funding, regardless of whether Federal funding constitutes all or only a portion of the financial support necessary to carry them out.

Grantee: The organization or individual awarded a grant or cooperative agreement by NIH that is responsible and accountable for the use of the funds provided and for the performance of the grant-supported project or activities. **The grantee is the entire legal entity even if a particular component is designated in the award document. The grantee is legally responsible and accountable to NIH for the performance and financial aspects of the grant-supported project or activity.**

Grants Management Officer (GMO):   An NIH official responsible for the business management aspects of grants and cooperative agreements, including review, negotiation, award, and administration, and for the interpretation of grants administration policies and provisions. Only GMOs are authorized to obligate NIH to the expenditure of funds and permit changes to approved projects on behalf of NIH. Each NIH Institute and Center that awards grants has one or more GMOs with responsibility for particular programs or awards.

Hospital: A nonprofit or for-profit hospital or medical care provider component of a nonprofit organization (for example, a foundation). The term includes all types of medical, psychiatric, and dental facilities, such as clinics, infirmaries, and sanatoria.

Indirect Costs: See "Facilities and Administrative Costs."

Institute/Center (IC):   The NIH organizational component responsible for a particular grant program(s) or set of activities. The terms "NIH IC" or "awarding office" are used throughout this document to designate a point of contact for advice and interpretation of grant requirements and to establish the focal point for requesting necessary prior approvals or changes in the terms and conditions of award. In the latter case, the terms refer specifically to the designated Grants Management Officer.

Institutional Base Salary: The annual compensation paid by an Applicant/grantee organization for an employee's appointment, whether that individual's time is spent on research, teaching, patient care, or other activities. The base salary excludes any income that an individual is permitted to earn outside of duties for the Applicant/grantee organization. Base salary may not be increased as a result of replacing organizational salary funds with NIH grant funds.

International Organization: An organization that identifies itself as international or intergovernmental, and has membership from, and represents the interests of, more than one country, without regard to whether the headquarters of the organization and location of the activity are inside or outside of the United States.

Key Personnel: Individuals who contribute in a substantive way to the scientific development or execution of a project, **whether or not they receive compensation from the grant supporting that project.** The Principal Investigator and Collaborators are included in this category.

Matching or Cost Sharing: The value of third-party in-kind contributions and the portion of the costs of a federally assisted project or program not borne by the Federal Government. Matching or cost sharing may be required by law, regulation, or administrative decision of an NIH Institute or Center. Costs used to satisfy matching or cost-sharing requirements are subject to the same policies governing allowability as other costs under the approved budget.

Modular Application: A type of Grant Application in which support is requested in specified increments without the need for detailed supporting information related to separate budget categories. When modular procedures apply, they affect not only Application preparation but also review, award, and administration of the Application/award.

Monitoring: A process whereby the programmatic and business management performance aspects of a grant are reviewed by assessing information gathered from various required reports, audits, site visits, and other sources.

New Investigator: An individual that has not previously served as a Principal Investigator on any Public Health Service-supported research project other than a small grant (e.g., an R15). If you have received any NIH funding, call NIH to determine whether or not you are considered a "new investigator."

Notice of Grant Award: The legally binding document that notifies the grantee and others that an award has been made, contains or references all terms and conditions of the award, and documents the obligation of Federal funds. The award notice may be in letter format and may be issued electronically.

Organization: A generic term used to refer to an educational institution or other entity, including an individual, which receives and/or applies for an NIH grant or cooperative agreement.

Principal Investigator/Program Director/Project Director: An individual designated by the grantee to direct the project or activity being supported by the grant. He or she is responsible and accountable to the grantee for the proper conduct of the project or activity.

Prior Approval: Written approval from the designated Grants Management Officer required for specified post-award changes in the approved project or budget. Such approval must be obtained prior to undertaking the proposed activity or spending NIH funds.

Program: A coherent assembly of plans, project activities, and supporting resources contained within an administrative framework, the purpose of which is to implement an organization's mission or some specific program-related aspect of that mission. For purposes of this policy statement, "program" refers to those NIH programs that carry out their mission through the award of grants or cooperative agreements to other organizations.

Program Income: Gross income earned by a grantee that is directly generated by the grant-supported project or activity or earned as a result of the award.

Program Official: The NIH official responsible for the programmatic, scientific, and/or technical aspects of a grant.

Project Period: The total time for which support of a project has been programmatically approved. The total project period is comprised of the initial competitive segment, any subsequent competitive segment(s) resulting from a competing continuation award(s), and non-competing extensions.

Real Property: Land, including land improvements, structures, and appurtenances, but not movable machinery and equipment.

Recipient: The organizational entity or individual receiving a grant or cooperative agreement. See "Grantee."

Research Misconduct: Fabrication, falsification, or plagiarism in proposing, performing, or reporting research, or in reporting research results. **Fabrication** is making up data or results and recording or reporting them. **Falsification** is manipulating research materials, equipment, or processes, or changing or omitting data or results such that research is not accurately represented in the research record. **Plagiarism** is the appropriation of another person's ideas, processes, results, or words without giving appropriate credit. The term does not include honest error or honest differences of opinion.

Significant Rebudgeting: A threshold that is reached when expenditures in a single direct cost budget category deviate (increase or decrease) from the categorical commitment level established for the budget period by more than 25 percent of the total costs awarded. Significant rebudgeting is one indicator of change in scope.

Small Business Concern: A business that is independently owned and operated and not dominant in its field of operation; has its principal place of business in the United States and is organized for profit; is at least 51 percent owned, or in the case of a publicly owned business, at least 51 percent of its voting stock is owned by U.S. citizens or lawfully admitted permanent resident aliens; has, including its affiliates, not more than 500 employees; and meets other regulatory requirements established by the Small Business Administration at 13 Code of Federal Regulations (CFR)Part 121.

State Government: The government of any state of the United States, the District of Columbia, the Commonwealth of Puerto Rico, any U.S. territory or possession, or any agency or instrumentality of a state exclusive of local governments. For purposes of NIH grants, federally recognized Indian tribal governments generally are considered state governments. State institutions of higher education and state hospitals are not considered state governments for purposes of the Department of Health and Human Services' general administrative requirements for grants and this policy statement.

Stipend: A payment made to an individual under a fellowship or training grant in accordance with pre-established levels to provide for the individual's living expenses during the period of training. A stipend is not considered compensation for the services expected of an employee.

Suspension: Temporary withdrawal of a grantee's authority to obligate grant funds, pending either corrective action by the grantee, as specified by NIH, or a decision by NIH to terminate the award.

Termination: Permanent withdrawal by NIH of a grantee's authority to obligate previously awarded grant funds before that authority would otherwise expire, including the voluntary relinquishment of that authority by the grantee.

Terms and Conditions of Award: All legal requirements imposed on a grant by NIH, whether based on statute, regulation, policy, or other document referenced in the grant award, or specified by the grant award document itself. The Notice of Grant Award may include both standard and special conditions that are considered necessary to attain the grant's objectives, facilitate post-award administration of the grant, conserve grant funds, or otherwise protect the Federal Government's interests.

Total Project Costs: The total allowable costs (both direct costs and facilities and administrative costs) incurred by the grantee to carry out a grant-supported project or activity. Total project costs include costs charged to the NIH grant and costs borne by the grantee to satisfy a matching or cost-sharing requirement.

Withholding of Support: A decision by NIH not to make a non-competing continuation award within the current competitive segment.

Acronyms and Abbreviations

CFR	Code of Federal Regulations
CSR	Center for Scientific Review
DCA	Division of Cost Allocation
DHHS	Department of Health and Human Services
EA	Expanded Authorities
F&A	Facilities and Administrative (costs)
FCTR	Federal Cash Transactions Report (SF-272)
FDP	Federal Demonstration Partnership
FSR	Financial Status Report (SF-269 or 269A)
GMO	Grants Management Officer
IC	Institute or Center
NGA	Notice of Grant Award
NIH	National Institutes of Health
NIHGPS	National Institutes of Health Grants Policy Statement
NRSA	National Research Service Award
OER	Office of Extramural Research
OFM	Office of Financial Management
OHRP	Office for Human Research Protections
OIG	Office of the Inspector General
OLAW	Office of Laboratory Animal Welfare
OMB	Office of Management and Budget
OPERA	Office of Policy for Extramural Research Administration
ORI	Office of Research Integrity
PA	Principal Investigator/Program Director/Project Director
PMS	Payment Management System
PO	Program Official
RFA	Request for Applications

SBIR	Small Business Innovation Research Program
SNAP	Streamlined Noncompeting Award Process
STTR	Small Business Technology Transfer Program

Other useful NIH sites:

http://www.niaid.nih.gov/ncn/grants/plan/plan.doc

At this site you will find some good advice from a specific NIH Institute, the National Institute of Allergy and Infectious Diseases, about how to plan an NIH grant Application. Topics covered are:

- Develop a Strategy for Planning an NIH Grant
- How to Choose an Application Topic
    —Should You Respond to an Institute Solicitation?
    —Comparing Investigator-Initiated Awards, RFAs, and PAs
    —Initiatives Can Be Advantageous, But Aren't Necessarily
    —RFAs and PAs May Have Special Requirements
- Develop a Solid Hypothesis
- Plan Your Application
- Decide Award Type and Duration
- Determine What Documentation You'll Need
- Develop a Modular Budget
- Send NIH Some Materials "Just in Time"
- Advice for New Investigators
    —Who Is a New Investigator?
    —Reviewers Have Different Expectations for New Applicants
    —Tips for New Applicants

http://www.niaid.nih.gov/ncn/grants/default.htm

At this site you will find the following Disclaimer and Tutorials:

These **"All About Grants" tutorials** help biomedical investigators, especially new ones, plan, write, and apply for the basic NIH research project grant, the R01. Our advice comes from the experience of NIAID staff, including former NIH grantees, and should be considered as opinion only. Differing opinions may exist.

We do not repeat instructions in the PHS 398 Grant Application Kit. **Before preparing an Application for an NIH grant, read all instructions, and follow the directions.** For changes in applying for a grant, **read weekly notices in the NIH Guide and articles in the Council News newsletter** at

http://www.niaid.nih.gov/ncn/newsletters/default.htm

- Annotated R01 Grant Application
- Grant Application Basics
- How to Plan a Grant Application

- How to Write a Grant Application
- How to Manage a Grant Award
- How to Write a Human Subjects Application
- Advice on Research Training Awards
- SBIR and STTR Advice
- Checklists for Applicants and Grantees
- Other Supplementary Materials

NIH extramural program

Grant	Cooperative Agreement	Contract
(NIH as Patron)	(NIH as Patron)	(NIH as Purchaser)
Project Conceived by Investigator NIH Supports or Assists	Project Conceived by Investigator or NIH NIH Supports or Assists	Project Conceived by NIH NIH Acquires Service or Product
Performer Defines Details and Retains Scientific Control	NIH Participates in Direction	NIH Exercises Direction and Control
NIH Maintains Cognizance Accomplishes a Public Purpose	NIH Monitors Accomplishes a Public Purpose	NIH Closely Monitors For Direct Benefit of Government

SUBMITTING YOUR APPLICATION

NOTE FROM AUTHOR: As I finish writing this book at the beginning of 2004, Applications to NIH are still being submitted on paper except at certain institutions that are test centers for electronic submission of Applications. When Applications are sent for review to a particular/appropriate Study Section, each member (Reviewer) of the Study Section receives a CD that contains (1) instructions for proposal review and (2) copies of all the Applications to be reviewed at the meeting. Reviewers are expected to bring the CD and a laptop computer to the Study Section meeting. For each Application, the 2 or 3 primary Reviewers for that Application also receive paper copies of the Applications and—usually—any related Appendix materials submitted by the PI.

Instructions

What to submit:
- Cover letter
- Original Application

- 5 **exact, single-sided copies** of the original Application
- 5 collated sets of Appendix material (A summary sheet, listing all of the items included in the Appendix, is helpful to the Reviewers.)
- Mailing label

What else is in the instructions
- Mailing address for Applications sent
  —USPS Regular mail
  —USPS Express
  —Courier service (non-USPS)
  —Applications delivered in-person are not accepted
  —For additional information, see

  http://grants.nih.gov/grants/guide/notice-files/NOT-OD-02-012.html

  —For particulars and exceptions see

  http://grants1.nih.gov/grants/funding/phs398/section_2.html#number

  - Table with PHS receipt, review, and award schedule for various types of Applications
  - Note about incomplete Applications
  - Information about vertebrate animals and other certifications
  - Notice about not submitting identical Applications to different agencies within the PHS or to different Institutes within an agency

---

A caution about Application assignment information

- Inquiries about assignment, review, or recommendation on funding of Applications are to be made **only to PHS officials. Be aware that it is inappropriate to contact consultants serving on advisory or review committees regarding these issues.**

INFORMATION ABOUT NIH GRANT APPLICATION REVIEW

The NIH Grants Policy Statement
Excerpted below are parts of the NIH Grants Policy Statement.
For the complete document, go to

http://216.239.41.104/search?q=cache:h6D3DjmEbvUJ:grants.nih.gov/grants/policy/nihgps_2001/nihgps_2001.pdf+&hl=en&ie=UTF-8

or to

http://grants.nih.gov/grants/policy/nihgps_2001/nihgps_2001.pdf

At the Web site, there is a complete Table of Contents on page 4.
A revised **NIH Grants Policy Statement** is available under "Grant Applications" at

http://www.niams.nih.gov/rtac/funding/grants/notlist.htm

Publication of the Revised NIH Grants Policy Statement (Rev. 12/03):
- Policy Changes
- Clarifications
- Enhancements

Release Date: November 26, 2003
Notice: NOT-OD-04-009
National Institutes of Health

NIH GRANTS POLICY STATEMENT

Introduction

The National Institutes of Health Grants Policy Statement (NIHGPS) is intended to make available to NIH grantees, in a single document, the **policy requirements that serve as the terms and conditions of NIH grant awards**. This document also is designed to be useful to those interested in NIH grants by providing information about NIH—its organization, its staff, and its grants process.

The NIHGPS is available on-line from the NIH Home Page at

http://www.nih.gov

- Click on "Funding Opportunities"
- In the left-most column (under "OER Site"), click on "Grant Topics"
- then click on "Grants Policy and Guidance"
- then click on "**Notice** – Updated NIH Grants Policy Statement ..."
- The Policy Statement is set up in 3 parts:
  - —**Part I** includes general information about NIH and its Grant Application and review processes
  - —**Part II** provides the standard terms and conditions of NIH grant awards as well as terms and conditions that apply to particular types of grants/grantees/activities that differ from or supplement the standard terms and conditions
  - —**Part III** includes a listing of pertinent offices and officials with their addresses and telephone numbers

This format allows general information, Application information, and other types of reference material to be separated from legally binding terms and conditions.

Part I

- Provides a glossary of commonly used terms
- Describes NIH and its relationship to other organizations within the Department of Health and Human Services (DHHS)
- Specifies grantee, NIH, and other DHHS staff responsibilities
- Outlines the Application and review processes
- Explains the various resources available to those interested in the NIH grants process

Part II

- Serves as the terms and conditions that are incorporated by reference in all NIH grant awards
- Includes generally applicable requirements, which may be in the form of full text or reference to or highlighting of statutory, regulatory, or Office of Management and Budget (OMB) requirements
- Specifies, in separate sections, requirements that pertain to
  —construction grants
  —training grants and fellowships
  —conference grants
  —consortium agreements
  —grants to foreign and international organizations
  —domestic grants with substantial foreign components
  —grants to Federal institutions
  —payments to (or on behalf of) Federal employees
  —grants to for-profit organizations
  —modular grants
  —research patient care activities

Part III

- Contains general contact information to aid the Reader
- Certain conventions are followed throughout this document
- The **term "Grant" is used to mean both "Grants and Cooperative Agreements"**
- The term "grantee" is used to refer to recipients of grants and awardees of cooperative agreements, unless the context requires use of a generic or alternate term, such as "recipient" or "awardee," for clarity
- "NIH" may be used in this document to refer to the entire organization or to its component organizations, or else to contrast an action by NIH, including actions by its Institutes or Centers, with an action by a grantee or other organization
- A reference to "Part II" or "Part III" without further elaboration means the corresponding part of this policy statement

Supersession

The NIHGPS was originally published with an effective date of October 1, 1998 for all NIH grants and cooperative agreements (hereafter, "grants") for budget periods beginning on or after that date. This version of the NIHGPS is an update of the 1998 publication. This revision of the NIHGPS is effective for all NIH grants and cooperative agreements for budget periods beginning on or after March 1, 2001, and supersedes the October 1998 NIHGPS in its entirety. It remains largely unchanged; however, it incorporates several new and modified requirements, clarifies certain policies, and emphasizes policies that require increased attention by grantees on the basis of recent developments. Among the changes are those that have been published since October 1998 as notices in the *NIH Guide for Grants and Contracts (NIH Guide)*. An explanation of the major changes from the NIHGPS that has been in effect since October 1, 1998 is included in the *NIH Guide* notice announcing the re-issuance of the NIHGPS.

- The *NIH Guide* is published on the NIH Home Page at

http://www.nih.gov

—access the link to "Grants and Funding Opportunities"

—then click on the "NIH Guide for Grants and Contracts")

- Maintenance: The **Office of Policy for Extramural Research Administration (OPERA)** is responsible for developing and maintaining this document. Interim changes will be published in the *NIH Guide*. Each change will be described, including its applicability and effective date; the affected section(s) of the NIHGPS specified; and the necessary language to implement it as a term or condition of award provided. Concurrently, conforming changes will be made in the electronic version of the NIHGPS (see access information above) with a date indicator showing the change's effective date.

- Grantees will be responsible for reviewing the *NIH Guide* for changes and for implementing them, as appropriate.

NIH Policy changes that are implemented with the 12/03 NIHGPS include:

- **Closely related work:** the option for grantees to pursue prior approval to account for multiple projects under a single cost objective has been eliminated. NIH will now apply the relatedness provision of OMB Circular A-21 (C., 4., d., (3)) to all NIH recipients that states **if a specific cost cannot be reasonably allocated to a specific project, it can be charged to any of the benefiting projects on any reasonable basis.**

- **Cost transfers:** policy now states that **transfers** of costs from one project to another or from one competitive segment to the next solely **to cover cost overruns are unallowable.**

- **Cost overruns:** included a definition to the glossary that states: "Any amount charged in access of the Federal share of costs for the project period (competitive segment)." Below are examples of NIH policy changes that have occurred since March 2001. Please note that the list below should not be considered all-inclusive; therefore, please refer to the *NIH Guide for Grants and Contracts* for details on other changes since March 2001:

http://grants.nih.gov/grants/policy/notices.htm

- **Expanded authorities:** Application of expanded authorities as a standard term and condition to all NIH awards.

- Examples of the **latest changes** in the Application submission policies: **NIH will continue to accept no more than 2 revised Applications after the submission of the original Application; however, the 2-year limitation has been eliminated.**

- **Resubmission of Application policy changed to allow grantees to resubmit unfunded Applications as new Applications in the following instances:**
  1) unsuccessful Applications for an RFA can be resubmitted as a **new** investigator-initiated Application
  2) previously unsuccessful investigator-initiated Applications can be resubmitted in response to an RFA as a new Application
  3) unfunded Applications that are reviewed for one research grant mechanism may be resubmitted for a different grant mechanism and should be prepared as a new Application

- **Data sharing:** Implementation of the NIH data-sharing policy.

- **Just-in-Time procedures:** Expanded to include option to submit IACUC approval.
- **NRSA Section Highlights:**
  —In accordance with the amendment of the Public Health Service Act, NIH renamed the National Research Service Awards to the Ruth L. Kirschstein National Research Service Awards
  —Includes the regulatory changes of NRSA part-time training
- **Audit: Threshold** for A-133 audits has increased from $300,000 to $500,000 for fiscal years ending on or after 12/31/2003.
- **Public Policy Changes that are discussed in the 12/03 NIHGPS:**
  —Stem Cell Research
  —USA PATRIOT Act
  —Public Health Security and Bioterrorism Preparedness and Response Act of 2002
  —HIPAA Privacy Rule

Policy clarifications since March 2001:

Clinical Practice Compensation (Institutional Base Salary): Compensation may be considered in the institutional base salary as long as all criteria are met:

1) clinical practice must be guaranteed by the university
2) clinical practice must be reported on the university's appointment form and paid by the university
3) clinical practice effort must be included and accounted for in the university's effort reporting

Key Personnel: Expanded definition to describe the contribution of key personnel as "measurable" whether or not salaries are requested. Zero percent effort and "as needed" are not acceptable for individuals that the grantee identifies as key personnel.

PI Eligibility: Elaborated on eligibility criteria for certain mechanisms/programs, no change in policy.
A discussion on the non-allowability of patent costs has been added to the NIHGPS. The policy now states that Invention, Patent, or Licensing Costs are not allowable as either direct or F&A costs because the creation of intellectual property is not a requirement of NIH grant awards. Such costs include licensing or option fees, attorney's fees for preparing or submitting patent Application, patent maintenance, or recording of patent-related information.

Consortium Written Agreements: Outlined that it is the responsibility of the grantees to include applicable requirements of the policy statement in their written agreements, and highlighted that agreements must also include a reference to the financial conflict of interest policy, intellectual property, and data-sharing requirements.

Document Enhancements: NIH Grants Policy Statement and the PHS 398 Application glossaries have been merged, where appropriate.

Other Support Policy: Previously located in the PHS 398 Application; has been included in the NIH Grants Policy Statement.

Glossary: Included in a table format.

Select Items of Cost: Section included in a table format.

Bayh-Dole Inventions reporting: Requirements are now included in a table format.

Cross Referencing Roles with eRA: NIH Grants Policy Statement role titles have been cross-referenced with the NIH eRA role titles, e.g.: authorized organizational official (also known as the signing official).

Abbreviations and acronyms are used throughout the policy statement without parenthetical definitions; therefore, readers should refer to the master list to identify unfamiliar terms, abbreviations, and/or acronyms.

Additional inquiries

Additional questions about the NIHGPS may be directed to:
NIH Division of Grants Policy
Tel: 301-435-0949

or

to the Grants Management Specialist that is identified on the NIH Notice of Grant Award.

The NIH Peer Review Process

To access the **National Advisory Environmental Health Sciences Council Orientation Handbook**, which contains a detailed description of the **NIH Peer Review Process**, go to

http://www.niehs.nih.gov/ecbinfo/council/councilorienthnbk/orientbook.html#_Toc432292873

NIH Integrated Review Groups (IRGs)

A list of the 20 CSR Integrated Review Groups (IRGs) and their descriptions is given at:

http://www.csr.nih.gov/review/IRGDESC.asp

A list of the Scientific Review Administrator (SRA) and the membership roster for each **Study Section** can be accessed from the above site or from

http://www.csr.nih.gov/Committees/rosterindex.asp

Check Web sites periodically to be sure you have the latest information. You may notice that specific items on the NIH Web site may be somewhat dated, but there are periodic updates at the main NIH Web site. Things are changing at NIH. It is important for you to keep up with the pertinent changes. For example, see

http://www.csr.nih.gov/events/implementplan.htm

NIH began a first comprehensive assessment of the organization and composition of CSR Study Sections in July 2001 in an attempt to align the review process with the "rapidly changing scientific landscape." The aim was to develop a system that provides the world's best peer review of health-related research Grant Applications submitted to NIH. After the Phase 1 report by the Panel on Scientific Boundaries for Review (PSBR) was accepted by the CSR Advisory Committee at the beginning of 2000, the Advisory Committee launched CSR into Phase 2.

To ensure that the NIH review process accommodates the ongoing emergence of new scientific opportunities and practices, PSBR recommended that

- formalized evaluations be carried out periodically to assess the structure and function of the CSR peer review process
- the Study Section design produced in Phase 2 of the project should be reviewed approximately every 5 years by the ad hoc external advisory groups for each IRG established that reported to the CSR Advisory Committee

In addition to intra-IRG evaluation, the PSBR recommended a periodic global assessment of the study sections, based on input from

—Applicants

—Reviewers

—NIH staff

Plans for intra- and inter-IRG evaluations are scheduled to begin when Phase 2 is complete.

Phase 2 should result in creation of specific Study Sections that will comprise the Integrated Review Groups (IRGs) proposed in the Panel's Phase 1 report, with some modifications. The Phase 2 implementation process will be gradual and will involve

—scientific research communities

—NIH program and review staff

—members of the PSBR

For additional discussion of the **implementation plan**, go to:

http://www.csr.nih.gov/events/implementplan.htm

You can access a large amount of information about NIH and the NIH grants process by starting at the NIH Web site

http://www.nih.gov

If you want to limit your search to information about the NIH Review Process, go to

http://www.csr.nih.gov

and click on:

"More Information on Writing Grants"

This will bring you to information about the NIH

—Application process

—review process

—funding components

—data on active grants

—special programs at NIH

INFORMATION YOU WILL NEED TO COMPLETE AN NIH GRANT APPLICATION

- Other support
- Personnel report
- Grant solicitations

- Start dates
- Inventions and patents
- Assurances and certifications
- Human subjects
- Research on transplantation of human fetal tissue
- Women and minority inclusion in clinical research policy
- Inclusion of children policy
- Research using human embryonic stem cells
- Vertebrate animals
- Debarment and suspension
- Drug-free workplace
- Restrictions on lobbying
- Non-delinquency on Federal debt
- Research misconduct
- Assurance of compliance (civil rights, handicapped individuals, sex discrimination, age discrimination)
- Responsibility of Applicants for promoting objectivity in research
- Use of metric system
- Smoke-free workplace
- Government use of information under privacy act
- Information available to the Principal Investigator
- Information available to the general public (Freedom of Information Act)
- Access to research data
- Recombinant DNA and human gene transfer research
- Information resources

For information about:

- Publications about NIH extramural research and research training programs, go to

    http://grants.nih.gov/grants/oer.htm

- Telephone numbers of NIH staff go to

    http://directory.nih.gov

or

    Telephone: 301-496-4000 (the NIH locator)
- NIH Extramural Research and Research Training Programs, go to

    http://grants.nih.gov/grants/oer.htm

or

    e-mail: GrantsInfo@nih.gov

or

    Telephone: 301-435-0714

- A specific Application, before review telephone or e-mail the Scientific Review Administrator named on the "notification of assignment."
- Receipt and referral of an Application, contact: Division of Receipt and Referral, Center for Scientific Review
    Telephone: (301) 435-0715
- Human Subject Protections, Institutional Review Boards, or related assurances (Office for Human Research Protections), go to

    http://ohrp.osophs.dhhs.gov/index.htm

- Animal Welfare and related regulations and assurances (Office of Laboratory Animal Welfare (OLAW)), go to

    http://grants.nih.gov/grants/olaw/olaw.htm

- What to submit in/with your Application and where to submit your Application to NIH go to

    http://grants1.nih.gov/grants/funding/phs398/section_2.html#number

NOTE: The above Web site has information (in greater detail than that given below) about the topics outlined below.

GUIDE FOR ASSIGNED REVIEWERS' PRELIMINARY COMMENTS ON RESEARCH GRANT APPLICATIONS (R01)

See

    http://www.csr.nih.gov/CDG/CD%20Guidelines/r01.pdf

OR

    http://www.google.com/search?q=cache:qrWyJMUEQcwJ:www.csr.nih.gov/CDG/C D%2520Guidelines/r01.pdf+&hl=en&ie=UTF-8

When Reviewers prepare written comments about Research Grant Applications to NIH that have been assigned to them for review, the Reviewers are asked to follow the NIH guidelines.
The goals of NIH-supported research are to
- **advance our understanding of biological systems**
- **improve the control of disease**
- **enhance health**

To judge the likelihood that the proposed research will have a substantial impact on the pursuit of these goals, Reviewers are asked
- to comment, in their written review of an Application, on each of the aspects listed below

- that the written reviews be devoid of any personal identifiers because the **unaltered comments of the Reviewers are sent to the Principal Investigator**

Format of the written reviewer's report

Description:
The **NIH scans the Abstract on page 2 of an Application for use in the Description section of the summary statement.** However, Reviewers must be prepared to present a summary of the goals of the Application to the Study Section so that all members can follow the critiques and discussion. Thus, any Description a Reviewer writes should be crafted keeping in mind the possibility of having to make such an oral presentation.

Critique:
Reviewers are asked to
- include as little DESCRIPTIVE information in this section as possible
- address, in 5 individual sections, each of the 5 criteria listed below:
  1. **Significance**
     - Does this study address an **important** problem?
     - If the aims of the Application are achieved, **how will scientific knowledge be advanced?**
     - What will be the **effect of these studies** on the concepts or methods that drive this field?
  2. **Approach**
     - Are the conceptual framework, design (including composition of study population), methods, and analyses
       - i adequately developed?
       - ii well-integrated?
       - iii appropriate to the aims of the project?
     - Does the Applicant
       - i acknowledge **potential problem** areas?
       - ii consider **alternative** tactics?
  3. **Innovation**
     - Does the project employ **novel** concepts, approaches or methods?
     - Are the **aims original and innovative?**
     - Does the project **challenge existing paradigms** or develop new methodologies or technologies?
  4. **Investigator**
     - Is the investigator **appropriately trained** and well suited to carry out this work?
     - Is the work proposed **appropriate** to the experience level of the principal investigator and other researchers (if any)?
     - PLEASE DO NOT INCLUDE descriptive biographical information unless it is important to the evaluation of merit.
  5. **Environment**
     - Does the **scientific environment** in which the work will be done contribute to the probability of success?
     - Do the proposed experiments take advantage of unique features of the scientific environment or employ useful collaborative arrangements?

- Is there evidence of **institutional support?**
- PLEASE DO NOT INCLUDE a description of available facilities or equipment unless it's important to the evaluation of merit.

Overall evaluation:

- In one paragraph, briefly summarize the most important points of the Critique, addressing the **strengths and weaknesses** of the Application **in terms of the 5 review criteria.**
- **Recommend a score** that reflects the overall impact of the project on the field, weighing the review criteria, as you consider appropriate for each Application. **An Application does not need to be strong in all categories to be judged likely to have a major scientific impact and, thus, deserve a high merit rating.** For example, an investigator may propose to carry out important work that by its nature is not innovative, but **is essential to move a field forward.**

In addition:

For **competing continuation (renewal) Applications, Reviewers are asked to:**
- Include an **evaluation of progress** over the past project period.

For **amended Applications, Reviewers are asked to:**
- Address **progress, changes, and responses to the critiques in the summary statement from the previous review,** indicating whether the Application is improved, the same as, or worse than the previous submission.
- Comments on progress and response to the previous review should be provided in a separate paragraph and/or under the appropriate criteria.

Protection of human subjects from research risks:

Evaluate the Application with reference to the following criteria:

- risk to subjects
- adequacy of protection of subjects against risks
- potential benefit to the subjects and to others
- importance of the knowledge to be gained

(Reviewers are asked to notify the SRA immediately if the Applicant fails to address all of these elements, so the SRA can determine if the Application should be withdrawn.)

If all of the criteria are adequately addressed, and there are no concerns, Reviewers are asked to write "Acceptable Risks and/or Adequate Protections," and, if possible, to provide a brief explanation.

If one or more criteria are inadequately addressed, Reviewers are asked to write, "Unacceptable Risks and/or Inadequate Protections" and document the actual or potential issues that create the human subjects concern.

If the Application indicates that the proposed human subjects research is exempt from coverage by the regulations, Reviewers are asked to determine if adequate justification is provided. If the claimed exemption is not justified, Reviewers should indicate "Unacceptable" and explain why they reached this conclusion.

If a clinical trial is proposed, Reviewers are asked to evaluate the Data and Safety Monitoring Plan. (If the plan is absent, Reviewers must notify the SRA immediately to determine if the Application should be withdrawn.) Reviewers should indicate if the plan is "Acceptable" or "Unacceptable", and, if unacceptable, explain why it is unacceptable.

Gender, minority, and children subjects:

Public Law 103-43 requires that women and minorities be included in all NIH-supported clinical research projects involving human subjects unless a clear and compelling rationale establishes that inclusion is inappropriate with respect to the health of the subjects or the purpose of the research.

> **NOTE:** NIH requires that children (defined by NIH as individuals under the age of 21) of all ages be involved in all human subjects research supported by the NIH unless there are scientific or ethical reasons for excluding them.

Each project involving human subjects must be assigned a code using the categories "1" to "5" below. Category 5 for minority representation in the project means that only foreign subjects are in the study population (no U.S. subjects). If the study uses both then codes 1 through 4 should be used.

Proposal writers should be sure that the minority and gender characteristics of the sample are scientifically acceptable, consistent with the aims of the project, and comply with NIH policy. **For each category, determine if the proposed subject recruitment targets are "A" (Acceptable) or "U" (Unacceptable).** If samples are rated as "U," NIH considers this a weakness in the research design that will be reflected in the overall score. Reviewers should explain the reasons for the recommended codes (see table below); this is particularly critical for any item coded "U."

Category	Gender (G)	Minority (M)	Children (C)
1	Both Genders	Minority & non-minority	Children & adults
2	Only Women	Only minority	Only children
3	Only Men	Only non- minority	No children included
4	Gender unknown	Minority representation	Representation of children unknown
5	Only Foreign Subjects		

Note: To the degree that acceptability or unacceptability affects the investigator's approach to the proposed research, such comments should appear under "Approach" in the 5 major review criteria detailed above, and should be factored into the score as appropriate.

Animal welfare:

Reviewers are asked to express any comments or concerns about the appropriateness of the responses to the 5 required points, especially whether the procedures will be limited to those that are **unavoidable** in the conduct of scientifically sound research.

Biohazards:

Reviewers are asked to note any materials or procedures that are potentially hazardous to research personnel and indicate whether the protection proposed will be adequate.

Budget:

Evaluate the direct costs only. Do NOT focus on detail. Reviewers are asked to determine whether the total budget is **appropriate** for the project proposed and to provide a rationale for suggested modification in amount or duration of support.

Other considerations (for Administrative Notes in the Summary Statement):
These comments are useful to NIH but should not influence your overall score.

Foreign:

If the Applicant organization is foreign, Reviewers are asked to comment on any special talents, resources, populations, or environmental conditions that are not readily available in the United States or that provide augmentation of existing U.S. resources. Reviewers are also asked to indicate whether similar research is being performed in the U.S. and whether there is a need for such additional research. These aspects do not apply to Applications from U.S. organizations for projects containing a significant foreign component.

Inclusion of minorities and women in clinical research study populations at NIH

For information about inclusion of minorities and women in clinical research study populations go to

http://www.nih.gov

and type "women and minorities" into the box at the upper right corner of the Web site, and then click on "Search." Note that there are many pages of choices at the Web site. Choose those that look promising for providing answers to your questions—but always make note of the date of the information provided and try to find the most recent entry that matches what you are trying to find. If in doubt, call NIH and ask whether there is any more recent information than that provided at the Web site.

Some of the sites provide answers to questions such as:

- What is the definition of clinical research?
- What is the definition of a clinical trial?
- What is sufficient and appropriate representation of women and minorities?
- Does the policy permit a study population that contains only one gender or minority group or sub-population?
- Can study populations in other related studies (research portfolio) be used to justify a study population that does not comply with the policy?
- What should Applicants do if they are in a geographic area that does not offer a study population with the diversity required by the policy?
- Is it acceptable to use existing cohorts that are deficient in women or minority participants?
- Is increased cost an acceptable justification for not including women, minorities, and minority sub-populations?
- What is the definition of minority groups and minority sub-populations?
- Do all minority groups and sub-populations have to be included in a study population?
- What is meant by outreach efforts to recruit women, minorities, and members of minority sub-populations?

You should contact NIH program staff

- to ask whether the policies about minorities and women in clinical research study populations that you find at the Web site are correct for the Institute to which you plan to apply for funding

- for additional guidance in interpreting the policy in the context of a specific NIH Institute, Center, or Division to which you plan to apply

CSR scoring procedures

Numerical rating

At NIH, each scored Grant Application is assigned a single, global score that reflects the overall impact that the project could have on the field based on consideration of 5 review criteria:

- Significance
- Approach
- Innovation
- Investigator
- Environment

with the emphasis on each criterion varying from one Application to another, depending on the nature of the Application and its relative strengths.

The best possible priority score is 100 and the worst score is 500. Individual Reviewers mark scores to 2 significant figures (e.g., 2.2), and the individual scores are averaged and then multiplied by 100 to yield a single overall **priority score** for each scored Application, e.g., 253.

Abstaining members and those NOT present during the discussion do NOT assign a numerical rating and are, thus, NOT counted in calculating the average of the individual ratings.

For Research Applications, Reviewers are asked to recommend that half of the Applications **NOT** be scored and to spread final scores to achieve a median score of 300. (If any member of the scientific review group requests that an Application be scored, all members **must** score the Application.) To the extent that the Study Section does not score some Applications, the scoring range is altered. If **50%** of the Applications are **NOT** scored, then the remaining Applications should be scored from 100 to 300. If only **25%** of the Applications are **NOT** scored then the remaining Applications should be scored from 100 to 400. Note that these procedures for scoring only 50% of the research Applications **do not apply to fellowships and career Applications; all fellowships and career Applications are scored.**

Percentile conversion

Research Grant Applications (R01s) reviewed in CSR Study Sections are assigned a percentile rank. **The conversion of priority scores to percentile rankings is based on scores assigned to Applications reviewed during the current plus the past two review rounds.** Applications reviewed by a standing Study Section are percentiled against all Applications reviewed by that same Study Section for the three consecutive rounds. Applications reviewed by Special Emphasis Panels (SEPs) are percentiled against the parent Study Section database if at least 30% of the Reviewers are current or recent (during the last two years) regular members of that Study Section. Applications reviewed by SEPs where fewer than 30% of the reviewers are current or recent members of a standing Study Section are given a percentile based on the distribution of scores assigned by all CSR Study Sections. **Note that at CSR, Applications OTHER than R01s (e.g., fellowships, small business Applications) are NOT percentiled.**

Calculation of percentiles

(The information below is taken from **NIH Peer Review Notes,** October, 1991, pages 2–3.)
Over years of use, percentiles have changed in a number of ways. These changes include:

- Which types of Applications are used to create the different percentile bases
- Which Applications are assigned a percentile
- Which Scientific Research Groups (SRGs) or IC review committees are eligible for percentile bases

See also:

**http://search.google.cit.nih.gov/search?q=cache:eJXDEgsu-fg:
http://impacii.info.nih.gov/pvdoc/PercentilesUserGuide_April2004.pdf+
calculation+of+percentiles&restrict=NIH&site=NIH_Master&output=xml_
no_dtd&client=NIH_Master&access=p&proxystylesheet=
http%3A%2F%2Fwww.nih.gov%2Fgoogle%2FNIH_Master.stylesheet.xslt#11**

The percentile value represents the relative rank for each priority score on a scale from 1.0 to 100.0. Following the NIH convention of assigning the order of priority scores for scientific merit inversely to the numerical scale, **the lowest percentile value represents the judgment of highest scientific merit.**

The calculated percentile value for a given Application specifies the percent of Applications with score equal to or better (lower number) than that Application, i.e., a cumulative percent distribution.

The formula for calculating the percentile is the following:

$$p = 100 (k - \tfrac{1}{2})/N$$

where

p = percentile value

100 = the percentile scale (a constant)

k = numerical rank of priority score

N = number of Applications in base

Consider the following set of scores as an example from a pool of 80 Applications, 14 of which were not scored:

Rank	Priority Score	Percentile
1	108	0.6
2	115	1.9
3	118	3.1
4	120	4.4
//	//	//
66	478	81.9

The percentile for priority score 118 above is calculated as follows:

$$p = 100(3 - \tfrac{1}{2})/80$$
$$= 100(2.5)/80$$
$$= 250/80$$
$$= 3.125$$
$$p = 3.1$$

Note that, for a given N, the percentile intervals are approximately equal, considering rounding to the nearest 0.1, and the interval (in this example, 1.25) × the number of Applications (80) = 100. This relationship holds without regard to the distribution of priority scores and without regard to the number of Applications left "unscored," because these are included in the percentile base.

Percentile payline and award rate

When an Institute indicates a particular percentile **payline**, it means that Applications with an equal or better (lower) percentile will generally be funded. Note, however, that one cannot relate the percent of approved Applications to be awarded (award rate) with the percentile payline. The award rate is the proportion of Applications assigned to a particular Institute, which were **actually** awarded. The award rate could be higher or lower than the percentile payline. For example, in one year, the award rate at NIEHS (27.5%) was lower than the percentile payline (30.3%) whereas, for NIDCD, the award rate (38.6%) was considerably greater than the percentile payline (27.9%).

A hypothetical example:

- National XYZ Institute (XYZ) has a percentile payline of 18.0 and among the many Applications reviewed by the Biology Study Section there were 6 XYZ Applications.

- If all 6 of those Applications had percentile ranks between 1 and 18, then all 6 probably would be funded by the XYZ for an award rate of 100%.

- If all 6 had percentile ranks numerically greater than 18, then none would be funded (award rate = 0%).

- If only 2 of the 6 Applications had percentiles between 0 and 18, and the other 4 had ranks greater than 18, then only 2 would be funded (award rate 33.3%).

Notes added by the Author:
All Applications reviewed, whether given a priority rating or left unscored, are included in the calculation of percentiles. Thus, in the equation shown earlier, N includes all Applications reviewed in the three last meetings of *that specific* Study Section, including those that were **NOT** scored and **NOT** given a percentile rank and were simply aligned below all scored Applications; it does not matter that they do not have a numerical score. Most Applications reviewed by ad hoc Study Sections, special committees, or NIH Institute/Center review groups are **ALSO** assigned percentiles. However, **Applications for set-aside funds, such as RFAs or SBIR grants, are NOT assigned percentiles.**

In the 1990s, about 5% to 7% of research project grants were paid out of percentile order for reasons of program priorities. It is important to note that Applications with *similar* percentiles, but assigned to different funding components, may have *different* funding outcomes because the different funding components may have different amounts of money with which to fund competing awards. (See "NIH Scientific Merit Review: Terminology and Practices," *NIH Peer Review Notes*, October 1993, pages 11–13.)

Salary limitation on grants, cooperative agreements, and contracts
See

http://www.niams.nih.gov/rtac/funding/grants/notice/notod02-030.htm

Release Date: January 25, 2002
NOTICE: NOT-OD-02-030
Concerning salary limitation on Grants, Cooperative Agreements, and Contracts.

NOTE from author: Check the above Web site before you start working on grant budget!

National Institutes of Health

This notice provides updated information regarding the **salary limitation** as it relates to NIH grant and cooperative agreement awards. This information also applies to extramural research and development contract awards.

Fiscal Year (FY) 2002 was the thirteenth consecutive year for which there was a legislatively mandated provision for the limitation of salary. Specifically, the Department of Health and Human Services (DHHS) Appropriation Act for FY 2002, Public Law 107-116, restricts the amount of **direct salary** of an individual under an NIH grant or cooperative agreement (hereafter referred to as a grant) or applicable contract to Executive Level I of the Federal Executive Pay scale. Effective January 1, 2002, the Executive Level I salary level was $166,700.

Direct salary is exclusive of Fringe benefits and Facilities and Administrative (F&A) expenses, also referred to as **indirect costs.** NIH grant/contract awards for Applications/Proposals that request direct salaries of individuals in excess of the applicable RATE per year will be adjusted in accordance with the legislative salary limitation and will include a notification such as the following:

According to the FY 2002 DHHS Appropriations Act, "None of the funds appropriated in this Act for the National Institutes of Health, the Agency for Healthcare Research and Quality, and the Substance Abuse and Mental Health Services Administration shall be used to pay the salary of an individual, through a grant or other extramural mechanism, at a rate in excess of Executive Level I" of the Federal Executive Pay Scale.

- **The term "salary" means "direct salary", which is exclusive of fringe benefits and F&A expenses.**
- **"Direct salary" has the same meaning as the term "institutional base salary."**
- An individual's **institutional base salary** is the annual compensation that the Applicant organization pays for an individual's appointment, whether that individual's time is spent on research, teaching, patient care, or other activities.
- Base salary excludes any income that an individual may be permitted to earn outside of duties to the Applicant Organization.

The Web site

http://www.niams.nih.gov/rtac/funding/grants/notice/notod02-030.htm

summarizes the time frames associated with existing salary caps.

Amended Applications

http://grants2.nih.gov/grants/policy/amendedapps.htm

New NIH Policy on Submission of Revised (Amended) Applications:
NIH GUIDE, Volume 25, Number 19, June 14, 1996
National Institutes of Health
As of 1996, NIH has NOT considered any A3 or higher amendments to an Application. The new policy applies to all mechanisms.

NIH data indicate that

- amended Applications now constitute more than 30% of all research project Grant Applications
- investigators who receive initial funding based on an amended Application, whether for a new submission (Type 1) or a competing renewal (Type 2), experience a lower success rate in subsequent efforts to secure funding for a competing renewal Application
- the probability of subsequent success in the competing renewal process diminishes with the number of amendments

NIH decided that after these three unsuccessful attempts at funding, it is preferable for all Applicants to take a fresh start at their research plans. The policy of limiting the number of amendments to **two** allows PIs sufficient time to generate preliminary data, if it is required by the reviewers, and to consider new findings in the area of research.

> **Author comments:** Be aware that amended Applications **may not** necessarily go to the **same** Study Section—and even if they do, the Study Section members who previously reviewed the Application may no longer be members of that Study Section. This may be to your advantage, but it is not uncommon for a different/new Reviewer to find new problems with the Application that were not found/discussed/commented on by the original Reviewer!

Data about NIH Awards (competing and non-competing) by Fiscal Year and Funding Mechanism can be accessed at:

http://grants2.nih.gov/grants/award/trends/fund9202.htm

Recruiting minorities for study sections and NIH minority programs: the pipeline for minorities

(This section is excerpted from NIH DRG Scientific Review & Information Systems, Advisory Committee Minutes, April 12 and 13, 1993, Item VII and VIII, pages 12 and 13.)

The statistics regarding minority science faculty are disturbing. Dr. Walter Massey, at NSF, indicated in the *Science* issue about Minorities that when he started at Brown University in 1970, there were 15 African-American faculty members. In 1993 that number had increased only to 17. At the University of Chicago in 1973 there were 17 tenured or tenure track African-American faculty members; some 20 years later, only 21 out of 1,266 faculty members were African-American. African-Americans comprise just slightly over 5 percent and Hispanics only about 2.5 percent of medical school faculty in the United States. In 1987, only 1 percent of full-time faculty in the natural sciences in the United States was African-American, and the statistics have not improved. From these statistics, one can see that there is clearly a pipeline problem that needs fixing.

NIH has been criticized for not awarding enough grants to minority investigators. **But NIH does not receive many Applications from minority researchers.** The low number of Applications and awards to minorities is a reflection of the output of the pipeline. In 1991, based on those who reported their race, 2.9 percent of the research project grants went to under-represented minorities. Their success rate did not differ significantly from that of the general pool of Applicants, but the Application rate is dismal.

Some NIH Awards

Institute and Center Coordinators for NIH Awards are listed at

http://www1.od.nih.gov/ohrm/Awards/Award-Coords.htm

The funding components at NIH use a variety of award mechanisms to support extramural research. However, **not all the components support all the award mechanisms.** NIH periodically publishes a list of **activity codes** for the awards. The list indicates which funding components support which award mechanisms. It's a good idea to keep up-to-date by reading **every** issue of the *NIH Guide for Grants and Contracts*. You can ask to have the Table of Contents of each issue e-mailed to you:

> *NIH Guide* **LISTSERV:**
>
> The *NIH Guide for Grants and Contracts* **is the official publication for NIH medical and behavioral research Grant Policies, Guidelines and Funding Opportunities.**
>
> Each week (usually on Friday afternoon), the NIH transmits an e-mail with the Table of Contents (TOC) information for that week's issue of the *NIH Guide*, via the NIH LISTSERV. The TOC includes a link to the **Current NIH Guide Weekly Index** as well as links to each *NIH Guide* article published for that week.
>
> **To Subscribe** to the *NIH Guide* LISTSERV, **send an e-mail to** listserv@list.nih.gov
>
> with the following text in the message body (**not in the "Subject" line**): **subscribe NIHTOC-L** *your name*
>
> *(Example: subscribe NIHTOC-L Joe Smith)*
>
> Your e-mail address will be automatically obtained from the e-mail message and added to the LISTSERV.
>
> **To UnSubscribe** to the *NIH Guide* LISTSERV, **send an e-mail to** listserv@list.nih.gov
>
> with the following text in the message body (**not in the "Subject" line**): **unsubscribe NIHTOC-L** *your name*
>
> *(Example: unsubscribe NIHTOC-L Joe Smith)*
>
> Your e-mail address will be automatically obtained from the e-mail message and removed from the LISTSERV.
>
> More information on using the NIH LISTSERV can be obtained from the NIH LISTSERV FAQ page.

NIH tries to reach communities that are under-funded. For example, there are a number of grant opportunities targeted to minorities. Also, although NIH funds medical research or research training in every state in the U.S., about 23 states plus Puerto Rico have not been participating in research as fully as NIH would like. To help these regions increase their capacity for medical research, NIH launched a pilot Institutional Development Award (IDeA) program in 2001 to determine if institutions in these areas have the potential to do good medical research.

For further information about grant opportunities, go to

http://grants1.nih.gov/grants/oer.htm

and look under "Grant Topics."

Also check

http://nihroadmap.nih.gov

SOME SPECIAL NIH AWARDS

Academic Research Enhancement Award (AREA) (R15)

See

http://www.ninds.nih.gov/funding/postdoc.htm#r15

NIH Program Announcement: PA-03-053
January 30, 2003
Use Application Form PHS 398
Application Receipt dates: January 25, May 25, September 25

and

http://grants2.nih.gov/grants/funding/area.htm

To stimulate research in educational institutions that provide baccalaureate or advanced training for a significant number of the nation's research scientists but have not been major recipients of NIH support, NIH has implemented the **Academic Research Enhancement Award (AREA)** program.

Congressional appropriations for the NIH have included funds for this initiative since 1985. Based on the expectation that funds will continue to be available each year, NIH invites Applications for AREA grants (R15) through an ongoing Program Announcement (PA). AREA funds are intended to support

- new = "type 1"

and

- continuing ("renewal" or "competing continuation") = "type 2"

health-related research projects proposed by faculty members of eligible schools and components of domestic institutions.

AREA grants enable qualified scientists to receive **support for small-scale research projects.** The grants are intended to create a research opportunity for scientists and institutions otherwise unlikely to participate extensively in NIH programs to support the nation's biomedical and behavioral research effort. **NIH anticipates that**

- investigators supported under the AREA program will benefit from the opportunity to conduct independent research

- the grantee institution will benefit from a research environment strengthened through AREA grants and furthered by participation in the diverse extramural programs of the NIH

- students will benefit from exposure to, and participation in, research and will be encouraged to pursue graduate studies in the health sciences

Salary and Research Costs: National Institute for Neurological Disorders and Stroke will provide up to a maximum of $150,000 in direct costs plus facilities and administrative costs for a period of up to 3 years. Allowable **direct costs** include:

- salaries for the Principal Investigator and other research personnel (including students)
- supplies
- equipment
- travel
- other items specifically associated with the proposed research project

Exploratory studies for high risk/high impact research (R21) (PA 97-049)

http://www.nigms.nih.gov/funding/pa/r21info.html

Purpose: to provide pilot-scale support for potentially ground-breaking ideas/methods/systems that meet the following criteria:

- They lack sufficient preliminary data for feasibility to be established, and therein lies the "risk."
- Their successful demonstration would have a major impact on biomedical research.
- They fall within areas supported by National Institute for General Medical Services.

All conditions must be satisfied. Therefore, gathering preliminary data for a proposal whose significance is already well established would not qualify. Similarly, projects that will provide incremental advances in knowledge, whether or not there is a lack of preliminary data, are likewise not eligible. Finally, only NIGMS is committed to accepting proposals in response to this Program Announcement, and will do so only if they fall within its purview. Potential Applicants are encouraged to call the NIGMS staff members listed in the program announcement regarding the areas of science that NIGMS supports.

Program highlights

- Applications will be reviewed in the Center for Scientific Review Study Sections, but will not receive percentile scores and will not be included in the base from which the percentiles of other Applications are calculated.
- Study Sections will be asked to take into account the requirements of NIGMS that the **project show "potential for ground-breaking, precedent-setting significance of the proposed research, with particular emphasis on novel and innovative approaches** that clearly require additional preliminary data for their value to be established."
- There is no "set-aside" for the program; NIGMS staff will recommend only those proposals clearly meeting the stated requirements.
- The **R21 cannot be renewed**; if sufficient data are generated during the term of the award, investigators could then apply for further funding through regular research grants, e.g., the R01 mechanism.

"RAPID" (Rapic Assessment Post-Impact of Disaster) Program—NIMH

A National Institute of Mental Health program. Grants are 1 to 2 years, nonrenewable and provide a maximum of $125,000 per year for study of the effects of catastrophic events on mental health. Accelerated review time for proposals is 5 to 6 weeks.

For information, go to

http://grants.nih.gov/grants/guide/pa-files/PAR-02-133.html

or call:
Farris Tuma, Sc.D.
Division of Mental Disorders, Behavioral Research and AIDS
National Institute of Mental Health
6001 Executive Boulevard, Room 6197, MSC 9617
Bethesda, MD 20892-9617
Rockville, MD 20852 (for express/courier service)
Telephone: (301) 443-5944
Fax: (301) 480-5514
e-mail: ftuma@nih.gov or ftuma@mail.nih.gov

Small Business Innovation Research (SBIR) Grant (At NIH these are called R43, R44)

The Small Business Innovation Research (**SBIR**) and the Small Business Technology Transfer (**STTR**) Programs support a broad spectrum of development by small businesses of **innovative technologies that have the potential to succeed commercially.** Scientists at research institutions, including colleges and universities, play important roles on SBIR and STTR grants, and obtain significant levels of funding for technology research and development under these programs.

Levels of Funding: **The SBIR and STTR Programs are mandated by the Congress of the United States, and funded by numerous agencies at levels specified by Federal law.**

The SBIR and STTR Programs are institute-wide programs that support development of innovative technologies and methodologies that **have commercial potential** and are **relevant to the broad research mission of NIH.**

Grants supported by the SBIR and the STTR Programs are awarded in 2 phases:

Phase I (1 year duration) is intended to

- establish the feasibility of a line of research and development
- permit construction of a prototype
- carry out feasibility tests of the prototype

A Phase I award is a prerequisite for a Phase II grant.

Phase II is similar to a competitive grant renewal, and is intended to support research and development continued from Phase I.

The Phase II grant is awarded on the basis of the

- results of the feasibility tests performed in Phase I
- research and development proposed in the Phase II Application

Phase III

Must be supported by NON-federal funding

The expectation is that after Phase II research and development:

- a product will be ready to introduce to the marketplace

or

- more likely, support for further development will be obtained from NON-federal sources (e.g., other businesses)

For both the **SBIR and STTR Programs, the Applicant organization must be a small business** that:

- is independently owned, controlled and operated for profit
- has its principal place of business in the United States
- has 500 or fewer employees

Under the **SBIR Program,** the Principal Investigator must be employed for more than 50% effort by the small business. But scientists at research institutions, including colleges and universities, may serve as consultants or as subcontractors to the project. Consultant and contractual costs may comprise up to 33% of the budget of a Phase I grant, and up to 50% of the budget of a Phase II grant in the SBIR Program. These arrangements:

- allow small businesses to take advantage of the wealth of expertise and facilities available outside of their own enterprise
- make it possible for scientists at research institutions to pursue research and development goals that might otherwise not be realized

For additional information see

http://www.nih.gov/grants/funding/sbir.htm

Sample SBIR Applications can be accessed via:

http://grants.nih.gov/grants/funding/sbirsttr_news.htm#20030916

Applications in response to

- the "Omnibus Solicitation" of the National Institutes of Health
- the Centers for Disease Control and Prevention
- the Food and Drug Administration

for the Small Business Innovation Research (SBIR) and Small Business Technology Transfer (STTR) Grant Applications must be received by April 1, August 1, and December 1, 2004. Check the above Web sites for possible changes of deadline dates in future years.

For other NIH awards:
Go to

http://www.nih.gov

or

http://search.nih.gov

and type "NIH awards" or the name of the award of interest in the "Search" box at the upper right corner of the site and then click on the word "Search" to the right of the box. Look through the list that appears and at the bottom of the page, click on the next underlined number to get to the next page of listings. As I write this Appendix there are more than 750 listings.

EXAMPLE OF AN NIH STUDY SECTION AGENDA

XYZ STUDY SECTION MEETING
ABC Hotel, Washington, DC
February X to X+1, 200Y

Agenda

February X, 200Y
I.   Call to order: 8:30 AM
II. Review of confidentiality, conflict of interest, and voting procedures. The meeting is closed to the public, in accordance with the provisions set forth in sections 552b(c)(4) and 552(c)(6), Title 5, U.S.C. and Section 10(d) of Public Law 92-463.
III. Review of Applications
     9:00 AM to Noon
IV. Lunch
     Noon to 1:00 PM
V.   Review of Applications
     1:00 PM to 5:30 PM

February X + 1, 200Y
Finish review of Applications: 8:30 AM to 5:00 PM
5:00 PM Adjourn

Notice of Grant Award
If you are awarded a grant you will receive a "Notice of Grant Award" that contains important information.

See

http://www.niaid.nih.gov/ncn/grants/manage/manage_c5.htm

The "Notice of Grant Award" is now **usually sent via e-mail**. If NIH sends your institution a "Notice of Grant Award," it means that all your Application information has been received and accepted by NIH, and the agency is going to award your grant. The "Notice of Grant Award" states

- the amount of funding for current and future years
- start and end dates
- terms and conditions of the award
- contact information for your Program Officer and grants management specialist

Sometimes NIH places **restrictions** on your actions until you have completed certain previous requirements.

For more information see the above Web site.

The peer review process
To find information about Office of Extramural Research (OER), Peer Review Policy and Issues, go to

http://grants1.nih.gov/grants/peer/peer.htm

You should be familiar with terms listed below used by CSR:
Taken from

http://www.csr.nih.gov/REVIEW/terms.htm

(1) **Integrated Review Group (IRG):** a cluster of Study Sections responsible for the review of Grant Applications in scientifically related areas. These Study Sections share common intellectual and human resources.

(2) **Percentile:** represents the relative position or rank of each priority score (along a 100.0 percentile band) among the scores assigned by a particular Study Section.

(3) **Priority score:** A numerical rating that reflects the scientific merit of the proposed research relative to the "state of the science."

(4) **Scientific Review Administrator (SRA):** NIH Health Scientist Administrators in charge of review and advisory groups.

(5) **Study Section:** A panel of experts established according to scientific disciplines or current research areas for the primary purpose of evaluating the scientific and technical merit of Grant Applications. Also called Scientific Review Groups (SRGs).

(6) **Summary statement:** a combination of the Reviewers' written comments and the SRAs summary of the members' discussion during the Study Section meeting. It includes the recommendations of the Study Section, a recommended budget, and administrative notes of special considerations.

For an Overview of Peer Review Practices and Guidelines and access to the topics listed below, go to

http://grants1.nih.gov/grants/peer/peer.htm

- Overview of Peer Review Process
- Glossary of Terms
- Review Procedures for Scientific Review Group Meetings
- Guidelines for Reviewers
- Guidelines for Review of Specific Applications
- Review of New Investigator R01s
- CSR Scoring Procedure
- Streamlined Review
- Review of Research Involving Natural Products Usually Prepared as Complex Mixtures
- Modular Grant Application and Award
- Inclusion of Children as Participants in Research Involving Human Subjects

For a description of what happens to your Research Project Grant Application (R01/R21) after it is received for Peer Review, go to

http://www.csr.nih.gov/REVIEW/peerrev.htm

More about the peer review process
- Overview
- Research Project Evaluation Criteria
- Dual-Level Peer Review:
  —**First level: Scientific Review** Group (SRG)
  —**Second level: Advisory Council** or Board of the potential awarding component (Institute, Center, or other unit). The review criteria can be found at

  http://grants.nih.gov/grants/peer/peer.htm

or can be obtained from
GrantsInfo:
Tel: 301-435-0714
e-mail: GrantsInfo@nih.gov

Interactions with NIH before submission of a Grant Application

- Additional information about the NIH peer review process and grant programs can be obtained from GrantsInfo@NIH.gov.
- Information about charters and membership of SRGs, Councils, and Boards can be obtained from the appropriate NIH agency.
- Applicants are encouraged to contact relevant Institute or Center staff for advice on preparing an Application and for information regarding programmatic areas of interest.
- Phone numbers for contacting Institute or Center staff are listed at:

http://grants1.nih.gov/grants/funding/phs398/section_2.html#number

Listings of Regular Standing Study Sections and Continuing Special Emphasis Panels (SEPs) are given at:

http://www.csr.nih.gov/Roster_proto/sectionl.asp

At the above Web site, you can also find links to other categories of rosters: Fellowships, SBIR/STTR, and other Study Sections.

Special Emphasis Panels (SEPs) are listed at:

http://era.nih.gov/roster/index.cfm

Interactions with NIH after submission

Applicants are encouraged to contact relevant Institute or Center staff for advice in preparing an Application and for information regarding programmatic areas of interest.

Interactions with NIH after review of a Grant Application

The Web site

http://grants2.nih.gov/grants/funding/phs398/section_2.html

has telephone numbers for all the NIH Institutes and Components and for:

- Agency for Healthcare Research and Quality
- Centers for Disease Control and Prevention
- National Institute for Occupational Safety and Health Procurement and Grants Office
- Food and Drug Administration
- Office of the Assistant Secretary for Health
- Office of Adolescent Pregnancy Programs
- Office of Family Planning
- Agency for Toxic Substances and Disease Registry
- Indian Health Service

NIH Institutes, Centers, and Divisions

A brief description of the mandate and activities of each of the **Institutes and Centers** is given at

> http://www.nih.gov/icd/

The information below is taken from the above Web site.

The **Office of the Director (OD)** is the central office at NIH for its **27 Institutes and Centers**. The OD is responsible for setting policy for NIH and for planning, managing, and coordinating the programs and activities of all the NIH components.

Telephone numbers for the agencies listed in the table below are given near the bottom of the Web site.

> http://grants1.nih.gov/grants/funding/phs398/section_2.html

2-Letter Code	Acronym	Institute	Year Established
Institutes			
CA	NCI	National Cancer Institute	1937
EY	NEI	National Eye Institute	1968
HL	NHLBI	National Heart, Lung, and Blood Institute	1948
HG	NHGRI	National Human Genome Research Institute	1989
AG	NIA	National Institute on Aging	1974
AA	NIAAA	National Institute on Alcohol Abuse and Alcoholism	1970
AI	NIAID	National Institute of Allergy and Infectious Diseases	1948
AR	NIAMS	National Institute of Arthritis and Musculoskeletal and Skin Diseases	1986
EB	NIBIB	National Institute of Biomedical Imaging and Bioengineering	2000
HD	NICHD	National Institute of Child Health and Human Development	1962
DC	NIDCD	National Institute on Deafness and Other Communication Disorders	1988
DE	NIDCR	National Institute of Dental and Craniofacial Research	1948
DK	NIDDK	National Institute of Diabetes and Digestive and Kidney Diseases	1948
DA	NIDA	National Institute on Drug Abuse	1973
ES	NIEHS	National Institute of Environmental Health Sciences	1969
GM	NIGMS	National Institute of General Medical Sciences	1962
MH	NIMH	National Institute of Mental Health	1949
NS	NINDS	National Institute of Neurological Disorders and Stroke	1950
NR	NINR	National Institute of Nursing Research	1986
LM	NLM	National Library of Medicine	1956

2-Letter Code	Acronym	Institute	Year Established
NIH Centers			
CT	CIT	Center for Information Technology (Formerly: Division of Computer Research and Technology 5 DCRT)	1964
RG	CSR	Center for Scientific Review (Formerly: Division of Research Grants 5 DRG)	1946
TW	FIC	John E. Fogarty International Center	1968
AT	NCCAM	National Center for Complementary and Alternative Medicine	1992
MD	NCMHD	National Center on Minority Health and Health Disparities	1993
RR	NCRR	National Center for Research Resources	1962
CC	CC	Warren Grant Magnuson Clinical Center	1953

Center for Scientific Review (CSR) *Review Sections*

The **Review Sections** of the **Referral and Review Branch** of the **Center for Scientific Review** are administrative groupings of **Initial Review Groups** which consist of sub-committees called **Study Sections**. See

http://www.csr.nih.gov/review/irgdesc.htm

and also

http://www.csr.nih.gov/Committees/rosterindex.asp

The CSR Regular Standing Study Section names and SRAs are listed at

http://www.csr.nih.gov/Roster_proto/sectionl.asp

If you click on the NAME of the Study Section, you will go to a list of the topics generally reviewed by that Study Section.

If you click on the [XXX-Roster, where XXX is the abbreviation of the names of the study section] (in blue print, under the name of the Study Section), you will go to a page that has a brief table with the headings:

Study Section / Membership Roster / SRA (E-MAIL) / Meeting Rosters

Click on "View Roster" under "Membership Roster" to see a list of the members of the Study Section, the member's affiliation, and the year each member's term on the Study Section ends. At the bottom of the roster is the date the roster was last updated.

Then click on "Study Section Information" (at the left), and return to

http://www.csr.nih.gov/Committees/rosterindex.asp

and click on "Study Section Information."

In the next window, click on "Study Section Reviewers"

In the window that opens, click on "How Scientists Are Selected For Study Section Service."

This will take you to

http://www.csr.nih.gov/events/studysectionservice.htm

If you want to be considered for service as a Reviewer, go to:

http://www.csr.nih.gov/events/studysectionservice.htm

The U.S. Department of Health and Human Services (DHHS)
200 Independence Avenue, S.W.
Washington, D.C. 20201
Toll Free Tel: 1-877-696-6775
Tel: 202-619-0257

- DHHS is one of the Executive Departments of the Executive Branch of the U.S. government.
- **DHHS is the largest grant-making agency in the Federal Government, providing some 60,000 grants per year.**
- The DHHS's Medicare program is the nation's largest health insurer, handling more than 900 million claims per year.
- In 2003, the DHHS had 65,500 employees and its budget for FY 2003 was $502 billion.

The Agencies that comprise DHHS are:
- Administration for Children and Families (ACF)
- Administration on Aging (AoA)
- Agency for Healthcare Research and Quality (AHRQ)
- Agency for Toxic Substances and Disease Registry (ATSDR)
- Centers for Disease Control and Prevention (CDC)
- Centers for Medicare & Medicaid Services (CMS)
- Food and Drug Administration (Food and Drug Administration)
- Health Resources and Services Administration (HRSA)
- Indian Health Service (IHS)
- **National Institutes of Health (NIH)**
- Program Support Center (PSC)
- Substance Abuse and Mental Health Services Administration (SAMHSA)

> **NOTE:** Although **the Public Health Service (PHS) has been discontinued as an entity,** the agencies that comprised the PHS continue to exist as part of DHHS.

Agencies of the former **Public Health Service (PHS) are:**
- Agency for Healthcare Research and Quality (AHRQ)
- Agency for Toxic Substances and Disease Registry (ATSDR)
- Centers for Disease Control and Prevention (CDC)
- Food and Drug Administration (FDA)
- Health Resources and Services Administration (HRSA)
- Indian Health Service (IHS)
- **National Institutes of Health (NIH)**

- Substance Abuse and Mental Health Services Administration (SAMHSA)

The position of NIH within DHHS is shown at

http://www.os.dhhs.gov/about/orgchart.html

NIH: An Agency of the Department of Health & Human Services
from

http://www.nih.gov/about/almanac/index.html

The National Institutes of Health (NIH), an agency of the United States (U.S.) Department of Health and Human Services, is one of the world's foremost medical research centers and is the steward of medical and behavioral research for the U.S.

The **mission of NIH** is to
- pursue science that increases our fundamental knowledge about the nature and behavior of living systems
- apply that knowledge to extend healthy life and reduce the burdens of illness and disability

The goals of NIH are to:
- **foster fundamental creative discoveries, innovative research strategies, and their Applications to advance the capacity of the U.S. to protect and improve health**
- **develop, maintain, and renew scientific human and physical resources that will assure the nation's capability to prevent disease**
- **expand the knowledge base in medical and associated sciences in order to enhance the nation's economic well-being and ensure a continued high return on the public investment in research**
- **exemplify and promote the highest level of scientific integrity, public accountability, and social responsibility in the conduct of science**

To realize the above goals, NIH provides leadership and direction to programs designed to improve the health of the nation by
- conducting and supporting research in the

—causes, diagnosis, prevention, and cure of human diseases
—processes of human growth and development
—biological effects of environmental contaminants
—understanding of mental, addictive, and physical disorders

and
- **directing programs** for the collection, dissemination, and exchange of information in medicine and health, including the development and support of medical libraries and the training of medical librarians and other health information specialists

Help for minority Applicants to NIH

The Division of Minority Opportunities in Research (MORE) has 3 components:
- Minority Access to Research Careers (MARC)
- Minority Biomedical Research Support (MBRS)
- Special Initiatives

> **NOTE:** Information about the "MORE" program—including "Grant Writing Tips"—can be found at
>
> **http://www.nigms.nih.gov/funding/moregrant_tips.html**

The above Web site has information about
- proposals for the following programs:
  - —MARC U*STAR
  - —MBRS RISE
  - —Bridges to the Baccalaureate Degree
  - —Bridges to the Doctoral Degree Programs
- important steps for preparing a competitive Grant Application

Below are excerpts of advice you will find at the above Web site. It is important that you visit this Web site and check for other information that may be useful and important for you.

Characteristics of a good Grant Application
- Important Steps in Preparing a Competitive Grant Application
- How to Develop a Good Research Plan
- The Grant Application Format and the Sequence of Topics in the Proposal
- Introduction (only for Revised Applications and Supplements)
- Specific Aims/Objectives
- Institutional Background and the Problem (need)
- Rationale for the Strategy (literature review)
- Progress Report (if competing renewal)
- Activity Plan (Research Design and Methods) to Achieve the Objectives
- The Proposed Intervention Activities to Remedy Identified Problems
- The Anticipated Impact of the Activities
- Who Will Implement the Plan?
- Possible Pitfalls and Probable Solutions
- How Are the Participants in the Activity Chosen?
- The Timeline for Implementation
- Evaluation Plan to Determine Program Outcomes
  See:

  http://www.theaps.org/education/promote/promote.html

- Administration of the Program
- Other Elements of the Grant Application
- Title Page (model pages)
- Description of the Project (Abstract)
- Budget (model budget)
- Biographical Sketches of Key Personnel
- Institutional Resources

Most common reasons for failure

- Lack of clear and well-defined measurable objectives
- Incomplete documentation of the need
- Missing or inadequate baseline data
- Activities poorly related to the objectives
- Poorly developed or missing evaluation plan
- Lack of institutional support
- Lack of coordination with other institutional programs aimed at accomplishing similar goals
- Lack of information on intellectual and physical resources available
- Lack of detailed specific schedules for implementation
- Lack of clarity in presentation

Some tips for preparing a good Application

- Write with the Reader in mind; remember that Readers do not simply read, they also interpret.
- Readers form opinions about the proposal from the clues they receive from the organization and emphasis you introduce.
- Information is interpreted more easily and correctly if it is placed in the expected place.
- Don't use jargon or buzz words.
- Include comments to convince the Reader of your convictions in the choice of activities.
- Let the proposal flow logically throughout.
- The Application should be easy to read and comprehend.
- Use simple declarative sentences—but avoid sounding like a first grader.
- Avoid non-precise use of words, poor syntax, and unusual abbreviations. Abbreviations should be defined at first use.

Goals and specific measurable objectives

NOTE: Conducting an activity is not an objective (i.e., organizing a GRE course, research seminars, workshops, science days, tutorials, or other pedagogical methods are not objectives).

What happens to proposals submitted to NIH?

- Scientific Review Administrator (SRA) assigns Reviewers.
- Institute assignment made for potential funding.
  The **MORE** Division has 3 components:
  —Minority Access to Research Careers (**MARC**)
  —Minority Biomedical Research Support (**MBRS**)
  —Special Initiatives.

- Study Section reviews Grant Applications and, after discussion of the Applications, makes recommendations at the Study Section meeting.
- Institute Staff are involved:
  —Program Administrator (also known as the Program Director)
  —Grants Management Specialist
  —National Advisory Council
  —Review Criteria
  —Priority Score
  —Funding Decision
  —Budgetary or Council Issues

MORE Division staff members administer programs in specific states.

http://www.nigms.nih.gov/news/announcements/more_listserv.html

To subscribe to the MORE LISTSERV, send an e-mail message to
LISTSERV@list.nih.gov
leave the subject line blank and, in the body of the message, type:
Subscribe MORECC-L Your Full Name (Program)
Your full name should consist of your first name, middle initial, and last name, followed by Ph.D., M.D., or other title, as appropriate. The program should be listed as MBRS, MARC, Bridges, or any combination of the three. An example of a completed message is: **Subscribe MORECC-L John M. Smith, Ph.D. (MARC).** For more information go to the above Web site or contact:
Dr. Clifton Poodry
Director, MORE Division, NIGMS
Room 2AS.37
45 Center Drive MSC 6200
Bethesda, MD 20892-6200
Tel: (301) 594-3900
Fax: (301) 480-2753
E-mail: poodryc@nigms.nih.gov

Section C of the Grant Application includes the Research Plan.

> **NOTE:** *Your outline should fit the needs of your project—but it must follow the NIH (or other agency) instructions.*

For information that may help you complete an NIH R01 Application, go to the Web sites listed below:

http://www.grants.nih.gov/grants/funding/phs398/section_1.html#8_research

http://www.niaid.nih.gov/ncn/grants/app/app.pdf

http://www.niaid.nih.gov/ncn/grants/app/default.htm

> **IMPORTANT:** NIH suggests that potential investigators bookmark
> **http://grants1.nih.gov/grants/funding/phs398/phs398.html#updates**
> and **ALWAYS check this site** for updated instructions and policy information **prior to submission of Applications.**

NIH also reminds Applicants to:

- Follow the type size and format specifications **or the Application will be designated as incomplete and will be returned** to the Applicant Organization **without peer review.**
- Prepare a succinct Research Plan. There is no requirement for Applicants to use the maximum allowable pages allotted to the Research Plan (Items a–d).
- Be cognizant of the required education about protection of human research subjects. Information about protection of human research subjects must be submitted prior to award. See

> **http://grants.nih.gov/grants/guide/notice-files/NOT-OD-00-039.html.**

Where can you find a good Grant Application?

It is not easy to find an example of a well-written NIH Grant Application. It's a good idea to ask colleagues who have been funded consistently for a decade or more if they might let you read their funded Application. If you cannot find a good model Application via a colleague, go to

> **http://www.niaid.nih.gov/ncn/grants/app/default.htm**

There you will find an Annotated R01 Grant Application to NIAID, which the NIH calls "an outstanding basic science Application" that Dr. Mark Smeltzer wrote as a new investigator in 1998. **Be aware that the Application is copyrighted. It may be used for nonprofit educational purposes provided the document remains unchanged and both Dr. Smeltzer and NIAID are credited.**

According to the above Web site, Dr. Smeltzer's Application appears as he submitted it to NIH except for changes NIH made to some forms to reflect PHS 398 version 5/01. For example, NIH (a) changed the budget request to a modular budget and (b) added annotations to explain how this Application reflects much of the advice that NIH give in their "All About Grants" Web tutorials. It should be noted that all the advice given is the opinion of NIAID staff scientists and should be taken as their advice only. Differing opinions may exist, including those of NIH peer reviewers.

A tutorial about how to write a Grant Application can be found at

> **http://www.niaid.nih.gov/ncn/grants/write/write.pdf**

The Web site

> **http://www.ninds.nih.gov/funding/write_grant_doc.htm**

has a lot of good advice about the topics listed below:

- How to Write a Research Project Grant Application
- Strategies for Getting an NIH Grant

- Writing an Application for a Research Project Grant
- Application Contents
- Developing Your Research Plan
- Writing and Formatting the Application
- Submitting Your Grant Application
- Problems and Concerns Commonly Cited by Reviewers
- Referral and Assignment of the Application
- Review of a Research Project Application
- How Funding Is Decided
- What to do when You Do Not Obtain Funding
- What to do when Your Application Is Approved for Funding
- Common Mistakes PIs make in their NIH Applications
- Writing a Grant Application: A "Technical" Checklist

A SAMPLE FORMAT for the "Table of Contents" for an NIH Grant Application is given at

http://www.nia.nih.gov/funding/researchsupport/P01GuideAttach.pdf

---

SPECIFIC INSTRUCTIONS FOR PREPARING THE RESEARCH PLAN

http://grants2.nih.gov/grants/funding/phs398/phs398.html

PHS 398 (REVISED May 2001) - Updated: 09/09/2003
See the 08/29/2003 NIH Guide Notice for information on the Update of the PHS 398 and PHS 2590 forms.
As stated earlier, there is **no Form Page for the Research Plan**.
The Research Plan should
- include sufficient information needed for evaluation of the project, independent of any other document
- be clear, specific, informative, and concise
- try to present the basic concepts and key ideas for your proposal as non-technical as possible
- try to anticipate questions that Reviewers might have about the project and supply the necessary information to answer these questions
- avoid redundancies
- be organized so that Parts a-d of the Research Plan answer the following 4 questions:
  —What do **you** intend to do?
  —Why is the work important?
  —What has already been done?
  —How are you going to do the work?

The Abstract
- Your Abstract must fit into the box/space provided using an allowable font style and size that is easy to read.

- The Abstract should be a succinct and accurate description of the work proposed in your Application which is comprehensible when separated from the rest of the Application.
- State the **broad, long-term objectives** of your project.
- State the **Specific Aims** in the form of hypotheses to be tested or objectives to be achieved.
- If appropriate, state the **Health-Relatedness** of the project.
- Describe the **Research Design and Methods** that will be used to achieve the Specific Aims/Objectives.
- State the **importance of the research.**
- Point out in what ways the research is **innovative.**
- Use language that can easily be understood by a broad audience.
- **Avoid summaries of past accomplishments.**
- **Do NOT use the first person.** This stricture applies only to the Abstract!
- Do NOT include any confidential or proprietary information in the Abstract. If your Application is funded, the Abstract will become public information.

Introduction

An Introduction is required only for

- Revisions (3 pages maximum)

or

- Supplements (1 page maximum)
    1. **Summary of substantial additions, deletions, and changes. (Highlight changes by brackets, indents, or change of type style.)**
        a. Addition: Page y, ¶x describes ...
        b. Addition: Page v, ¶w describes ...
        c. Deletion: Page x, ¶z has been deleted because ...
        d. Change: Page m, ¶n has been changed to reflect ...
    2. Responses to criticisms in previous Summary Statement
        a. Response to pink sheet ¶x
        b. Response to pink sheet ¶y
    3. Work done since prior version of Application was submitted (Describe experiments and results)
        a. Set of experiments # 1: completed since prior submission
        b. Set of experiments # 2: begun since prior submission

Research Plan

- **Maximum of 25 pages total for Parts a–d of the Research Plan.**
- All tables, graphs, figures, diagrams, and charts must be included WITHIN the 25-page limit.
- **NIH recommends how to apportion the space among the sub-sections. Unless there is a good reason not to follow the NIH recommendations, it is probably wise to use the suggested page distribution.**
- **NIH (a) encourages Applicants to be succinct and (b) reminds Applicants that it is not necessary to use all 25-pages allotted to Parts a–d of the Research Plan.**
- **NIH warns Applicants that the 25-page limit is strictly enforced. Applications that exceed this limit or do not conform to the type size limitations (spelled out**

at the NIH Web site) **will constitute grounds for the PHS to return the Application without review.**

A. Specific Aims:

1 page recommended by NIH

- **First:** state the **Broad, Long-term Objective(s)** of the proposal. The Broad, Long-term Objectives are sort of the "carrot at the end of a stick." It represents where you are heading—what you expect to accomplish in one or more project periods (perhaps 6 to 10 years).
- **Then,** for **EACH** Specific Aim:
    i.   Specific Aim 1
    ii. Specific Aim 2
    iii. Specific Aim 3
    state what the research proposed in this Specific Aim is intended to accomplish; e.g.,
    —test a stated hypothesis
    —create a novel design
    —solve a specific problem
    —develop a new technology

B. Background and Significance:

2–3 pages recommended by NIH

Address each of the 4 items listed below. "Background," will generally be the longest part of this section, but it is the **least important from the perspective of the Reviewer's ability to judge your quality as a scientist.** Any bright high school student can probably write a good Background section given enough time in the library. It takes the knowledge and experience of a good scientist in the field to **evaluate** the existing knowledge!

- Background

    Throughout the Background section, you should cite **pertinent** references and list them in the Bibliography, "Section 9: Literature Cited."

- **Critically evaluate** the existing knowledge in the field.
- Discuss the **gaps in current knowledge** that this project is intended to fill
- **Explain the importance of the research** by relating the Specific Aims to the Broad, Long-term Objectives and to the Health Relevance, e.g.,

    —Specific Aim 1 will . . . toward the Broad, long-term objectives. The Health Relevance of this Specific Aim is ...
    —Specific Aim 2 will . . . toward the Broad, long-term objectives. The Health Relevance of this Specific Aim is ...
    —Specific Aim 3 will . . . toward the Broad, long-term objectives. The Health Relevance of this Specific Aim is ...

*Keep in mind that "NIH" stands for the "National Institutes of **HEALTH**" and that the mandate of the agency is to improve the health of the people of the United States. Thus, it is good if you have a "Health Relevance." However, do not "manufacture" a Health Relevance for your project if there really is none. But if there is no Health Relevance, you should seriously consider whether NIH is the right agency to which to submit your Application! It pays to call and determine whether the agency is interested in your project before you begin work on the Application.*

C. **Progress Report/Preliminary Studies:**

6–8 pages recommended by NIH for the narrative portion of this section of the Application.

(i) Progress Report for Competing Continuation and Supplemental Applications:

- A "Progress Report" is required for

  —**competing continuation** Applications

  and for

  —**supplemental** Applications

If the competing continuation or supplemental Application involves **clinical research,** then you must report on the enrollment of research subjects and their distribution by ethnicity/race and sex/gender. Use the "5/01 Inclusion Enrollment Report" (MS Word or PDF) to provide this information for each relevant funded study and for each relevant study that will be continued. **If the Application contains more than one study, provide a separate table for each study.** Also report on any sub-populations as an attachment to the table. If, during the previous project period, information on ethnicity/race and sex/gender was collected using an earlier NIH reporting format involving a single-question format to capture both ethnicity and race, then the former "4/98 Version of the Inclusion Table" (MS Word or PDF) may be used in the Progress Report section. **Tables on inclusion will not be counted in the Research Plan page limitation.** For more detailed instructions on using the 5/01 Inclusion Enrollment Report and the 4/98 Version of the Inclusion Table, see

http://grants.nih.gov/grants/guide/notice-files/NOT-OD-01-053.html

- Provide the beginning and ending dates for the period covered since the project was last reviewed competitively.
- Summarize the Specific Aims of the previous Application and give a **succinct account of published and unpublished results,** indicating progress toward the achievement of each Specific Aim.
  - —Include small but readable and well-labeled figures, tables, and copies of photos; provide original full-size photos in the Appendix.
  - —Cite your own publications in the text, and list them in the appropriate section at the end of the Progress Report.
- Discuss briefly the **importance of each finding.**

Write the Progress Report in a format such as the following:

(1) Specific Aim (SA) 1 (from the previous Application)

   (a) Summary of SA 1 (from previous Application)

   (b) Progress toward achievement of SA 1 (from previous Application)

   (c) Importance of findings related to achievement of SA 1 (from previous Application)

(2) Specific Aim (SA) 2 (from the previous Application)

   (a) Summary of SA 2 (from previous Application)

   (b) Progress toward achievement of SA 2 (from previous Application)

   (c) Importance of findings related to achievement of SA 2 (from previous Application)

(3) Repeat the above for each SA listed in the original Application

(4) Discuss any changes in Specific Aims since the project was last reviewed competitively and provide a rationale for the change

- List the **titles and complete references** to all

—Publications
—Manuscripts **accepted** for publication
—Patents
—Other printed materials that have resulted from the project since it was last reviewed competitively
List the above as follows:
- (1) Published materials
    - (a) Original research reports
        - (i)   Hokum, J. and Pokum, L., ...1995
        - (ii) Hokum, J. and Pokum, L., ...1994
        - (iii) Hokum, J. and Pokum, L., ...1993
    - (b) Review articles
    - (c) Books
    - (d) Abstracts
- (2) Manuscripts accepted for publication
    - (a) Original research reports
    - (b) Review articles
    - (c) Books
    - (d) Abstracts
- (3) Patents
- (4) Invention reports
- (5) Other printed materials
    - **—Reprints of up to 10 of the publications listed above may be included in the 5 collated sets of Appendices.**

NOTE: The **publications** portion of the Competing Continuation and Supplemental Applications Progress Report **is NOT considered as part of the 25-page limit.**
Personnel Report: Do not submit the Personnel Report **with** the **Application.**

When the Personnel Report is requested by the awarding component, use the Personnel Report Form Page.

(ii) New Applications:

- For **NEW Applications,** a "Preliminary Studies" section is required in place of the "Progress Report."

  For new Applications, use the Preliminary Studies section to provide

  —an account of the Principal Investigator/Program Director's **preliminary studies pertinent to the Application**
  and
  —**information** that will help to establish the
  > **EXPERIENCE**
  > **and**
  > **COMPETENCE**

  of the investigator **to pursue the proposed project.**
- Include preliminary data you have obtained. Present such data in the form of small but readable and well-labeled figures, tables, and copies of photos; provide original full-size photos in the Appendix.

—Cite, in the text, any **pertinent publications** you have, and list them in the appropriate section at the end of the Preliminary Studies section.

Peer review committees generally view preliminary data as an essential part of a Research Grant Application. Preliminary data often help the Reviewers assess the likelihood of the success of the proposed project.

D. Research Design and Methods:

13–16 pages recommended by NIH (keep in mind that the maximum length of the first 4 Sections of the Research Plan a–d must not exceed 25 pages)

Cite pertinent references in this section, and include them in the bibliography section (Literature Cited).

If there is an overall Research Design for the total project, describe it at the beginning of this section. Then describe the Research Design and Methods for each Specific Aim as indicated below.

Research Design to accomplish Specific Aim 1

- Procedures (Methods) to carry out the Research Design for Specific Aim **1**.
- Include all pertinent **control experiments** for all procedures.
- Means by which data will be
  —Collected
  —Analyzed
  —**Interpreted**
- For any new methodologies: Explain **advantage(s)** over existing methodologies.
- Discuss **potential limitations and difficulties** of proposed procedures.
- Discuss **alternative approaches** to achieve the aim.

Research Design to accomplish Specific Aim 2

- Procedures (Methods) to carry out the Research Design for Specific Aim **2**.
- Include all pertinent **control experiments** for all procedures.
- Means by which data will be
  —Collected
  —Analyzed
  —Interpreted
- For any new methodologies: Explain **advantage(s)** over existing methodologies.
- Discuss **potential limitations and difficulties** of proposed procedures.
- Discuss **alternative approaches** to achieve the aim.

Repeat the bulleted items above for each Specific Aim.

NOTE: In some proposals it may be more appropriate to discuss some of these items together for two or more Specific Aims. The decision should be made on the basis of, first, clarity and, second, brevity. General procedures (Methods) that apply to more than one Research Design should be grouped together under the heading "General procedures (Methods)," described once (rather than being repeated), placed at the end of the "Research Design and Methods" section, and referred to as necessary.

- Give a tentative sequence or timetable for the studies. (Be brief. The Reviewers want to know that you have planned the project carefully and that you know what you are doing. They do NOT want to know at what time you plan to take a coffee break!!!)
- Point out procedures, situations, or materials that may be hazardous to personnel. For each case, specify the precautions to be exercised.

E. Human Subjects Research

For guidance in determining whether the proposed research involves Human Subjects Research as defined in part A of the human subjects regulations (45 CFR 46), use the decision charts on OHRP's Web site

http://ohrp.osophs.dhhs.gov/humansubjects/guidance/decisioncharts.htm

If you marked "Yes" for Item 4, "Human Subjects," on the Face Page of the Application, create a section heading entitled, "Human Subjects Research" immediately following the last entry in the Research Design and Methods section. There is no specific page limit for the "Human Subjects" section of the Application, but try to be succinct.

You will need to discuss inclusion of women, minorities, and children among other items. For additional information/instructions, go to:

http://www.grants.nih.gov/grants/funding/phs398/section_1.html#8_research

F. Vertebrate Animals

"Animals" are defined as any live, vertebrate animal used or intended for use in:
- Research
- Research training
- Experimentation
- Biological testing
- Any related purposes

The **Policy about Humane Care and Use of Laboratory Animals** requires that Applicant organization(s) that propose to use vertebrate animals, file a **written** Animal Welfare Assurance with the Office for Laboratory Animal Welfare (OLAW), establishing appropriate policies and procedures to ensure the humane care and use of live vertebrate animals involved in research activities supported by NIH.

Institutions are required to comply with the Animal Welfare Act as amended (7 USC 2131 et sec.) and other Federal statutes and regulations relating to animals.

These documents are available from the Office for Laboratory Animal Welfare, National Institutes of Health, Bethesda, MD 20892, (301) 496-7163.

No award to an individual will be made unless that individual is affiliated with an assured organization that accepts responsibility for compliance with the PHS policy for humane care and use of animals.

Foreign Applicant organizations applying for PHS awards for activities involving vertebrate animals are also required to comply with policy or provide evidence that acceptable standards for the humane care and use of animals will be met.

Tutorial: "How to Write An Application Involving Research Animals"

The National Institute of Allergy and Infectious Diseases (NIAID) and the Office of Laboratory Animal Welfare (OLAW) have developed a Web tutorial that provides a step-by-step guide to the preparation of an Application and covers such topics as

- considering alternatives
- obtaining assurances and IACUC approval
- just in time processes
- NIH review of animal subjects Applications
- grant awards
- IACUC monitoring of awards
- reporting requirements

Although the tutorial is designed specifically for NIAID Applicants, the information is relevant to investigators submitting Applications to the NIH for activities involving animals. The tutorial is available at

http://www.niaid.nih.gov/ncn/clinical/researchanimals/tutorial/index.htm

G. **Consultants**
   Provide letters and Biosketches for each such person; place the letters in this subsection. *The letters from Consultants should contain specific and substantive information about the role the Consultants and/or Collaborators will play in the project.*

H. **Consortium/Contractual agreements**
   See the NIH instructions.

I. **Literature Cited**
   - There is **no page limit** for this section but check the NIH Web site for possible changes.
   - Refer to the literature thoroughly and thoughtfully. Choose wisely!
   - The publication list need not be exhaustive. NIH suggests, "less than 100 of the most relevant citations."
   - List all publications that support your hypothesis and methods.
   - If there are alternative points of view about your subject matter, show Reviewers that you are knowledgeable about these and that you are an unbiased but discerning person by referencing them if appropriate.
   - Use a consistent format. Each citation must have—in the same order:
     —the names of ALL authors (do NOT use "*et al.*")
     —complete title of book or journal
     —volume number
     —page numbers (first AND last page)
     —year of publication

Citations show Reviewers your breadth of knowledge of your field. Research proposals do not fare well when Applicants fail to reference relevant published research, particularly if it indicates that the proposed approach has already been attempted or the methods were found to be inappropriate for answering the questions posed.

WHAT TO PUT INTO THE APPENDIX

Appendix
- Does your Application have the necessary Appendices?
- Does your Appendix include a table of contents?

- Are all the manuscripts that you have listed in the Appendix either published or in press?
- NOTE: Manuscripts that are "In preparation" or have been submitted but have not yet been accepted for publication may NOT be listed.
- Each manuscript listed should clearly indicate whether it is "In press" or has already been published.
- Specify how many manuscripts are provided in the Appendix. There is a limit of 10 unless otherwise specified in the RFA or PA.
- Are images, photos, graphs, etc., that are provided in the Appendix, also included—in reduced form—in the Research Plan?
- If hard-to-copy or color images or photos are included in the Research Plan, are the originals provided in the Appendix?

NOTE: **Do not use the Appendix to circumvent the page limitations of the Research Plan.** Graphs, diagrams, tables, and charts that do not need to be in a glossy format to show details must not be included in the Appendix. **An Application that does not observe these limitations will be returned.** These Appendix limitations may not apply to specialized Grant Applications. Request and follow the additional instructions for those Applications.

NOTE: The Appendix will not be duplicated with the Application and will usually be sent only to certain members of the SRG who will serve as the Primary Reviewers of the Application.

SAMPLE BUDGET JUSTIFICATIONS

You may or may not be required to submit a Budget and Budget Justification as part of a Grant Application. At NIH, with its modular budgets for more modest financial requests, a Budget and Budget Justification are required only if you are requesting funds greater than $250,000 **per year**. However, wise proposal-writers will prepare a carefully thought-out budget for themselves to get a fairly accurate idea about how many modules to request.

Thinking through a Budget **Justification** is also a good exercise to justify to yourself that you are actually requesting an amount of funding that will be appropriate and sufficient to carry out your project. Thus, despite the seeming expedience of Modular budgets for many NIH Grant Applications, savvy proposal-writers realize that

- Modular Budgets are intended to save the Reviewers' time
- **Modular Budgets don't really save the PI much time**
- It does take somewhat less time to create an **informal** Budget and Budget Justification for your own needs than to write a carefully crafted **formal** Budget and Budget Justification.

This Appendix contains excerpts from Budget Justifications from 2 actual grant Applications. Example B is from a proposal that the Reviewers considered to be "an extremely well-written grant proposal." I have taken the liberty of making a few minor changes to improve the text.

Keep in mind that the examples of Budget Justifications shown here are not the only way to write a Budget Justification. But they serve to illustrate a format that I considered effective after listening to about 600 budget discussions (3 meetings per year for 2 years with about 100 proposals per meeting = 600!) during the time I was a member of an NIH Study Section.

Also, be aware that rules and procedures at NIH and other funding agencies change periodically. Thus, you should use the information in this Appendix (as in the other parts of this book!) only as a guide. ALWAYS read and respond to the MOST CURRENT IN-STRUCTIONS of the agency to which you plan to apply!

In the "mock" Budget Justifications given below, please be aware that I have used letters arbitrarily to represent numbers (amounts); please do **NOT** assume, for example, that $X always stands for the same specific numeral/number of dollars.

BUDGET JUSTIFICATION: EXAMPLE A

(1) **Personnel** $XYZ,ZYX

   (a) Dr. Jones, Principal Investigator (salary + fringe) $XY,XYZ

   Dr. Jones has planned this project, including the specific experiments to be carried out. He will be responsible for managing the project and for analyzing and interpreting the data with the help of Dr. Smith. He and Dr. Smith will jointly develop manuscripts for publication as is warranted. Dr. Jones has specific expertise in .... He will spend 100% of his time on this project year round. He has a long track record in the field of . . . .

   (b) Dr. Smith, Investigator (salary + fringe) $AB,CDE

   Dr. Smith is an established investigator in the field of . . ., and will provide the "hands on" experience for the . . . aspects of the project. She will be responsible for carrying out the XYZ experiments described in the methods section of the proposal. This project requires a person with the expertise and competence of Dr. Smith for successful completion of these experiments, which are described on page X. Dr. Smith has been with the University of ABC for 6 years and has collaborated with Dr. Jones for the last 3 years. They have been a very successful team and have published 11 papers in peer-reviewed journals during their collaboration. Dr. Smith's salary is based on $45,800 for full time. She has a three-quarter-time appointment at the university during the academic year and plans to devote 75% of her time to this research project. ($3/4 \times 9/12 = 0.56 \times 0.75 = 0.42 \times \$45,800 = \$19,236$). During the 3 summer months, she will work full time at the university and devote 100% of her time to this project. ($1.0 \times 3/12 = 0.25 \times 1.0 = 0.25 \times \$45,800 = \$11,450$). Fringe benefits have been calculated at 30%.

   (c) Mr. West, Research Assistant (salary + fringe) $FG,HIJ

   Mr. West will devote 100% effort to this project year-round. He has been working with Dr. Jones for the last 9 years and has developed unique expertise in the field of .... Mr. West has been a co-author on 15 publications during his time in Dr. Jones's laboratory. His full-time effort is essential for carrying out the experiments on ..., which are an integral part of the total research project.

(d) Technician (To be named) (salary + fringe) $KL,MNP

In addition to Mr. West, the research assistant, a medium level technician is essential for carrying out this project. The laboratory currently does not have a technician in this category. We intend to hire someone with a B.A. degree who has extensive experience in carrying out the experiments described on pp. X–Y of this proposal. We will specifically look for a person who has had hands-on experience working with a system similar to the one in which we propose to work in this project.

(2) Consultant Costs $0

Dr. Northstar, consultant, is a full professor at the University of . . . , department of . . . . She is a nationally known expert in . . . and is currently writing a book on this subject. She has agreed to be a consultant at no charge for the part of the project dealing with . . . . She will advise on . . . , and will also provide help with data analysis (see letter in "consultants" **Section** of the Research Plan).

(3) Equipment $XXX

(a) Zeiss microscope, model XYZ $ZZZ

We have been using a microscope that belongs to Dr. M in the department of . . . . Dr. M will be leaving the University of . . . at about the time that this project is scheduled to begin if it is funded. Dr. M will take his microscope with him to the University of . . . . Because a good-quality microscope is essential to carrying out this research project, we are requesting $ZZZ to purchase a model XYZ Zeiss microscope.

(b) Diamond knife $YY

Dr M. will be taking his diamond knife with him when he leaves this department. Therefore, we are requesting $YY to purchase a diamond knife for cutting thin sections for these experiments.

(c) Embedding oven $Z

We have been using Dr. M's embedding oven. He has received permission to take the oven to the University of . . . when he moves there next semester. We are therefore requesting $Z to purchase an embedding oven.

(4) Supplies $ZZZ

(a) Rats (including maintenance) $ZZZ
    etc.

BUDGET JUSTIFICATION: EXAMPLE B

This Budget Justification is from a grant proposal that Reviewers considered to be "an extremely well-written grant proposal." Example B in Appendix V is the Summary Statement for this proposal.

(1) Personnel $XX

    (a) PI $YY

    See justification under "Collaborating Investigator"

    (b) Collaborating Investigator $ZZ

    Dr. A and Dr. B have planned this project and will, for the most part, plan the specific experiments to be carried out. We will be entirely responsible for analyzing and interpreting the biochemical data; we will also plan the morphological experiments, but because neither of us have "hands-on" experience in this area, the work will of necessity be done by someone experienced in morphological techniques and the anatomy of the . . . .

    (b) Research Associate (To be named) $Z

    This is the person who will provide the "hands-on" experience and will (with the help of the research assistant) be responsible for carrying out all the morphological aspects of the experiments described in the "Methods" section of the proposal. This project cannot be carried out without a morphologist of this level of competence and someone to help with the more routine aspects of the lengthy experimental work-up. A search cannot be initiated for this individual unless and until funding is obtained. The Research Associate would be responsible for carrying out and helping to interpret the morphological experiments. This individual will have to be experienced in both light and electron microscopy and must be familiar with anatomy in particular. He/she should have had 3 or more years of postdoctoral experience in morphology.

    (c) Research Assistant $X

    The Research Assistant, Mr. X, will assist with both the morphological and biochemical experiments. He is familiar with tissue work-up, sectioning, and photographic techniques. He will also assist with handling of animals, as well as the more routine aspects of the biochemical assays. He will be primarily responsible to the Research Associate morphologist, and also help the PI and Co-investigator set up certain experiments and run the necessary assays.

(2) Consultant $0

Dr. X at the XYZ Hospital, Department of . . . is a known expert in . . . and is currently finishing a chapter on this subject. He has agreed to be a consultant, at no charge, and will also provide materials from . . . , as they become available (see letter in "consultants" **Section** of the Research Plan). In addition, he will help us procure such material from other sources.

(3) Equipment $XXX

    (a) Zeiss microscope $YYY

    See justification under "Diamond knife"

    (b) Diamond knife $ZZZ

The Morphology Unit at X is a well equipped, but heavily used facility. Most equipment necessary to carry out this project is available through the Z-Unit; however, Dr. Y, the Unit head, has indicated that because of the heavy use required for carrying out this project, a separate light microscope and diamond knife will be essential for our work. Fluorescence optics will be necessary for the . . . experiments to localize and quantify various . . ., e.g., ... We estimate that both the Research Associate Morphologist and the Research Assistant will use this microscope substantially on a daily basis. In addition, it will be used frequently by the PI and Collaborating Investigator to review the results of experiments and discuss the interpretations with the Research Associate morphologist.

(c) Embedding oven $X

Although embedding ovens are available in the Morphology Unit, we have been advised by the Unit to have our own for the purposes of optimal curing of plastic sections.

(d) Supplies $YY

(e) Animals $ZZ

A full-time Morphologist with a full-time Research Assistant will be able to carry out 2 experiments (each having 10– to 12– morphological samples and an equivalent number of biochemical samples)/week, for 3 weeks of every month. The 4th week will be used to record and assess the results, including taking and processing photographs. We are thus calculating costs on the basis of 38 weeks for experiments, taking into account 3 weeks vacation time/year.

(i) Eggs $A

We estimate 2.5 dozen eggs/week at $X/dozen plus $Y delivery charge = $Z/week. With X% inflation by the beginning of the project period, this cost would be $A for the first year of the project.

(ii) Other Animals $B

The second experiment each week will involve bovine . . . half of the time, and in vitro experiments in newborn and young rats during the remaining weeks.

- Cow organs $38XY
  The current price of . . . is $X each. We anticipate using Y per week for 38 weeks of the year. $X \times Y \times 38 = \$38XY$

- Rats (Cost and care) $D
  Current price of one litter of rats (newborn) = $X. We project $Y by the beginning of the project period. One litter/week for Y weeks = $Z. Animal room charge for maintenance of one cage of rats at $X/year/cage = $YY. Total for rats and care = $ZZ.

(f) Medium and serum $XX

  (i) Medium $YZ
       We estimate a total of . . . chick embryo organ cultures/week to obtain the requisite number of morphological and biochemical samples. These samples
       require 20 mL of medium/flask, i.e., one 500-mL bottle of medium/week. (. . . will be maintained in
       reusable glass flasks and will require only . . . mL
       of medium.) We project the cost of medium will be
       $Y/bottle by the beginning of the project period.
       $Y × Z weeks = $YZ.

  (ii) Serum $12X
       Fetal calf serum, essential for the maintenance of
       chick embryo in culture, is $X/100 mL bottle. We
       estimate 12 bottles/year.
       $X × 12 = $12X.

(g) Chemicals, glassware, plastic-ware $XXX

  (i) Chemicals $YY
       Antibiotics, buffers, assay reagents for biochemical experiments, radioactive precursors for uptake
       and incorporation studies, etc. We estimate $YY.

  (ii) Plastic flasks $912X
       We have found ABC flasks to be optimal for cultures: 24 flasks/week at $X/flask for 38 weeks =
       $912X.

  (iii) Counting vials and scintillation fluid $ZZ
       The project will require approximately X incorporation and uptake studies. We estimate $ZZ in
       this category.

(h) Microscopy supplies $XX

  (i) Dissecting instruments $Y
       Microdissecting scissors cost approximately $X.
       We estimate $Y in this category.

  (ii) Fixatives $Z
       Glutaraldehyde, paraformaldehyde, osmium tetroxide, dehydrating agents, embedding compounds,
       and stains for light microscopy. We estimate $Z.

  (iii) Other supplies $Y
       This category includes grids, grid holders, and stains
       for electron microscopy and embedding molds, disposable beakers, disposable gloves, slides, cover
       slips, and vials required for light microscopy.

(i) Photo supplies $ZZZ

  (i) Black and white film $XX
       2 rolls/experiment, $Y/roll,
       2 experiments/week × 38 weeks = $XX.

(ii) Color slides $YY
1 roll/week × $Y/roll for film and processing ×
38 weeks = $YY

(iii) Paper for printing black and white photos $X
We plan to use multigrade resin paper, 50 sheets/
experiment (including test sheets).
2 experiments/week = 100 sheets/week. $Y/100
sheets × 38 weeks = $38Y.

(iv) Photochemicals $Z
For processing black and white film and prints. We
estimate $Z/year.

(5) Travel $XX

Because of the nature of the proposed work, which involves ... as a
model of . . . , it will be important for the Research Associate to go to
both the . . . meeting and the . . . meeting. In addition, it will be important for the PI to attend conferences specifically concerned with the
latest development on . . . once a year to keep up with both the clinical and research areas related to this disease. In November, 20XX, a
_____ symposium took place in _____. Another _____ Symposium is
scheduled in early 20YY (see _____ Newsletter, Vol. X, No. Y, page Z,
Sept. 20XX).

The total figure for travel is based on $ZZ for this year's _____ travel
budget. (This figure was arrived at by the _____ Committee at _____,
calculated on the basis of budget airfares and double room occupancy.)
Assuming similar costs for the other 2 meetings, in the same geographic
area, and allowing a small increment for inflation, we are estimating
$XX in the travel category for the first year.

(6) Other expenses $YYY

(a) Publication costs $YZY
These include drafting, photography, photocopy charges, etc.
Publications resulting from this project will of necessity involve
numerous photographic plates. The current page charge for half
tones, for example, in the *Journal of XYZ* is $XY/page for short
papers and $XZ/page for longer papers. 300 reprints for a 6-page
article will cost at least $ZYX. We estimate at least one major
publication/year:

(i)   Drafting $ X
(ii)   Photographs $ Y
(iii) Page charges (6 × $Z) $ 6Z
(iv)   Reprints (500) $ YY
       Total Publication Costs   **$YZY**

(b) Users' fee for the Morphology Unit $XXX
Because of increased expenses and decreased funding, the
Morphology Unit at . . . has instituted a $Z-per-hour "use fee" for
all users.

The items included in the user's fee do not cover any supplies requested in the above budget; the user's fee does include service contracts, use of available instruments, liquid nitrogen, etc. The requested amount is based on 20 hours of use/week.

(7) **Budget for subsequent years**

   (a) Each category is increased by X% per year to account for inflation.

   (b) No additional equipment is requested in years 02 and 03.

   (c) "Other Expenses" is increased by $YYY in year 03 for sharpening the diamond knife.

■ APPENDIX IV ■

ABOUT GRANT APPLICATIONS TO THE NATIONAL SCIENCE FOUNDATION (NSF)

INFORMATION ABOUT NSF

National Science Foundation (NSF)

National Science Foundation
4201 Wilson Blvd.
Arlington, VA 22230
Tel: 703-292-5111
NSF Division of Grants and Agreements: 703-292-8210
Assistance with FastLane: e-mail: fastlane-comments@nsf.gov
Office of Grants & Contracts: 202-357-7880

> **NOTE:** A new version of the NSF Grant Proposal Guide (GPG) (NSF 04-2) was made available in 2003 and has been effective for proposals submitted on or after October 1, 2003. GPG-NSF 04-2 supercedes all prior versions of the GPG. See
>
> **http://www.nsf.gov/pubs/2004/nsf042/faqs04_2.pdf**

On February 22, 2004, Arden L. Bement, Jr. became Acting Director of the National Science Foundation. He joins NSF from the National Institute of Standards and Technology (NIST), where he had been director since December 2001. Prior to his appointment as NIST director, Bement served as the David A. Ross Distinguished Professor of Nuclear Engineering and head of the School of Nuclear Engineering at Purdue University.

To access NSF publications, go to

http://www.nsf.gov/home/menus/publications.htm

More about NSF

Reproduced below is the "Preface" from Draft 3.1 (NSB-03-70), June 5, 2003 of the NSF GPRA (Government Performance and Results Act of 1993) Strategic Plan for FY 2003–2008. To access the entire draft document, go to

http://www.nsf.gov/od/stratplan_03-08/draft-stratplan.htm

scroll to the bottom and click on either
[Adobe Acrobat PDF]
or
[Microsoft Word document]

The role of NSF

Created in 1950, NSF is an independent U.S. government agency responsible for advancing science and engineering (S&E) in the United States across a broad and expanding frontier. NSF plays a critical role in supporting
- fundamental research
- education
- infrastructure

at colleges, universities, and other institutions throughout the country. Although NSF represents about 4% of the total Federal budget for research and development, it accounts for approximately 20% of all Federal support for basic research and 40% of non-life-science basic research at U.S. academic institutions. NSF's broad support for basic research, particularly at U.S. academic institutions, provides not only a key source of funds for discovery in many fields, but also unique stewardship in developing the next generation of scientists and engineers. NSF is also the principal Federal agency charged with promoting **science and engineering education** at all levels and in all settings, from pre-kindergarten through career development. This helps ensure that the United States has world-class scientists, mathematicians, and engineers, and well-prepared citizens.

Except for the South Pole Station and the other Antarctic Program facilities, NSF operates no laboratories or research facilities itself. NSF carries out its mission primarily by making merit-based Grants and Cooperative Agreements to individual researchers and groups, in partnership with colleges, universities, and other institutions—public, private, state, local, and Federal—throughout the United States. NSF uses merit review to select about 10,000 new awards each year from more than 32,000 competitive proposals submitted by the science and engineering research and education communities.

NSF works with its partner institutions and organizations to chart new paths for science and engineering research and education. For example, NSF fosters strategic collaborations with key national and international counterparts that address national and global science and engineering priorities. NSF has been designated to lead interagency initiatives in such areas as information technology research and nanotechnology.

The **National Science Board** (NSB) is NSF's policymaking board and serves as **adviser to the President and Congress on policy matters related to science and engineering research and education.** The Board is composed of 24 part-time members, who are appointed by the President and confirmed by the Senate. They are selected on the basis of their eminence in science, engineering, education, and public affairs.

National Science Foundation (NSF) Awards
See the two Web sites below

http://nsf.gov
http://nsf.gov/home/grants.htm

The NSF funds research and education in science and engineering, via
- grants
- contracts
- cooperative agreements

The NSF accounts for about 20% of Federal support to academic institutions for basic research.

To receive e-mail or Internet alerts of new program announcements, go to the NSF Web site or subscribe to the NSF Custom News Service at

http://www.nsf.gov/home/cns/

A list of recent awards made by NSF may be seen via FastLane at

http://www.fastlane.nsf.gov/servlet/A6RecentWeeks

For case-specific help with policy and procedural questions related to an award that **YOU have received,** contact:
- your Sponsored Programs Office
- the NSF grants official identified in your award letter
- NSF Division of Grants and Agreements (Tel: 703-292-8210)

The Policy Office, in the NSF Division of Grants and Agreements, provides general policy guidance for proposers and for awardees. The Policy Office page includes NSF regulations, other Federal regulations, notices of important policies, and other information for proposers and awardees.

Since October 1, 2000, all proposals to NSF must be submitted using FastLane. For guidance on how to prepare a FastLane proposal in 10 easy steps, go to

http://www.fastlane.nsf.gov/a0/about/10steps.htm

For assistance with using FastLane, e-mail

fastlane@nsf.gov

> **NOTE** that on February 23, 1999, the National Science Board issued a Statement on the Sharing of Research Data.
> The National Science Board is an independent policy body established by Congress in 1950 with dual responsibilities to:
> - Oversee and guide the activities of, and establish policies for, the National Science Foundation; and
> - Serve as an independent national science policy body that provides advice to the President and the Congress on policy issues related to science and engineering that have been identified by the President, Congress or the Board itself.
> The Board has 24 members appointed by the President and confirmed by the Senate, plus the NSF Director as an *ex officio* member.
> See
> http://www.nsf.gov/nsb/
> http://www.nsf.gov/nsb/aboutmore.htm
> A Statement by the National Science Board on the Sharing of Research Data (Date: February 23, 1999) can be found at http://www.nsf.gov/search97cgi/vtopic

WORDS OF WISDOM FROM SCIENTISTS WITH EXPERIENCE WITH NSF

> **NOTE:** This Appendix was originally written by Dr. Bruce Trumbo, Professor of Statistics and Mathematics at California State University, Hayward, for one of my earlier books. It was subsequently revised for later editions by Dr. Trumbo, Dr. Sherwin S. Lehrer, Senior Scientist at Boston Biomedical Research Institute (BBRI), who served on a National Science Foundation review panel from 1985 to 1988, and Dr. Hartmut Wohlrab, also of BBRI and also a member of an NSF grant review panel in 1993. The current Appendix was revised by me and subsequently read by Dr. Stephen H. Vessey, Acting Deputy Division Director, Division of Integrative Biology & Neuroscience, Biology Directorate, NSF, and by his Science Assistant, Amanda Voight, whose suggested changes I have incorporated.

Almost all of the general principles and many of the specific suggestions in this book apply to writing an effective proposal for submission to many agencies or foundations. However, because the National Science Foundation (NSF) is another major source of support for scientific research, I thought it important to point out the ways in which NSF differs from NIH.

Differences in Mission of NIH and NSF

Congress assigned NSF and NIH different scientific missions.

- NSF supports basic research in almost all scientific fields, such as sociology, physics, biology, economics, psychology, chemistry, mathematics, engineering, science education, etc.
- NSF does **not** support research primarily focused on clinical medicine. However, some projects involving basic scientific research may have potential clinical Applications and may, thus, fulfill the missions of both agencies.
- For proposals submitted to the Biology Directorate at NSF, you may NOT submit the same proposal to NIH **unless** you are a beginning investigator.
- If you submit a proposal that was **not** funded by one agency to the **other** agency, you must restructure the text to **conform** to the instructions of the agency to which you are submitting the application.
- Sometimes, NIH and NSF agree to **jointly fund** a project that is of interest to both agencies.

NSF programs and proposals

If you access the NSF Web site at

http://www.nsf.gov/

and click on "Grants and Awards," you will access a page called "Overview of Grants and Awards." Alternatively, you can click on "Grant Proposal Guide," which is published periodically. These sites will lead you to further information about the NSF grants process.

Grant-seekers should be aware that although NSF is doing some pilot programs that are totally paperless, to date (March 2004), the paper copy is still the official copy. However, most of the review process is already done electronically: NSF no longer sends paper copy to reviewers unless requested, and reviews and panel summaries are returned to Principal Investigators (PI's) via the FastLane Web site.

Grant-seekers should also be aware that NSF **supports a broader variety of research fields than does NIH, where the topics tend ultimately to be health-related.** Thus, the details of processing and reviewing proposals differ more from section to section of NSF than from Institute to Institute at NIH. However, as is the case at NIH, it is important for proposal-writers to NSF to be aware of deadlines and of any special proposal-writing suggestions of the NSF section that handles their area of science. Such information is available in

- the NSF Bulletin
  To subscribe go to
  http://www.nsf.gov/home/ebulletin/
  or directly to
  http://www.nsf.gov/cgi-bin/ebulletin/mailit.pl
- professional journals
- university research offices

Although NSF officers are not official consultants in grantsmanship, a telephone call or e-mail to the appropriate NSF official may help an Applicant define or clarify the relevance of a particular project to a specific NSF program before the Applicant spends a lot of time "barking up the wrong tree."

NSF

- Provides general research grants
- Supports a variety of cooperative international and exchange programs
- Periodically establishes special programs to meet specific needs e.g., support for a conference in an expanding research area or for a particular kind of instrumentation

NSF programs also include:

- Research opportunities for women (advance program)
- Instructional and research instrumentation programs
- Various fellowships

NSF programs are announced on the NSF Web site and include details about the application process. It is important to understand that the required machinations of government procedures sometimes leave as little as 90 days between the formal announcement of these programs and the deadline for applying. However, many of these programs continue essentially unchanged for several fiscal years and those "in the know" are generally aware of programs under consideration at NSF. Thus, scientists and students who know their own research needs and capabilities, and who make it their business to follow trends of NSF support can often guess the general thrust of possible proposals for special program funds. Nonetheless, it is important, before deciding to apply to a particular program, to read—very carefully—the specific program announcement and determine the

- purposes for which the program was established
- exact eligibility requirements
- specific contractual requirements

Subscribe to the NSF Custom New Service at

http://www.nsf.gov/home/cns/

or via

http://www.nsf.gov/home/cns/helpOne/whatsnew.cfm?ref=/index.cfm

It is important to remember that far-fetched rationalizations that attempt to squeeze a proposal (however sound scientifically) into an ill-fitting mold waste the time of proposers, Reviewers, and Program Officers.

Potential Applicants should be aware that different agencies have different formats for proposal submission and different matters that are important to the agency. For example, NSF tends to be somewhat less formal than NIH with respect to the form of the Research Plan (except for very strict page limits), but the NSF budget pages are prescribed and are somewhat different from those of NIH. In addition, **cost-sharing** is mandated in certain specific NSF programs, especially those involving equipment. **Cost-sharing** should be summarized on the **Budget Form** and explained in the **Budget Justification**. Issues of **cost-sharing** are often discussed with administrators of grantee institutions in the course of NSF budget negotiations. **Cost-sharing** is **not**, however, required for most Applications. Also, be aware that at NSF, **indirect costs are included in the total award and are not negotiated separately.**

DIFFERENCES BETWEEN NSF AND NIH IN METHODS OF PROPOSAL REVIEW

Another major difference between NIH and NSF is the review process

- The use of Initial Review Groups by NIH is described in detail in the main part of this book.
- NSF uses a variety of review procedures, less uniform than the NIH process with its review groups.

Many NSF programs use mail reviews. Typically, the Program Director will initially select several outside Reviewers for a proposal, following guidelines to ensure a balanced review.

Some NSF programs arrange panel meetings of Reviewers, for which panel members and/or outside Reviewers have submitted written reviews to NSF before the panel meets. Thus, the essence of an NSF panel meeting is a summary of the proposal by experts in the field that is generally followed by a round-table discussion that focuses initially on many individual reactions to each proposal.

Sometimes, NSF panels are asked to rank proposals or to sort them into several categories as to merit, but anything approaching the detailed scorekeeping approach used at NIH is rare in an NSF panel meeting.

Even when NSF Reviewers meet in face-to-face discussions, their interaction is likely to be structured somewhat more loosely than at an NIH Study Section, with each review panel having its own flavor that is set by the Program Director.

Reviewers are asked to comment on all aspects of the proposal and to rate it with one of the following descriptors:

- Excellent
- Very Good
- Good
- Fair
- Poor

NSF merit review criteria

NSF merit review criteria are listed below. Following each criterion are potential considerations that the Reviewer may employ in the evaluation. These are suggestions and not all of them will apply to any given proposal. Each Reviewer will be asked to address only those that are relevant to the proposal and for which she/he is qualified to make judgments.

Criterion 1: What is the intellectual merit of the proposed activity?

- How important is the proposed activity to advancing knowledge and understanding within its own field or across different fields?
- How well qualified is the proposer (individual or team) to conduct the project? (If appropriate, the Reviewer will comment on the quality of prior work.)
- To what extent does the proposed activity suggest and explore creative and original concepts?
- How well conceived and organized is the proposed activity?
- Is there sufficient access to resources?

Criterion 2: What are the broader impacts of the proposed activity?

- How well does the activity advance discovery and understanding while promoting teaching, training, and learning?

- How well does the proposed activity broaden the participation of underrepresented groups (e.g., gender, ethnicity, disability, geographic, etc.)?
- To what extent will it enhance the infrastructure for research and education, such as facilities, instrumentation, networks, and partnerships?
- Will the results be disseminated broadly to enhance scientific and technological understanding?
- What may be the benefits of the proposed activity to society?

PIs should address the following elements in their proposal to provide Reviewers with the information necessary to respond fully to the NSF merit review criteria described above. NSF staff will give these elements careful consideration in making funding decisions.

Integration of research and education

One of the principal strategies in support of NSF's goals is to foster integration of research and education through the programs, projects, and activities that NSF supports at academic and research institutions. These institutions provide abundant opportunities where individuals may concurrently assume responsibilities as researchers, educators, and students, and where all can engage in joint efforts that infuse education with the excitement of discovery and enrich research through the diversity of learning perspectives.

Integrating diversity into NSF programs, projects, and activities

Broadening opportunities and enabling the participation of all citizens—women and men, under-represented minorities, and persons with disabilities—are essential to the health and vitality of science and engineering. NSF is committed to this principle of diversity and deems it central to the programs, projects, and activities it considers and supports (NSF 99-172).

NSF often seeks additional reviews to:
- reconcile differences in Reviewer reaction

  or
- pursue issues raised by the first round of Reviewers

Based on the relative merit determined by the panel and/or mail reviews, the panel may informally recommend either
- **funding**

  or
- **"declination" of the project**

The mandate of the panel/Reviewers is to assign a merit descriptor to Applications. Although panel members may—and often do—recommend funding or "declination" of a project, **the ultimate decision about funding is the responsibility of the NSF staff.**

Reviewers at NSF
- provide the balanced body of opinion and evaluation needed for a prompt and fair decision
- make sure that the essence and importance of the proposal are clear
- look for a bibliography that is neither skimpy and skewed towards publications of the PI and her/his colleagues, nor padded and expansive

For projects recommended for funding, the **Program Director** attempts to fund as many proposals as possible with the available funds. Often, a smaller budget, consistent with the requirements of the reviewed project, is recommended, which may then permit funding of additional projects.

Anonymous verbatim copies of Reviewers, comments—and, in most cases, a verbatim summary of the panel discussion—are sent to the Principal Investigator after final action on the proposal has been taken. These comments can be educational for both successful and unsuccessful Applicants. The PI may also receive a context statement that provides information about how the panel was conducted, the number of proposals reviewed, and the number in each merit category.

> **NOTE: Because the initial impression of each panel Reviewer—and the only impression of a mail Reviewer—is the solitary one of a fellow scientist reading the proposal, the NSF review system places a heavy responsibility on the proposer to communicate ideas in a clear and organized way and to document the budget adequately.**

Some Reviewers are researchers in the same sub-field as the proposer. Other Reviewers may view the proposal from some scientific distance. It is important for proposal writers to

- explain exactly what they propose to do

and

- show the place and importance of the project in the context of the field as a whole

The latter point takes on added significance when one considers that the Program Director, who cannot possibly be an expert in the specific sub-field of each proposal s/he handles, selects the Reviewers based largely on information contained within the proposal.

FastLane provides an opportunity for the Applicant to suggest names of Reviewers, and the names of Reviewers **not** to be used. The most important way for an Applicant to help ensure that the Reviewers chosen to assess the proposal will provide a fair evaluation is to write the proposal so that the

- basis/background of the proposal is clearly detailed
- importance of the proposed work is clearly established and documented and the possible/likely outcomes are discussed
- bibliography is ample but not "padded" and that it is not skewed towards publications of the PI and her/his colleagues

Dr. Bruce Trumbo, who wrote the first version of "Part B" of this Appendix for an earlier edition of this book, wrote, "I have had a few opportunities to compare the NSF and NIH review processes for essentially identical proposals. In each of these instances the procedural differences mentioned here, while important, were of far less practical significance than the astonishing similarities in results. The same issues were discussed, the same objections offered, the sam e strengths noted, the same budget items questioned, and the same conclusions reached. The main manuscript begins with the comment that a good proposal requires, above all else, a good idea. By bad presentation it is possible to obscure a good idea from Reviewers either at NSF or NIH. A routine or mediocre idea will look no better than routine or mediocre when viewed through either pair of spectacles."

AN OUTLINE OF THE NSF GRANT PROPOSAL GUIDE (GPG)

http://www.nsf.gov/pubs/2004/nsf042/start.htm

The GPG provides guidance for the preparation and submission of proposals to NSF. Some NSF programs have program solicitations that modify the general provisions of this Guide, and, in such cases, the guidelines provided in the solicitation must be followed. Contact with NSF program personnel prior to proposal preparation is encouraged.

Below is the **Table of Contents (TOC) of the GPG** as given at the above Web site. **In some places** I have included some of the text provided in the GPG. However, it is the responsibility of a potential Applicant to NSF to go to the relevant Web site and read **ALL** the instructions for preparing a grant Application to NSF. Do **NOT** rely solely on the excerpts I have provided below. Go to

http://www.nsf.gov/pubs/2004/nsf042/2.htm

and read and respond to ALL the pertinent instructions at this site.

The NSF FastLane system uses Internet/Web technology to facilitate the way NSF does business with the research, education, and related communities. All FastLane functions are accessed by using a Web browser on the Internet. The NSF FastLane system should be used for

- proposal preparation
- submission
- status checking
- project reporting
- post-award administrative activities

The Grant Proposal Guide (GPG)
Table of Contents

About the National Science Foundation

Foreword

I. Introduction
   A. Overview
   B. The Proposal
      Proprietary or Privileged Information
         The proposal should present the
         - objectives and scientific, engineering, or educational significance of the proposed work;
           suitability of the methods to be employed;
         - qualifications of the investigator and the grantee organization;
         - effect of the activity on the infrastructure of science, engineering, and education;
         - amount of funding required.

         The proposal should **present the merits of the proposed project** clearly and should be prepared with the care and thoroughness of a paper submitted for publication. Sufficient information should be provided so that Reviewers will be able to evaluate the proposal in accordance with the two merit review criteria established by the National Science Board.

NSF expects strict adherence to the rules of proper scholarship and attribution. The responsibility for proper attribution and citation rests with authors of a proposal; all parts of the proposal should be prepared with equal care for this concern. Serious failure to adhere to such standards can result in findings of research misconduct.

C. Who May Submit Proposals

Scientists, engineers, and educators usually initiate proposals that are officially submitted by their employing organization. **Before formal submission, the proposal may be discussed with appropriate NSF program staff.**

Graduate students are NOT encouraged to submit research proposals, but should arrange to serve as research assistants to faculty members.

Some NSF divisions accept proposals for Doctoral Dissertation Research Grants when submitted by a faculty member on behalf of the graduate student.

The Foundation also provides support specifically for women and minority scientists and engineers, scientists and engineers with disabilities, and faculty at primarily undergraduate academic institutions.

For Categories of Proposers See:

http://www.nsf.gov/pubs/2004/nsf042/1.htm#bfn1

D. When to Submit Proposals

Many NSF programs accept proposals at any time. Other programs, however, establish target dates, deadlines, or submission windows for submission of proposals to allow time for their consideration by review panels that meet periodically. These target dates, deadlines, and submission windows are published in specific program announcements and solicitations that can be obtained from the NSF Clearinghouse at **pubs@nsf.gov** or electronically through the NSF Web site. Proposers should allow up to six months for programmatic review and processing.

E. How to Submit Proposals

Proposals to NSF must be submitted electronically via the FastLane system. For proposers who cannot submit electronically, a deviation must be approved in advance of submission of the paper proposal.

Proposals received by NSF are generally converted to hard copy for distribution to the Reviewer community because the wide variety of equipment available to Reviewers may not, at this time, assure that an all-electronic review process would be successful or totally fair to proposers. In the near future, NSF envisions that it will be possible to avoid this printing step and send proposals out for review by electronic means.

1. Electronic Requirements

   Special Instructions for Proposals That Contain High Resolution Graphics or Other Graphics Where Exact Color Representations are Required for Proper Interpretation by the Reviewer

2. Submission Instructions

   Once the proposal is submitted, PIs can access the number assigned to the proposal via the "Submitted Proposals" list in the FastLane Proposal Preparation module.

If a proposal number is not in the FastLane System, contact the FastLane Help Desk:

Tel: 800-673-6188 or 703-292-8142

e-mail: fastlane@nsf.gov

3. Acknowledgement of Proposal Receipt

Once the proposal is assigned to an NSF program, the cognizant program information is available via the FastLane "Proposal Status Inquiry" function for PIs and through the "Recent Proposals" report for sponsored projects offices. Communications about the proposal should be addressed to the cognizant Program Officer with reference to the proposal number. **Proposers are strongly encouraged to use FastLane to verify the status of their submission to NSF.**

II. Proposal Preparation Instructions

http://www.nsf.gov/pubs/2004/nsf042/2.htm

A. Conformance with Instructions for Proposal Preparation

Note: A proposal will not be processed until NSF has received the complete proposal.

Note: There is a Proposal Preparation Checklist at

http://www.nsf.gov/pubs/2004/nsf042/appa.htm

B. Format of the Proposal

1. Proposal Pagination Instructions

Note: Each section of the proposal that is uploaded as a file must be individually paginated before uploading to FastLane.

2. Proposal Margin and Spacing Requirements

- Proposals must have 2.5 cm margins at the top, bottom, and on each side.
- The type size must be clear and readily legible, and conform to the following 3 requirements:
    - the height of the letters must not be smaller than 10 point;
    - type density must not exceed 15 characters per 2.5 cm (for proportional spacing, the average for any representative section of text must not exceed 15 characters per 2.5 cm);
    - no more than 6 lines must be within a vertical space of 2.5 cm.

    Line spacing (single-spaced, double-spaced, etc.) is at the discretion of the proposer, but established page limits must be followed unless the specific program solicitations eliminate this option.

The guidelines specified above establish the minimum type size requirements. However, PIs are advised that readability is most important and should take precedence in selection of an appropriate font for use in the proposal.

C. Proposal Contents

    1. Single Copy Documents

        a. Information About Principal Investigators/Project Directors and co-Principal Investigators/co-Project Directors

        b. Deviation Authorization (if applicable)

        c. List of Suggested Reviewers or Reviewers

- Proposers may include a list of suggested Reviewers who they think are especially well qualified to review the proposal.
- Proposers may also designate persons they would prefer not review the proposal, indicating why. **These suggestions are optional.**
- The GPG contains information on conflicts of interest that may be useful in preparation of this list.

    The Program Officer handling the proposal considers these suggestions and may contact the proposer for further information. However, the decision whether or not to use the suggestions remains with the Program Officer.

        d. Proprietary or Privileged Information (if applicable)

        e. Proposal Certifications

- Certification for Authorized Organizational Representative or Individual Applicant
- Certification Regarding Conflict of Interest
- Drug-Free Workplace
- Debarment and Suspension
- Certification Regarding Lobbying

    2. Sections of the Proposal

        a. Cover Sheet

        b. Project Summary

    The proposal must contain a summary of the proposed activity suitable for publication, not more than one page in length. It should **NOT** be an abstract of the proposal, but rather a self-contained description of the activity that would result if the proposal were funded. **The summary should be written in the third person** and include a **statement of objectives** and **methods** to be employed. It must clearly address in separate statements (within the one-page summary):

- The intellectual merit of the proposed activity.
- The broader impacts resulting from the proposed activity.
- It should be informative to other persons working in the same or related fields and, insofar as possible, understandable to a scientifically or technically literate lay reader.
- **Proposals that do not separately address both merit review criteria (the first 2 items above) within the one page Project Summary will be returned without review.**

c. Table of Contents

Note: A Table of Contents is automatically generated for the proposal by the FastLane system. The proposer cannot edit this form.

d. Project Description (Including Results from Prior NSF Support)

   i. Content

The project Description should provide a clear statement of the work to be undertaken. It must include:

- objectives for the period of the proposed work and expected significance;
- relation to longer-term goals of the PI's project;
- relation to the present state of knowledge in the field, to work in progress by the PI under other support, and to work in progress elsewhere.
- For further details see

http://www.nsf.gov/pubs/2004/nsf042/2.htm

   ii. Page Limitations and Inclusion of Universal Resource Locators (URLs) within the Project Description

   iii. Results from Prior NSF Support

See specific instructions at

http://www.nsf.gov/pubs/2004/nsf042/2.htm

   iv. Unfunded Collaborations

   v. Group Proposals

   vi. Proposals for Renewed Support

e. References Cited

Each reference must include

- names of all authors (in the same sequence in which they appear in the publication)
- article title
- journal title
- book title
- volume number
- page numbers
- year of publication

If the document is available electronically, the Web site address also should be given.

Proposers must be especially careful to follow accepted scholarly practices in providing citations for source materials relied upon when preparing any section of the proposal.

There is no page limitation for the references, but this section must include bibliographic citations only and **must not be used to provide parenthetical information outside of the 15-page Project Description.**

f. Biographical Sketch(es)

A biographical sketch (limited to two pages) is required for each individual identified as senior project personnel. The following information must be provided in the order and format specified below:

i. Professional Preparation

ii. Appointments

iii. Publications

A list of no more than 5 publications most closely related to the proposed project; and up to 5 other significant publications, whether or not related to the proposed project. Each publication listed must include

- names of all authors (in the same sequence in which they appear in the publication)
- article title
- journal title
- book title
- volume number
- page numbers
- year of publication
- If the document is available electronically, the Web site address should be provided

For unpublished manuscripts, list only those **submitted or accepted** for publication (along with most likely date of publication).

Patents, copyrights and software systems developed may be substituted for publications.

Additional lists of publications, invited lectures, etc., must **NOT** be included. Only the list of 10 will be used in the review of the proposal.

iv. Synergistic Activities

A list of up to 5 examples that demonstrate the broader impact of the individual's professional and scholarly activities that focus on the integration and transfer of knowledge as well as its creation. Examples could include, among others:

- innovations in teaching and training (e.g., development of curricular materials and pedagogical methods);
- contributions to the science of learning;
- development and/or refinement of research tools;
- computation methodologies, and algorithms for problem-solving;
- development of databases to support research and education;
- broadening the participation of groups underrepresented in science, mathematics, engineering, and technology;
- service to the scientific and engineering community outside of the individual's immediate organization.

v.   Collaborators & Other Affiliations
   (a) Collaborators and Co-Editors
   (b) Graduate and Postdoctoral Advisors
   (c) Thesis Advisor and Postgraduate-Scholar Sponsor
g. Budget

Each proposal must contain a budget for each year of support requested, unless a particular program solicitation stipulates otherwise.

Completion of the budget does not eliminate the need to **document and justify the amounts requested in each category**. A budget justification of **up to 3 pages** is authorized to provide the necessary justification and documentation.

The proposal may request funds under any of the categories listed so long as the item and amount are considered **necessary to perform the proposed work** and are not precluded by specific program guidelines or applicable cost principles.

i.   Salaries and Wages (Lines A and B on the Proposal Budget)
   (a) Policies

As a general policy, NSF recognizes that salaries of faculty members and other personnel associated directly with the project constitute appropriate direct costs and may be requested in proportion to the effort devoted to the project.

NSF regards research as one of the normal functions of faculty members at institutions of higher education. Compensation for time normally spent on research within the term of appointment is deemed to be included within the faculty member's regular organizational salary. **Grant funds may NOT be used to augment the total salary or rate of salary of faculty members during the period covered by the term of faculty appointment or to reimburse faculty members for consulting or other time in addition to a regular full-time organizational salary covering the same general period of employment.** Exceptions may be considered under certain NSF science and engineering education program solicitations for weekend and evening classes or for administrative work done as overload.

Summer salary for faculty members on academic-year appointments **is limited** to no more than two-ninths of their regular academic-year salary. This limit includes summer salary received from all NSF-funded grants.

These same principles apply to other types of non-academic organizations, such as research institutes. Since their employment periods are usually annual, salary must be shown under "calendar months." **For such persons, "summer salary" is normally inappropriate under an NSF grant.**

Sometimes an independent institute or laboratory proposes to employ college or university faculty members on a part-time basis. In such cases, the general intent of the policies above apply, so that an individual's total income will not be augmented in ways that would not be possible under a grant to an academic institution.

In most circumstances, particularly for institutions of higher education, salaries of administrative or clerical staff are included as part of indirect costs [also known as Facilities and Administrative Costs (F&A) for Colleges and Universities]. Salaries of administrative or clerical staff may be requested as direct costs, however, for a project requiring an extensive amount of administrative or clerical support and where these costs can be readily and specifically identified with the project with a high degree of accuracy. The circumstances for requiring direct charging of these services must be clearly described in the budget justification. NSF may delete such costs, if they are not clearly justified.

(b) Procedures

List the names of the PI(s), faculty, and other senior personnel and the estimated number of full-time-equivalent academic-year, summer, or calendar-year person-months for which NSF funding is requested and the total amount of salaries per year. For postdoctoral associates and other professionals, list the total number of persons for each position, with the number of full-time-equivalent person-months and total amount of salaries per year. For graduate and undergraduate students, secretarial, clerical, technical, etc., whose time will be charged directly to the project, only the total number of persons and total amount of salaries per year in each category is required. **Salaries requested must be consistent with the organization's regular practices.** The budget justification should detail the rates of pay by individual for senior personnel, postdoctoral associates, and other professionals.

The budget may request funds for support of graduate or undergraduate research assistants to help carry out the proposed research. Compensation classified as salary payments must be requested in the salaries and wages category. Any direct costs requested for tuition remission must be listed in the "Other" category under "Other Direct Costs."

(c) Confidential Budgetary Information

The proposing organization may request that salary data on senior personnel not be released to persons outside the Government during the review process. See the GPG for specifics on how to accomplish this.

ii. Fringe Benefits (Line C on the Proposal Budget)

If the grantee's usual accounting practices provide that its contributions to employee benefits (social security, retirement, etc.) be treated as direct costs, NSF grant funds may be requested to fund fringe benefits as a direct cost.

iii. Equipment (Line D on the Proposal Budget)

Equipment is defined as an item of property that has an acquisition cost of $5,000 or more (unless the organization has established lower levels) and an expected service life of more than one year. Items of needed equipment must be listed individually by description and estimated cost, including tax, and adequately justified. Allowable items ordinarily will be limited to research equipment and apparatus not already available for the conduct of the work. General-purpose equipment, such as a personal computer, is not eligible for support unless primarily or exclusively used in the actual conduct of scientific research.

iv. Travel (Line E on the Proposal Budget)

(a) General

Travel and its relation to the proposed activities must be specified and itemized by destination and cost. Funds may be requested for

- field work
- attendance at meetings and conferences
- other travel associated with the proposed work

Subsistence may be included.

To qualify for support, attendance at meetings or conferences must enhance the PI's ability, with respect to one of the items below

- perform the work
- plan extensions of it
- disseminate the results

Allowance for air travel normally will not exceed the cost of round-trip, economy airfares.

Persons traveling under NSF grants must travel by U.S.-flag carriers, if available.

(b) Domestic Travel

Includes travel in the U.S., its possessions, Puerto Rico, and travel to Canada and Mexico.

(c) Foreign Travel

For travel to areas other than those listed above. See

http://www.nsf.gov/pubs/2004/nsf042/2.htm

v. Participant Support (Line F on the Proposal Budget)

vi. Other Direct Costs (Lines G1 through G6 on the Proposal Budget)

(a) Materials and Supplies (Line G1 on the Proposal Budget)

(b) Publication/Documentation/Dissemination (Line G2 on the Proposal Budget)

Funds for the costs of documenting, preparing, publishing or otherwise making available to others the findings and products of the work conducted under the grant. This generally includes the following types of activities:

- Reports
- Reprints
- Page charges or other journal costs (except costs for prior or early publication)
- Necessary illustrations
- Cleanup, documentation, storage, and indexing of data and databases
- Development, documentation, and debugging of software
- Storage, preservation, documentation, indexing, etc., of physical specimens, collections or fabricated items

 (c) Consultant Services (Line G3 on the Proposal Budget)

 Anticipated consultant services must be justified and information furnished on each individual's

- expertise
- primary organizational affiliation
- normal daily compensation rate
- number of days of expected service
- consultants' travel costs, including subsistence
- payment for a consultant's services, exclusive of expenses, which may not exceed the consultant's normal rate or the daily maximum rate established annually by NSF, whichever is less

 (d) Computer Services (Line G4 on the Proposal Budget)

 (e) Sub-awards (Line G5 on the Proposal Budget)

 (f) Other (Line G6 on the Proposal Budget)

vii. Total Direct Costs (Line H on the Proposal Budget)

viii. Indirect Costs [also known as Facilities and Administrative Costs (F&A) for Colleges and Universities; Line I on the Proposal Budget]

ix. Total Direct and Indirect Costs (F&A; Line J on the Proposal Budget)

x. Residual Funds

xi. Amount of this Request

xii. Cost Sharing

 (a) Statutory Cost-Sharing Requirement

 (b) Cost-Sharing Requirements Under NSF Program Solicitations

xiii. Unallowable Costs

 (a) Entertainment

 (b) Meals and Coffee Breaks

 (c) Alcoholic Beverages

Proposal Preparation Instructions can be found at

http://www.nsf.gov/pubs/2004/nsf042/2.htm

Each proposing organization that has not received an NSF grant within the previous two years should be prepared to submit basic organization and management information and certifications, when requested, to the Division of Grants and Agreements. The information required is contained in the NSF Prospective New Awardee Guide, available electronically on the NSF Web site. The information contained in this Guide will assist the organization in preparing documents that the National Science Foundation requires to conduct administrative and financial reviews of the organization. This Guide also serves as a means of highlighting the accountability requirements associated with Federal awards.

    To facilitate proposal preparation, Frequently Asked Questions (FAQs) regarding proposal preparation and submission are available electronically on the NSF Web site.

FOLLOWING AGENCY INSTRUCTIONS FOR PROPOSAL PREPARATION

It is important that all proposals conform to the instructions provided in the GPG. Conformance is required and will be strictly enforced unless a deviation has been approved. NSF may return proposals without review if they are not consistent with these instructions. NSF must authorize any deviations from these instructions in advance. Deviations may be authorized in one of two ways:

1. through specification of different requirements in an NSF solicitation;

or

2. by the written approval of the cognizant NSF Assistant Director/Office Head or designee. These deviations may be in the form of a "blanket deviation" for a particular program or programs or, in rare instances, an "individual" deviation for a particular proposal.

Proposers may deviate from these instructions only to the extent authorized. Proposals must identify the deviation in one of the following ways as appropriate:

(a) by identifying the solicitation number that authorized the deviation in the appropriate block on the proposal Cover Sheet;

or

(b) for individual deviations, by identifying the name, date, and title of the NSF official authorizing the deviation. Further instructions are available on the FastLane Web site.

FORMAT OF THE PROPOSAL

Prior to electronic submission, it is strongly recommended that proposers conduct an administrative review to ensure that proposals comply with the proposal preparation guidelines established in the GPG. A proposal preparation checklist that may be used to assist in this review is given on the NIH Website.

To access the "Checklist" page:

- Go to

    http://grants.nih.gov/grants/funding/phs398/phs398.html

- Scoll down to
    "Microsoft Word (MS Word and Portable Document Format (PDF) Forms"
- In the table entitled **"Individual Form Files,"** scroll down to **"Checklist Form Page"**
- Click on either
    MS Word Format
    or
    PDF Format

This checklist is not intended to be an all-inclusive repetition of the required proposal contents and associated proposal preparation guidelines. It is, however, meant to highlight certain critical items so they will not be overlooked when the proposal is prepared.

1. Proposal Pagination Instructions

Proposers are advised that FastLane does not automatically paginate a proposal. Each section of the proposal that is uploaded as a file must be individually paginated before upload to FastLane.

2. Proposal Margin and Spacing Requirements

   Proposals must have 2.5 cm margins at the top, bottom, and on each side. The type size must be clear and readily legible, and conform to the following 3 requirements:

   - the height of the letters must not be smaller than 10 point;
   - type density must be no more than 15 characters per 2.5 cm (for proportional spacing, the average for any representative section of text must not exceed 15 characters per 2.5 cm);
   - no more than 6 lines must be within a vertical space of 2.5 cm.

   The type size used throughout the proposal must conform to all 3 requirements. Line spacing (single-spaced, double-spaced, etc.) is at the discretion of the proposer, but **established page limits must be followed**. (Individual program solicitations may eliminate this requirement.)

   While the guidelines specified above establish the minimum type size requirements, PIs are advised that **readability is of paramount importance and should take precedence in selection of an appropriate font for use in the proposal.**

PROPOSAL CONTENTS

1. Single-Copy Documents

   Certain categories of information that are submitted in conjunction with a proposal are for "NSF Use Only." As such, the information is not provided to reviewers for use in the review of the proposal. With the exception of proposal certifications (which are submitted via the Authorized Organizational Representative function 15), these documents should be submitted electronically via the Proposal Preparation module in the FastLane system. A summary of each of these categories follows:

   (a). Information About Principal Investigators/Project Directors and co-Principal Investigators/co-Project Directors

   NSF is committed to providing equal opportunities for participation in its programs and promoting the full use of the Nation,s research and engineering resources. To aid in meeting these objectives, NSF requests information on the gender, race, ethnicity, and disability status of individuals named as PIs/co-PIs on proposals and awards. Except for the required information about current or previous Federal research support and the name(s) of the PI/co-PI, submission of the information is voluntary, and individuals who do not wish to provide the personal information should check the box provided for that purpose.

   (b). Deviation Authorization (if applicable)

   Instructions for obtaining a deviation from NSF proposal preparation instructions are provided in Chapter II Section A: Conformance with Instructions for Proposal Preparation.

(c). List of Suggested Reviewers or Reviewers (optional)

Proposers may include a list of suggested reviewers who they believe are especially well qualified to review the proposal. **Proposers also may designate persons they would prefer not review the proposal, indicating why.** These suggestions are optional. GPG Appendix B, Potentially Disqualifying Conflicts of Interest, contains information on conflicts of interest that may be useful in preparation of this list.

The cognizant Program Officer handling the proposal considers the suggestions and may contact the proposer for further information. However, the decision whether or not to use the suggestions remains with the Program Officer.

The cognizant Program Officer handling the proposal considers the suggestions and may contact the proposer for further information. However, the decision of whether to use the suggestions remains with the Program Officer.

(d). Proprietary or Privileged Information (if applicable)

Instructions for submission of proprietary or privileged information are provided in Chapter I Section B: The Proposal.

(e). Proposal Certifications

With the exception of the Disclosure of Lobbying Activities identified below, the procedures for submission of the proposal certifications differ from those used with other single-copy documents. The Authorized Organizational Representative (AOR) must use the "Authorized Organizational Representative function" in the FastLane system to electronically sign and submit the proposal certifications. It is the proposing organization's responsibility to assure that only properly authorized individuals sign in this capacity.

The required proposal certifications are as follows:

- Certification for Authorized Organizational Representative or Individual Applicant: The AOR is required to complete certifications regarding the accuracy and completeness of statements contained in the proposal, as well as to certify that the organization (or individual) agrees to accept the obligation to comply with award terms and conditions.

- Certification Regarding Conflict of Interest: The AOR is required to complete certifications stating that the institution has implemented and is enforcing a written policy on conflicts of interest. The policy must be consistent with the provisions of GPM Section 510: that, to the best of his/her knowledge, all financial disclosures required by the conflict of interest policy were made; and that conflicts of interest, if any, were, or prior to the institution's expenditure of any funds under the award, will be, satisfactorily managed, reduced, or eliminated in accordance with the institution's conflict of interest policy. Conflicts that cannot be satisfactorily managed, reduced, or eliminated must be disclosed to NSF via use of the Notifications and Requests Module in the NSF FastLane System.

- Drug-Free Workplace: The AOR is required to complete a certification regarding the Drug-Free Workplace Act.

- Debarment and Suspension: The AOR is required to complete a certification regarding Debarment and Suspension.
- Certification Regarding Lobbying: The AOR is required to complete a certification regarding lobbying restrictions. The Certification for Contracts, Grants, Loans and Cooperative Agreements is included in full text on the FastLane submission screen. This certification is applicable when the proposal exceeds $100,000. The box for "Disclosure of Lobbying Activities" must be checked on the proposal Cover Sheet only if, pursuant to paragraph 2 of the certification, submission of the SF LLL is required.

2. Sections of the Proposal

The sections described below represent the body of a proposal submitted to NSF. With the exception of "Special Information and Supplementary Documentation" and "Appendices," all sections are required parts of the proposal. These documents must be submitted electronically via the Proposal Preparation module in the FastLane system.

(a). Cover Sheet

Proposers are required to select the applicable program announcement, solicitation or program description. If the proposal is not submitted in response to a specific program announcement, solicitation, or program description, proposers should select "Grant Proposal Guide." Compliance with this requirement is critical to determining the relevant proposal processing guidelines. Proposers must then follow instructions for selection of an applicable NSF Division and Program(s) to which the proposal should be directed.

A block is included for the proposer to enter its organization's Data Universal Numbering System (DUNS) number. The DUNS number is a nine-digit number assigned by Dun and Bradstreet Information Services. If the proposer does not have a DUNS number, it must contact Dun and Bradstreet by telephone directly at (800) 333-0505 to obtain one. A DUNS number will be provided immediately by telephone at no charge.

Should the project be performed at a place other than where the award is to be made, that should be identified in the block entitled, "Name of Performing Organization."

Examples are as follows:

Grantee Organization

Performing Organization

Northern Virginia University

Northern Virginia University Health Center

Southern Virginia University Research Foundation

Southern Virginia University

The title of the project must be brief, scientifically or technically valid, intelligible to a scientifically or technically literate reader, and suitable for use in the public press. NSF may edit the title of a project prior to making an award.

The proposed duration for which support is requested must be consistent with the nature and complexity of the proposed activity. Grants are normally awarded for up to 3 years but may be awarded for periods of up to 5 years. The Foundation encourages PIs to request awards for durations of 3 to 5 years when such durations are necessary for completion of the proposed work and when such durations are technically and managerially advantageous. Specification of a desired starting date for the project is important and helpful to NSF staff; however, requests for specific effective dates may not be met. Except in special situations, requested effective dates must allow at least 6 months for NSF review, processing and decision. Should unusual situations (e.g., a long lead time for procurement) create problems regarding the proposed effective date, the PI should consult his/her organization's sponsored projects office.

Some NSF program solicitations require submission of both a preliminary and full proposal as part of the proposal process. In such cases, the following instructions apply:

- During the preliminary proposal stage, the proposing organization should identify the submission as a preliminary proposal by checking the block entitled, "Preliminary Proposal" on the proposal Cover Sheet;
- During the full proposal submission stage, the proposing organization should identify in the block entitled, "Show Related Preliminary Proposal Number", the related preliminary proposal number assigned by NSF.

Should any of the listed items on the proposal Cover Sheet apply to a proposal, the applicable box(es) must be checked.

Profit-making organizations must identify their status by completing each of the appropriate submitting organization boxes on the Cover Sheet, using the following guidelines:

a. A small business must be organized for profit, independently owned and operated (not a subsidiary of or controlled by another firm), have no more than 500 employees, and not be dominant in its field. The appropriate box also must be checked when the proposal involves a cooperative effort between an academic institution and a small business.

b. A minority business must be:

   (i) at least 51% owned by one or more minority or disadvantaged individuals or, in the case of a publicly owned business, have at least 51% of the voting stock owned by one or more minority or disadvantaged individuals;

   and

   (ii) one whose management and daily business operations are controlled by one or more such individuals.

c. A woman-owned business must be at least 51% owned by a woman or women, who also control and operate it. "Control" in this context means exercising the power to make policy decisions. "Operate" in this context means being actively involved in the day-to-day management.

(b). Project Summary

The proposal must contain a summary of the proposed activity suitable for publication, not more than one page in length. It should not be an abstract of the proposal, but rather a self-contained description of the activity that would result if the proposal were funded. The summary should be written in the third person and include a statement of objectives and methods to be employed. It must clearly address in separate statements (within the one-page summary): (1) the intellectual merit of the proposed activity; and (2) the broader impacts resulting from the proposed activity. (See Chapter III for further descriptive information on the NSF merit review criteria.) It should be informative to other persons working in the same or related fields and, insofar as possible, understandable to a scientifically or technically literate lay reader. Proposals that do not separately address both merit review criteria within the one page Project Summary will be returned without review.

(c). Table of Contents

A Table of Contents is automatically generated for the proposal by the FastLane system. The proposer cannot edit this form.

(d). Project Description (including Results from Prior NSF Support)

   (i)   Content

All proposals to NSF will be reviewed utilizing the two merit review criteria described in greater length in Chapter III.

The Project Description should provide **a clear statement of the work to be undertaken** and must include:

- objectives for the period of the proposed work;
- expected significance;
- relation to longer-term goals of the PI's project;
- relation to the present state of knowledge in the field;
- relation to work in progress by the PI under other support;
- relation to work in progress elsewhere.

The Project Description should outline the general plan of work, including the broad design of activities to be undertaken, and, where appropriate, provide a clear description of experimental methods and procedures and plans for preservation, documentation, and sharing of data, samples, physical collections, curriculum materials, and other related research and education products. It must describe as an integral part of the narrative, the broader impacts resulting from the proposed activities, addressing one or more of the following as appropriate for the project:

- how the project will integrate research and education by advancing discovery and understanding while at the same time promoting teaching, training, and learning;
- ways in which the proposed activity will broaden the participation of underrepresented groups (e.g., gender, ethnicity, disability, geographic, etc.);
- how the project will enhance the infrastructure for research and/or education, such as facilities, instrumentation, networks, and partnerships;
- how the results of the project will be disseminated broadly to enhance scientific and technological understanding;

- potential benefits of the proposed activity to society at large.

Examples illustrating activities likely to demonstrate broader impacts are available electronically on the NSF Web site.

(ii) Page Limitations and Inclusion of Universal Resource Locators (URLs) within the Project Description

Brevity will assist Reviewers and Foundation staff in dealing effectively with proposals. Therefore, the Project Description (including Results from Prior NSF Support, which is limited to 5 pages) may not exceed 15 pages. Visual materials, including charts, graphs, maps, photographs and other pictorial presentations are included in the 15-page limitation. PIs are advised that the project description must be self-contained and are cautioned that URLs (Internet addresses) that provide information necessary to the review of the proposal should not be used because Reviewers are under no obligation to view such sites.

Conformance to the 15-page limitation will be strictly enforced and may not be exceeded unless a deviation has been specifically authorized. (Chapter II, Section A, Conformance with Instructions for Proposal Preparation, contains information on deviations.)

(iii) Results from Prior NSF Support

If any PI or co-PI identified on the project has received NSF funding in the past 5 years, information on the award(s) is required. Each PI and co-PI who has received more than one award (excluding amendments) must report on the award most closely related to the proposal. The following information must be provided:

(a) the NSF award number, amount and period of support;

(b) the title of the project;

(c) a summary of the results of the completed work, including, for a research project, any contribution to the development of human resources in science and engineering;

(d) publications resulting from the NSF award;

(e) a brief description of available data, samples, physical collections, and other related research products not described elsewhere; and

(f) if the proposal is for renewed support, a description of the relation of the completed work to the proposed work.

Reviewers will be asked to comment on the quality of the prior work described in this section of the proposal. Please note that the proposal may contain up to 5 pages to describe the results. Results may be summarized in fewer than 5 pages, which would give the balance of the 15 pages for the Project Description.

(iv) Unfunded Collaborations

Any substantial collaboration with individuals not included in the budget should be described and documented with a letter from each collaborator, which should be provided in the supplementary documentation section of the FastLane Proposal Preparation module. Collaborative activities that are identified in the budget should follow the instructions in Chapter II, Section D.3.

(v)　Group Proposals

NSF encourages submission of proposals by groups of investigators; often these are submitted to carry out interdisciplinary projects. Unless stipulated in a specific program solicitation, however, such proposals will be subject to the 15 page Project Description limitation established in Section (ii) above. PIs who wish to exceed the established page limitations for the Project Description must request and receive a deviation in advance of proposal submission. (Chapter II, Section A, Conformance with Instructions for Proposal Preparation, contains information on deviations.)

(vi)　Proposals for Renewed Support

A proposal for renewed support may be either

a "traditional" proposal in which the proposed work is documented and described as fully as though the proposer were applying for the first time;

or

an "Accomplishment-Based Renewal" (ABR) proposal, in which the project description is replaced by copies of no more than 6 reprints of publications resulting from the research supported by NSF during the preceding 3 to 5 year period, plus a brief summary of plans for the proposed support period. See GPG for additional information on preparation of Renewal Proposals.

(e)　References Cited

Reference information is required. Each reference must include the names of all authors (in the same sequence in which they appear in the publication), the article and journal title, book title, volume number, page numbers, and year of publication. If the document is available electronically, the Web site address also should be identified. Proposers must be especially careful to follow accepted scholarly practices in providing citations for source materials relied upon when preparing any section of the proposal. While there is no established page limitation for the references, this section must include bibliographic citations only and must not be used to provide parenthetical information outside of the 15-page project description.

(f)　Biographical Sketch(es)

A biographical sketch (limited to 2 pages) is required for each individual identified as senior project personnel. (See Appendix F for the definition of Senior Personnel.) The following information must be provided in the order and format specified below:

(i)　Professional Preparation

- A list of the individual's undergraduate and graduate education and postdoctoral training as indicated below:
- **Undergraduate Institution(s)**
  —Major
  —Degree & Year

- **Graduate Institution(s)**
  —Major
  —Degree & Year
- **Postdoctoral Institution(s)**
  —Area
  —Inclusive Dates (years)

(ii) Appointments

A list, in **reverse chronological order,** of all the individual's academic/professional appointments beginning with the current appointment.

(iii) Publications

A list of:

—up to 5 publications most closely related to the proposed project;

—up to 5 other significant publications, whether or not related to the proposed project.

Each publication identified **must include:**

- names of **ALL** authors (in the same sequence in which they appear in the publication)
- title of article
- title of journal
- title of book
- volume number
- page numbers
- year of publication
- if the document is available electronically, the Web site address also should be identified

For unpublished manuscripts, list only those submitted or accepted for publication (along with most likely date of publication). Patents, copyrights, and software systems developed may be substituted for publications. Additional lists of publications, invited lectures, etc., must **not** be included. Only the list of 10 will be used in the review of the proposal.

(iv) Synergistic Activities

A list of up to 5 examples that demonstrate the broader impact of the individual's professional and scholarly activities that focus on the integration and transfer of knowledge as well as its creation. Examples could include, among others:

- innovations in teaching and training (e.g., development of curricular materials and pedagogical methods);
- contributions to the science of learning;
- development and/or refinement of research tools;
- computation methodologies, and algorithms for problem-solving;

- development of databases to support research and education;
- broadening the participation of groups underrepresented in science, mathematics, engineering and technology;
- service to the scientific and engineering community outside of the individual's immediate organization.

(v) Collaborators and Other Affiliations

(a) Collaborators and Co-Editors. A list of all persons in alphabetical order (including their current organizational affiliations) who are currently, or who have been collaborators or co-authors with the individual on a project, book, article, report, abstract, or paper during the 48 months preceding the submission of this proposal. Also include those individuals who are currently or have been co-editors of a journal, compendium, or conference proceedings during the 24 months preceding the submission of the proposal. If there are no collaborators or co-editors to report, this should be so indicated.

(b) Graduate and Postdoctoral Advisors. A list of the names of the individual's own graduate advisor(s) and principal postdoctoral sponsor(s), and their current organizational affiliations.

(c) Thesis Advisor and Postgraduate-Scholar Sponsor. A list of all persons (including their organizational affiliations), with whom the individual has had an association as thesis advisor, or with whom the individual has had an association within the last 5 years as a postgraduate-scholar sponsor. The total number of graduate students advised and postdoctoral scholars sponsored also must be identified.

The information in section 5 of the biographical sketch is used to help identify potential conflicts or bias in the selection of Reviewers. See GPG Appendix B, Potentially Disqualifying Conflicts of Interest for additional information on Reviewer conflicts.

For the personnel categories listed below, the proposal also may include information on exceptional qualifications that merit consideration in the evaluation of the proposal.

Postdoctoral associates

Other professionals

Students (research assistants)

For equipment proposals, the following must be provided for each auxiliary user:

Short biographical sketch;

List of up to 5 publications most closely related to the proposed acquisition.

(g). Budget

Each proposal must contain a budget for each year of support requested, unless a particular program solicitation stipulates otherwise. Completion of the budget does not eliminate the need to document and justify the amounts requested in each category. A budget justification of up to three pages is authorized to provide the necessary justification and documentation.

The proposal may request funds under any of the categories listed so long as the item and amount are considered necessary to perform the proposed work and are not precluded by specific program guidelines or applicable cost principles.

A full discussion of the budget and the allowability of selected items of cost are contained in the following sections, the GPM as well as other NSF program solicitations. Allowability of costs is determined in accordance with OMB Circulars regarding Cost Principles available at

http://www.whitehouse.gov/omb/circulars/index.html

(i)   Salaries and Wages (Lines A and B on the Proposal Budget)

    (a)   Policies

As a general policy, NSF recognizes that salaries of faculty members and other personnel associated directly with the project constitute appropriate direct costs and may be requested in proportion to the effort devoted to the project.

NSF regards research as one of the normal functions of faculty members at institutions of higher education. Compensation for time normally spent on research within the term of appointment is deemed to be included within the faculty member's regular organizational salary. Grant funds may not be used to augment the total salary or rate of salary of faculty members during the period covered by the term of faculty appointment or to reimburse faculty members for consulting or other time in addition to a regular full-time organizational salary covering the same general period of employment. Exceptions may be considered under certain NSF science and engineering education program solicitations for weekend and evening classes or for administrative work done as overload. (See GPM Section 611.)

Summer salary for faculty members on academic-year appointments is limited to no more than two-ninths of their regular academic-year salary. This limit includes summer salary received from all NSF-funded grants.

These same principles apply to other types of non-academic organizations, such as research institutes. Since their employment periods are usually annual, salary must be shown under "calendar months." For such persons, "summer salary" is normally inappropriate under an NSF grant.

Sometimes an independent institute or laboratory proposes to employ college or university faculty members on a part-time basis. In such cases, the general intent of the policies above apply, so that an individual's total income will not be augmented in ways that would not be possible under a grant to an academic institution.

In most circumstances, particularly for institutions of higher education, salaries of administrative or clerical staff are included as part of indirect costs [also known as Facilities and Administrative Costs (F&A) for Colleges and Universities]. Salaries of administrative or clerical staff may be requested as direct costs, however, for a project requiring an extensive amount of administrative or clerical support and where these costs can be readily and specifically identified with the project with a high degree of accuracy. The circumstances for requiring direct charging of these services must be clearly described in the budget justification. NSF may delete such costs, if they are not clearly justified.

(b) Procedures

The names of the PI(s), faculty, and other senior personnel, and the estimated number of full-time-equivalent academic-year, summer, or calendar-year person-months for which NSF funding is requested and the total amount of salaries per year must be listed. For postdoctoral associates and other professionals, the total number of persons for each position must be listed, with the number of full-time-equivalent person-months and total amount of salaries per year. For graduate and undergraduate students, secretarial, clerical, technical, etc., whose time will be charged directly to the project, only the total number of persons and total amount of salaries per year in each category is required. Salaries requested must be consistent with the organization's regular practices. The budget justification should detail the rates of pay by individual for senior personnel, postdoctoral associates, and other professionals.

The budget may request funds for support of graduate or undergraduate research assistants to help carry out the proposed research. Compensation classified as salary payments must be requested in the salaries and wages category. Any direct costs requested for tuition remission must be listed in the "Other" category under "Other Direct Costs."

(c) Confidential Budgetary Information

The proposing organization may request that salary data on senior personnel not be released to persons outside the Government during the review process. In such cases, the item for senior personnel salaries in the proposal may appear as a single figure and the person-months represented by that amount omitted. If this option is exercised, senior personnel salaries and person-months must be itemized in a separate statement, and forwarded to NSF in accordance with the instructions specified in Chapter I, Section B, Proprietary or

Privileged Information. This statement must include all of the information requested on the proposal budget for each person involved. NSF will not forward the detailed information to reviewers and will hold it privileged to the extent permitted by law. The information on senior personnel salaries will be used as the basis for determining the salary amounts shown in the grant budget. The box for "Proprietary or Privileged Information" must be checked on the proposal Cover Sheet when the proposal contains confidential budgetary information.

(ii) Fringe Benefits (Line C on the Proposal Budget)

If the grantee's usual accounting practices provide that its contributions to employee benefits (social security, retirement, etc.) be treated as direct costs, NSF grant funds may be requested to fund fringe benefits as a direct cost.

(iii) Equipment (Line D on the Proposal Budget)

Equipment is defined as an item of property that has an acquisition cost of $5,000 or more (unless the organization has established lower levels) and an expected service life of more than one year. Items of needed equipment must be listed individually by description and estimated cost, including tax, and adequately justified. Allowable items ordinarily will be limited to research equipment and apparatus not already available for the conduct of the work. General-purpose equipment, such as a personal computer, is not eligible for support unless primarily or exclusively used in the actual conduct of scientific research. (See also GPG Chapter VI, Section D, Equipment, for further information on title to equipment.)

(iv) Travel (Line E on the Proposal Budget)

(a) General

Travel and its relation to the proposed activities must be specified and itemized by destination and cost. Funds may be requested for field work, attendance at meetings and conferences, and other travel associated with the proposed work, including subsistence. In order to qualify for support, however, attendance at meetings or conferences must enhance the PI's ability to perform the work, plan extensions of it, or disseminate its results.

Allowance for air travel normally will not exceed the cost of round-trip, economy airfares. (See also GPM Section 614.) Persons traveling under NSF grants must travel by U.S.-flag carriers, if available.

(b) Domestic Travel

For budget purposes, domestic travel includes travel in the U.S., its possessions, Puerto Rico, and travel to Canada and Mexico.

(c) Foreign Travel

For budget purposes, travel outside the areas specified above is considered foreign. The proposal must include relevant information, including countries to be visited (also enter names of countries on the proposal budget), dates of visit, if known, and justification for any foreign travel planned in connection with the project.

Travel support for dependents of key project personnel may be requested only when all of the following conditions apply:

(i) the individual is a key person who is essential to the research on a full-time basis;

(ii) the individual's residence away from home and in a foreign country is for a continuous period of six months or more and is essential to the effective performance of the project;

(iii) the dependent's travel allowance is consistent with the policies of the organization administering the grant.

(iv) participant support (Line F on the Proposal Budget)

This budget category refers to costs of transportation, per diem, stipends, and other related costs for participants or trainees (but not employees) in connection with NSF-sponsored conferences, meetings, symposia, training activities and workshops. (See Chapter II, Section D.7) Generally, indirect costs (F&A) are not allowed on participant support costs. The number of participants to be supported must be entered in the parentheses on the proposal budget. These costs also must be justified in the Budget Justification section of the proposal. Some programs, such as Research Experiences for Undergraduates have special instructions for treatment of participant support.

(v) other direct costs (Lines G1 through G6 on the Proposal Budget)

Any costs charged to an NSF grant must be reasonable and directly allocable to the supported activity. The budget must identify and itemize other anticipated direct costs not included under the headings above, including materials and supplies, publication costs, computer services and consultant services. Examples include aircraft rental, space rental at research establishments away from the grantee organization, minor building alterations, payments to human subjects, service charges, tuition remission, and construction of equipment or systems not available off the shelf. Reference books and periodicals may be charged to the grant only if they are specifically required for the project.

(a) Materials and Supplies (Line G1 on the Proposal Budget)

The proposal budget must indicate the general types of expendable materials and supplies required, with their estimated costs. The breakdown should be more detailed when the cost is substantial.

(b) Publication/Documentation/Dissemination (Line G2 on the Proposal Budget)

The proposal budget may request funds for the costs of documenting, preparing, publishing or otherwise making available to others the findings and products of the work conducted under the grant. This generally includes the following types of activities:

- reports
- reprints
- page charges or other journal costs (except costs for prior or early publication)
- necessary illustrations
- cleanup
- documentation
- storage and indexing of data and databases
- development
- documentation and debugging of software
- storage, preservation, documentation, indexing, etc., of physical specimens, collections, or fabricated items.

(c) Consultant Services (Line G3 on the Proposal Budget)

Anticipated consultant services must be justified and information furnished on each individual's expertise, primary organizational affiliation, normal daily compensation rate, and number of days of expected service. Consultants' travel costs, including subsistence, also may be included. Payment for a consultant's services, exclusive of expenses, may not exceed the consultant's normal rate or the daily maximum rate established annually by NSF, whichever is less.

(d) Computer Services (Line G4 on the Proposal Budget)

The cost of computer services, including computer-based retrieval of scientific, technical and educational information, may be requested. A justification based on the established computer service rates at the proposing organization must be included. The proposal budget also may request costs, which must be shown to be reasonable, for leasing of computer equipment. Special purpose computers or associated hardware and software, other than general purpose PCs, may be requested as items of equipment and justified in terms of their necessity for the activity proposed.

(e) Sub-awards 26 (Line G5 on the Proposal Budget)

Except for the procurement of such items as commercially available supplies, materials, equipment or general support services allowable under the grant, no significant part of the research or substantive effort under an NSF grant may be contracted or otherwise transferred to another organization without prior NSF authorization. The intent to enter into such arrangements must be disclosed in the proposal. At a minimum, the disclosure must include a clear description of the work to be performed, and the basis for selection of the sub-awardee (except for collaborative/joint arrangements) and a separate budget for each sub-award.

(f) Other (Line G6 on the Proposal Budget)

Any other direct costs not specified in Lines G1 through G5 must be identified on Line G6. Such costs must be itemized and justified in the budget justification.

(vii) Total Direct Costs (Line H on the Proposal Budget)

The total amount of direct costs requested by the proposer, to include Lines A through G, must be entered on Line H.

(viii) Indirect Costs [also known as Facilities and Administrative Costs (F&A) for Colleges and Universities; Line I on the Proposal Budget]

The applicable indirect cost rate(s) negotiated by the organization with the cognizant Federal negotiating agency must be used in computing indirect costs (F&A) for a proposal. If an organization has no established indirect cost rate, it should contact the Cost Analysis/Audit Resolution Branch of NSF's Division of Acquisition and Cost Support. An organization may obtain guidelines for submitting rate proposals from that Branch, telephone (703) 292-8244.

Within Government guidelines, unless otherwise indicated in a specific program solicitation, it is NSF policy that grantees are entitled to reimbursement from grant funds for indirect costs (F&A) allocable to the NSF share of allowable direct costs of a project, except grants:

- solely for the support of travel, equipment, construction of facilities, or doctoral dissertations;
- for participant support costs;
- to foreign grantees; and
- to individuals (i.e., Fellowship awards).

(ix) Total Direct and Indirect Costs (F&A; Line J on the Proposal Budget)

The total amount of direct and indirect costs (F&A; sum of Lines H and I) must be entered on Line J.

(x) Residual Funds (Line K on the Proposal Budget)

This line is used only for budgets for incremental funding requests on continuing grants. Grantees must provide a rationale for residual funds in excess of 20% as part of the annual project report.

(xi) Amount of This Request (Line L on the Proposal Budget)

The total amount of funds requested by the proposer will be the same as the amount entered on Line J unless the Foundation disapproves the carry-over of residual funds. If disapproved, Line L will be equal to Line J minus Line K.

(xii) Cost Sharing (Line M on the Proposal Budget)

(a) Statutory Cost Sharing Requirement. In accordance with Congressional requirements (see GPM 330), NSF requires that each grantee share in the cost of research projects resulting from unsolicited proposals. In addition to proposals submitted solely in response to the Grant Proposal Guide, proposals submitted in response to NSF program announcements are considered unsolicited and are subject to the statutory cost sharing requirement.

The grantee may meet the statutory cost sharing requirement by choosing either of two alternatives:

- by cost sharing a minimum of one percent on the project;

or

- by cost sharing a minimum of one percent on the aggregate costs of all NSF-supported projects requiring cost sharing.

The statutory cost sharing is not required for grants that provide funds solely for the following purposes (not considered to be support of "research"), although such awards may be subject to other cost sharing requirements identified in a specific solicitation:

- international travel;
- construction, improvement or operation of facilities;
- acquisition of research equipment;
- ship operations;
- education and training;
- publication, distribution and translation of scientific data and information;
- symposia, conferences and workshops;
- special studies authorized or required by Subsections 3a(5) through 3a(7) of the NSF Act, as amended.

In accordance with Important Notice 128, Revision of the NSF Cost Sharing Policy, for unsolicited proposals submitted in response to the Grant Proposal Guide and for proposals submitted in response to NSF program announcements, only the statutory cost sharing amount (1%) is required. In such cases, proposers are advised NOT to identify cost sharing amounts on Line M of the proposal budget. A set of Frequently Asked Questions (FAQs) regarding the cost sharing issue is available for use by the proposer and awardee community on the NSF Web site.

(b) Cost Sharing Requirements Under NSF Program Solicitations. Proposals submitted in response to NSF solicitations may be subject to special cost sharing requirements. In cases where cost sharing is required, NSF has determined that proposals submitted in response to the solicitation provide a tangible benefit to the award recipient(s) (normally beyond the immediate term or scope of the NSF-supported activity). Benefit is defined in terms of capacity building, potential dollar revenues, time frames, or third party users. NSF-funded activities that are characterized by such benefits are awards for infrastructure-building purposes (instrumentation/equipment/centers/facilities) or for awards where there is clear potential to make profit or generate income (e.g., curriculum development). In accordance with Important Notice 128, proposers are advised not to exceed the cost sharing level or amount specified in the solicitation.

When cost sharing is required, it is considered an eligibility rather than a review criterion. In order to retain this concept, NSF has modified the FastLane system to ensure that Line M is masked from peer reviewers during the review process.

Proposers are advised that all proposed cost sharing commitments, if incorporated into the award, are subject to audit. When applicable, the estimated value of any in-kind contributions should be included on Line M. An explanation of the source, nature, amount, and availability of any proposed cost sharing also must be provided in the budget justification. It should be noted that contributions derived from other Federal funds or counted as cost sharing toward projects of another Federal agency may not be counted towards meeting the specific cost sharing requirements of the NSF grant. Failure to provide the level of cost sharing reflected in the approved grant budget may result in termination of the NSF grant, disallowance of grant costs and/or refund of grant funds to NSF by the grantee.

(xiii) Unallowable Costs

Proposers should be familiar with the complete list of unallowable costs that is contained in the applicable cost principles. Because of their sensitivity, the following categories of unallowable costs are highlighted:

(a) Entertainment

Costs of entertainment, amusement, diversion and social activities and any costs directly associated with such activities (such as tickets to shows or sporting events, meals, lodging, rentals, transportation, and gratuities) are unallowable. Expenses of grantee employees who are not on travel status are unallowable. This includes cases where they serve as hosts or otherwise participate at meals that are primarily social occasions involving speakers or consultants. Costs of employees on travel status are limited to those allowed under the governing cost principles for travel expenses. (See GPM Section 614.)

(b) Meals and Coffee Breaks

No NSF funds may be spent on meals or coffee breaks for intramural meetings of an organization or any of its components, including, but not limited to, laboratories, departments, and centers.

(c) Alcoholic Beverages

No NSF funds may be spent on alcoholic beverages.

(h). Current and Pending Support

This section of the proposal calls for required information on all current and pending support for ongoing projects and proposals, including subsequent funding in the case of continuing grants. All current project support from whatever source (e.g., Federal, State, local, or foreign government agencies, public or private foundations, industrial or other commercial organizations) must be listed. The proposed project and all other projects or activities requiring a portion of time of the PI and other senior personnel must be included, even if they receive no salary support from the project(s). The total award amount for the entire award period covered (including indirect costs) must be shown as well as the number of person-months per year to be devoted to the project, regardless of source of support. Similar information must be provided for all proposals already submitted or submitted concurrently to other possible sponsors, including NSF. Concurrent submission of a proposal to other organizations will not prejudice its review by NSF. Note the Biological Sciences Directorate exception to this policy, however, delineated in Chapter I Section A: Overview.

If the project now being submitted has been funded previously by a source other than NSF, the information requested in the paragraph above must be furnished for the last period of funding.

(i). Facilities, Equipment and Other Resources

This section of the proposal is used to assess the adequacy of the organizational resources available to perform the effort proposed. Proposers must describe only those resources that are directly applicable.

(j). Special Information and Supplementary Documentation

Except as specified below, special information and supplementary documentation must be included as part of the project description (or part of the budget justification), if it is relevant to determining the quality of the proposed work. Information submitted in the following areas is not considered part of the 15-page project description limitation. This Special Information and Supplementary Documentation section also is not considered an appendix. Specific guidance on the need for additional documentation may be obtained from the organization's sponsored projects office or in the references cited below.

- Rationale for performance of all or part of the project off-campus or away from organizational headquarters (GPM Section 633).

- Documentation of collaborative arrangements of significance to the proposal through letters of commitment (GPG Chapter II, Section D.3).

- Environmental impact statement for activities that have an actual or potential impact on the environment (GPM Section 830).

- Work in foreign countries. Some governments require nonresidents to obtain official approval to carry out investigations within their borders and coastal waters under their jurisdiction. PIs are responsible for obtaining the required authorizations and for advising NSF that they have been obtained or requested. Advance coordination should minimize disruption of the research (GPM Section 763 and GPM 715).

- Research in Greenland (GPM Section 763).

- Antarctic proposals to any NSF program require operational worksheets by the first Wednesday of June in the year before any proposed fieldwork. See "proposals with fieldwork" and "Special budget considerations" under "Antarctic Research."

- Research in a location designated, or eligible to be designated, a registered historic place (GPM Section 840). Where applicable, the box for "Historic Places" must be checked on the proposal Cover Sheet.

- Research involving field experiments with genetically engineered organisms (GPM Section 712).

- Documentation regarding research involving the use of human subjects, hazardous materials, vertebrate animals, or endangered species. (GPM Section 710, GPG Chapter II, Sections D.5 and D.6) Where applicable the box for "Human Subjects" or "Vertebrate Animals" must be checked on the proposal Cover Sheet.

- Projects that involve technology utilization/transfer activities, that require a management plan, or that involve special reports or final products.

- Special components in new proposals or in requests for supplements, such as Facilitation Awards for Scientists and Engineers with Disabilities (FASED), Research Opportunity Awards or Research Experiences for Undergraduates. (See GPG Chapter II, Section D.2 for information on FASED, and for the other programs identified, consult the relevant program solicitation.)

- Research in Undergraduate Institutions. (See program solicitation for information.)

- Research Experiences for Undergraduates (REU). (See program solicitation for REU site proposals for further information.)

In addition, the supplementary documentation section should alert NSF officials to unusual circumstances that require special handling, including, for example:

- proprietary or other privileged information in the proposal

- matters affecting individual privacy

- required intergovernmental review under E.O. 12372 (Intergovernmental Review of Federal Programs) for activities that directly affect State or local governments

- possible national security implications.

(k). Appendices

All information necessary for the review of a proposal must be contained in Sections A through I of the proposal. Appendices may not be included unless a deviation has been authorized. Chapter II, Section A. Conformance with Instructions for Proposal Preparation, contains further information.

SPECIAL GUIDELINES

1. Small Grants for Exploratory Research (SGER) Proposals

Proposals for small-scale, exploratory, high-risk research in the fields of science, engineering, and education normally supported by NSF may be submitted to individual programs. Such research is characterized as:

- preliminary work on untested and novel ideas;
- ventures into emerging and potentially transformative research ideas;
- Application of new expertise or new approaches to "established" research topics;
- having a severe urgency with regard to availability of, or access to data, facilities or specialized equipment, including quick-response research on natural or anthropogenic disasters and similar unanticipated events;

or

- efforts of similar character likely to catalyze rapid and innovative advances.

Investigators are strongly encouraged to contact the NSF program(s) most germane to the proposal topic before submitting an SGER proposal. This will facilitate determining whether the proposed work meets the guidelines described above and availability and appropriateness for SGER funding, or whether the work is more appropriate for submission as a fully reviewed proposal. The project description must be brief (no more than 2 to 5 pages) and must include clear statements as to

- why the proposed research should be considered particularly exploratory and high risk
- the nature and significance of its potential impact on the field
- why an SGER grant would be a suitable means of supporting the work.

Brief biographical information is required for the PI and co-PI(s) only, and must list no more than 5 significant publications or other research products. The box for "Small Grant for Exploratory Research" must be checked on the proposal Cover Sheet.

These proposals will be subject to **internal** NSF merit review only. Renewed funding of SGER awards may be requested only through submission of a non-SGER proposal that will be subject to full merit review. The maximum SGER award amount will not exceed $200,000. Although the maximum award amount is $200,000, the award amount usually will be substantially less than a given program's average award amount. The project's duration will normally be 1 year, but may be up to 2 years.

At the discretion of the Program Officer, and with the concurrence of the Division Director, a small fraction of especially promising SGER awards may be extended for a period of 6 additional months and supplemented with up to $50,000 in additional funding. The SGER award extensions will be possible for awards of 2-year initial duration as well as for those of shorter initial duration. Requests for extensions must be submitted 1 to 2 months before the expiration date of the initial award. A project report and outline of proposed research, not to exceed 5 pages, must be included.

2. Facilitation Awards for Scientists and Engineers with Disabilities (FASED)

   As part of its effort to promote full utilization of highly qualified scientists, mathematicians, and engineers, and to develop scientific and technical talent, the Foundation has the following goals:

   - to reduce or remove barriers to participation in research and training by physically disabled individuals by providing special equipment and assistance under awards made by NSF;

- to encourage disabled individuals to pursue careers in science and engineering by stimulating the development and demonstration of special equipment that facilitates their work performance.

Individuals with disabilities eligible for facilitation awards include principal investigators, other senior project personnel, and graduate and undergraduate students. The cognizant NSF Program Officer will make decisions regarding what constitutes appropriate support on a case-by-case basis. The specific nature, purpose, and need for equipment or assistance should be described in sufficient detail in the proposal to permit evaluation by knowledgeable reviewers.

There is no separate program for funding of special equipment or assistance. Requests are made in conjunction with regular competitive proposals, or as a supplemental funding request to an existing NSF award. Specific instructions for each type of request are provided below.

a.   Requests as part of a competitive proposal submission

Funds may be requested to purchase special equipment, modify equipment, or provide services required specifically for the work to be undertaken. Requests for funds for equipment or assistance that compensate in a general way for the disabling condition are not permitted. For example, funds may be requested to provide:

- prosthetic devices to manipulate a particular apparatus
- equipment to convert sound to visual signals, or vice versa, for a particular experiment
- access to a special site or to a mode of transportation (except as defined below)
- a reader or interpreter with special technical competence related to the project
- other special-purpose equipment or assistance needed to conduct a particular project.
    - However, items such as standard wheel chairs, prosthetics, hearing aids, TDD/text-phones, or general readers for the blind would **NOT** be supported because the need for them is not specific to the proposed project.
    - Similarly, ramps, elevators, or other structural modifications of research facilities are **NOT** eligible for direct support under this program.

There is no maximum funding amount that has been established for such requests. It is expected, however, that the cost (including equipment adaptation and installation) will not be a major component of the total proposed budget for the project. Requests for funds for special equipment or assistance to facilitate the participation of individuals with disabilities should be included in the proposed budget for the project and documented in the budget justification. The specific nature, purpose, and need for such equipment or assistance should be described in sufficient detail in the Project Description to permit evaluation of the request by knowledgeable reviewers.

b. Supplemental Funding Requests to existing NSF grants

Supplemental funds for special equipment or assistance to facilitate participation in NSF-supported projects by persons with disabilities may be provided under existing NSF grants. Normally, title is vested in the grantee organization for equipment purchased in conjunction with NSF-supported activities. In accordance with the Grant General Conditions (GC-1), the grantee organization guarantees use of the equipment for the specific project during the period of work funded by the Foundation, and assures its use in an appropriate manner after project completion. In instances involving special equipment for persons with disabilities, the need for such may be unique to the individual. In such cases, the grantee organization may elect to transfer title to the individual to assure appropriate use after project completion.

Supplemental requests should be submitted electronically by using the "Supplemental Funding Request" function in FastLane and should include a brief description of the request, a budget, and a budget justification. Requests must be submitted at least 2 months before funds are needed. Funding decisions will be made on the basis of the justification and availability of program funds with any resultant funding provided through a formal amendment of the existing NSF grant.

3. Collaborative Proposals

A collaborative proposal is one in which investigators from 2 or more organizations wish to collaborate on a unified research project. Collaborative proposals may be submitted to NSF in 1 of 2 methods: as a single proposal, in which a single award is being requested (with sub-awards administered by the lead organization); or by simultaneous submission of proposals from different organizations, with each organization requesting a separate award. In either case, the lead organization's proposal must contain all of the requisite sections as a single package to be provided to reviewers (that will happen automatically when procedures below are followed.) All collaborative proposals must clearly describe the roles to be played by the other organizations, specify the managerial arrangements, and explain the advantages of the multi-organizational effort within the project description. **PIs are strongly encouraged to contact the cognizant NSF Program Officer prior to submission of a collaborative proposal.**

a. Submission of a single proposal

The single proposal method allows investigators from 2 or more organizations who have developed an integrated research project to submit a single, focused proposal. A single investigator bears primary responsibility for the administration of the grant and discussions with NSF, and, at the discretion of the organizations involved, investigators from any of the participating organizations may be designated as co-PIs.

By submission of the proposal, the organization has determined that the proposed activity is administratively manageable. NSF may request a revised proposal, however, if it considers that the project is so complex that it will be too difficult to review or administer as presented. (See Chapter II, Section C.2.g.(6)(e) for additional instructions on preparation of this type of proposal.)

b. Simultaneous submission of proposals from different organizations

In many instances, simultaneous submission of proposals that contain the same project description from each organization might be appropriate. For these proposals, the project title must begin with the words, "Collaborative Research." The lead organization's submission will include a proposal Cover Sheet, project summary, project description, references cited, biographical sketches, budgets and budget justification, current and pending support, and facilities, equipment, and other resources for their organization. Non-lead organization submissions will include all of the above for their organization except the project summary, project description, and references cited that are the same for all collaborating organizations. FastLane will combine the proposal submission for printing or electronic viewing. To submit the collaborative proposal, the following process must be completed.

(i) Each non-lead organization must assign their proposal a proposal PIN. This proposal PIN and the temporary proposal ID generated by FastLane when the non-lead proposal is created must be provided to the lead organization before the lead organization submits its proposal to NSF.

(ii) The lead organization must then enter each non-lead organization(s) proposal PIN and temporary proposal ID into the FastLane lead proposal by using the "Link Collaborative Proposals" option found on the FastLane "Form Preparation" screen.

Given that such separately submitted collaborative proposals constitute a "single" proposal submission to NSF, it is imperative that the proposals be submitted within a reasonable timeframe to one another. Failure to submit all components of the collaborative proposal on a timely basis may impact the review of the proposal.

4. Proposals for Equipment

Proposals for specialized equipment may be submitted by an organization for:

(1) individual investigators;

(2) groups of investigators within the same department;

(3) several departments;

(4) organization(s) participating in a collaborative or joint arrangement;

(5) any components of an organization;

(6) a region.

One individual must be designated as PI. Investigators may be working in closely related areas or their research may be multidisciplinary.

Note: Many organizations within NSF have formal instrumentation programs that may include special guidelines such as cost sharing or other requirements. It is important to use the applicable guidelines in these competitions. The appropriate program should be consulted.

Instrumentation and equipment proposals must follow the format of research proposals. Each potential major user must describe the project(s) for which the equipment will be used. These descriptions must be succinct, not necessarily as detailed as in an individual research proposal, and must emphasize the intrinsic merit of the activity and the importance of the equipment to it. A brief summary will suffice for auxiliary users.

Equipment to be purchased, modified or constructed must be described in sufficient detail to allow comparison of its capabilities with the needs of the proposed activities. Equipment proposals also must describe comparable equipment already at the proposing organization(s) and explain why it cannot be used. This includes comparable government-owned equipment that is on-site.

Equipment proposals must discuss arrangements for acquisition, maintenance and operation, including:

- overall acquisition plan;
- biographical sketch of the person(s) who will have overall responsibility for maintenance and operation and a brief statement of qualifications, if not obvious;
- description of the physical facility, including floor plans or other appropriate information, where the equipment will be located;
- statement of why the equipment is severable or non-severable from the physical facility;
- annual budget for operation and maintenance of the proposed equipment, indicating source of funds, and particularly related equipment;
  and
- brief description of other support services available and the annual budget for their operation, maintenance and administration.

The terms of a grant require that special-purpose equipment purchased or leased with grant funds be subject to

- reasonable inventory controls
- maintenance procedures
- organizational policies that enhance its multiple or shared use on other projects, if such use does not interfere with the work for which the equipment was acquired.

If the government retains title, those items must be included in the annual inventory submitted to the NSF Property Administrator. Equipment proposals must include the information described above within the 15-page project description. These proposals normally compete with proposals for research or education projects.

5. Proposals Involving Vertebrate Animals

For proposals involving the use of vertebrate animals, sufficient information must be provided within the 15-page project description to enable reviewers to evaluate the choice of species, number of animals to be used, and any necessary exposure of animals to discomfort, pain, or injury.

Consistent with the requirements of the Animal Welfare Act [7 U.S.C. 2131 et seq] and the regulations promulgated by the Secretary of Agriculture [9 CFR, 1.1-4.11], NSF requires that proposed projects involving use of any vertebrate animal for research or education be approved by the submitting organization's Institutional Animal Care and Use Committee (IACUC) before an award can be made. For this approval to be accepted by NSF, the organization must have a current Institutional Animal Welfare Assurance established with the Public Health Service (PHS).

If the organization does not have such an Assurance in place, then approval of the project by the IACUC of an organization with a current PHS Assurance will be acceptable, if the IACUC agrees to provide the required oversight of facilities and activities during the award. Alternatively, the submitting organization may create its own IACUC by establishing a single-project Institutional Animal Welfare Assurance with NSF. In any case, IACUC approval must be received prior to an award. Proposers with questions regarding this requirement should contact the cognizant NSF Program Officer.

The box for "Vertebrate Animals" must be checked on the proposal Cover Sheet with the IACUC approval date (if available) identified in the space provided. If IACUC approval has not been obtained prior to submission, the proposer should indicate "Pending" in the space provided for the approval date.

These same rules apply to awards to individuals (fellowships) for activities that involve use of vertebrate animals. The "Vertebrate Animals" box should be checked on the proposal Cover Sheet. Evidence of IACUC approval can be provided in a letter giving the date of IACUC approval with the appropriate organizational signature.

6. Proposals Involving Human Subjects

Projects involving research with human subjects must ensure that subjects are protected from research risks in conformance with the relevant Federal policy known as the Common Rule (Federal Policy for the Protection of Human Subjects, 45 CFR 690). All projects involving human subjects either must have approval from the organization's Institutional Review Board (IRB) before issuance of an NSF award, or affirm that the IRB has declared the research exempt from continued oversight, in accordance with the applicable subsection of section 101(b) of the Common Rule. The box for "Human Subjects" must be checked on the proposal Cover Sheet with the IRB approval date (if available) or exemption subsection from the Common Rule identified in the space provided. If IRB approval has not been obtained prior to submission, the proposer should indicate "Pending" in the space provided for the approval date.

Additional information, including Frequently Asked Questions and Vignettes, for use in interpreting the Common Rule for Behavioral and Social Science Research, is available on the NSF Web site at

http://www.nsf.gov/bfa/dga/policy/guidance.htm#human

7. Proposals for Conferences, Symposia and Workshops

NSF supports conferences, symposia and workshops in special areas of science and engineering that bring experts together to discuss recent research or education findings or to expose other researchers or students to new research and education techniques. NSF encourages the convening in the U.S. of major international conferences, symposia, and workshops. Conferences will be supported only if equivalent results cannot be obtained at regular meetings of professional societies. Although requests for support of conferences, symposia, and workshops ordinarily originate with educational institutions or scientific and engineering societies, they also may come from other groups. Shared support by several Federal agencies, States, or private organizations is encouraged. Because proceedings of such conferences normally should be published in professional journals, requests for support may include publication costs. Proposals for Conferences, Symposia, and Workshops should generally be made at least a year in advance of the scheduled date. Conferences or meetings, including the facilities in which they are held, funded in whole or in part with NSF funds, must be accessible to participants with disabilities. A conference, symposium or workshop proposal (that complies with the page and font size instructions in Chapter II, Section B, Format of the Proposal) must contain the following elements:

- Cover Sheet;
- Summary of one page or less indicating the objectives of the project;
- Statement of the need for such a gathering and a list of topics;
- Recent meetings on the same subject, including dates and locations;
- Names of the chairperson and members of organizing committees and their organizational affiliations;
- Information on the location and probable date(s) of the meeting and the method of announcement or invitation;
- Statement of how the meeting will be organized and conducted, how the results of the meeting will be disseminated, and how the meeting will contribute to the enhancement and improvement of scientific, engineering, and/or educational activities;
- A plan for recruitment of and support for speakers and other attendees, that includes participation of groups underrepresented in science and engineering (e.g., underrepresented minorities, women, and persons with disabilities);
- Estimated total budget for the conference, together with an itemized statement of the amount of support requested from NSF (the NSF budget may include participant support for transportation (when appropriate), per diem costs, stipends, publication, and other conference-related costs. (Note: participant support costs must be excluded from the indirect cost base.)
- Support requested or available from other Federal agencies and other sources. (Chapter II, Section C.2.h should be consulted to prepare this portion of the proposal.)

For additional coverage on allowability of costs associated with meetings and conferences, proposers should consult GPM Section 625.

8. Proposals to Support International Travel

Proposals for travel support for U.S. participation in international scientific and engineering meetings held abroad are handled by the NSF organizational unit with program responsibility for the area of interest.

Group travel awards are encouraged as the primary means of support for international travel. A university, professional society, or other non-profit organization may apply for funds to enable it to coordinate and support U.S. participation in one or more international scientific meeting(s) abroad.

Proposals submitted for this purpose should address the same items as those indicated for conferences, symposia, and workshops (see Section 7 above), with particular attention to plans for composition and recruitment of the travel group. Information on planned speakers should be provided where available from the conference organizer.

Group travel proposals may request support only for the international travel costs of the proposed activity. However, in addition, group travel proposals also may include as compensation for the grantee, a flat rate of $50 per traveler for general administrative costs of preparing announcements, evaluating proposals, and handling travel arrangements customarily associated with this type of project (See GPM Section 765).

Group travel grantees are required to retain supporting documentation that funds were spent in accordance with the original intent of the proposal. Such documentation may be required in final reports and is subject to audit.

9. Proposals for Doctoral Dissertation Research

   NSF awards grants in support of doctoral dissertation research in some disciplines, primarily field research in the environmental, behavioral, and social sciences. Support may be sought through those disciplinary programs and, in cases involving research abroad, through the Office of International Programs. The thesis advisor or concerned faculty member submits proposals on behalf of the graduate student. Further information can be obtained from the cognizant program office.

10. The NSF Prospective New Awardee Guide is available electronically on the NSF Web site at

    http://www.nsf.gov/pubsys/ods/getpub.cfm?nsf03054

11. FAQs regarding FastLane proposal preparation and submission also are available electronically on the FastLane Web site.

12. Requests for approval of a deviation from NSF's electronic submission requirement must be forwarded to the cognizant NSF program for review and approval prior to submission of the paper proposal.

13. Further instructions for this process are available electronically on the FastLane Web site.

14. Detailed instructions for completion of this process are available electronically on the FastLane Web site.

15. For consistency with the Department of Health and Human Services conflict of interest policy, in lieu of "organization," NSF is using the term "institution," which includes all categories of proposers.

16. Detailed instructions for submission of the SF LLL are available on the FastLane Web site.

17. Requests for approval of a deviation from NSF's electronic submission requirement must be forwarded to the cognizant NSF program for review and approval prior to submission of the paper proposal.

18. Examples illustrating activities likely to demonstrate broader impacts are available electronically on the NSF Web site at

    http://www.nsf.gov/pubs/2004/nsf042/bicexamples.pdf

19. If the proposer has a Web site address readily available, that information should be included in the citation, as stated above. It is not NSF's intent, how-

ever, to place an undue burden on proposers to search for the URL of every referenced publication. Therefore, inclusion of a Web site address is optional. A proposal that includes reference citation(s) that do not specify a URL address is not considered to be in violation of NSF proposal-preparation guidelines and the proposal will still be reviewed.

20. Detailed instructions for submission of confidential budgetary information are available on the FastLane Web site.

21. See also the NSF Grant General Conditions for additional information on use of US Flag Air-Carriers at

http://www.nsf.gov/home/grants/grants_gac.htm

23. Proposers are advised that the NSF Grant General Conditions require the grantee to obtain written authorization from the cognizant NSF program officer prior to the reallocation of funds budgeted for participant support.

24. The current maximum consultant daily rate is available electronically on the NSF Web site at

http://www.nsf.gov/bfa/dga/policy/start.htm

25. The term "sub-award" also includes contracts, subcontracts and other arrangements.

26. Proposals submitted in response to program solicitations are considered "solicited." This means that the resulting awards are not subject to statutory cost sharing.

27. Section .23 of OMB Circular A-110 describes criteria and procedures for the allowability of cash and in-kind contributions in satisfying cost sharing and matching requirements.

28. See the NSF Grant General Conditions, Article 6.

29. Detailed instructions for the electronic preparation and submission of collaborative proposals are available on the FastLane Web site at

http://www.fastlane.nsf.gov/a1/newstan.htm#collaborative

30. See GPM 542 for additional information on vesting of title to equipment.

31. In addition to vertebrate animals covered by the Animal Welfare Act, the requirements specified in this GPG coverage also are extended to rats, birds, and mice.

32. Such letters should be provided as supplementary documentation and should be submitted electronically via the Proposal Preparation module in the FastLane system.

NSF proposal processing and review

http://www.nsf.gov/pubs/2004/nsf042/3.htm

Proposals received by the NSF Proposal Processing Unit are assigned to the appropriate NSF program for acknowledgement and, if they meet NSF requirements, for review. All proposals are carefully reviewed by a scientist, engineer, or educator serving as an NSF

Program Officer, and usually by three to ten other persons outside NSF who are experts in the particular fields represented by the proposal. **Proposers are invited to suggest names of persons they believe are especially well qualified to review the proposal and/or persons they would prefer not review the proposal.** These suggestions may serve as one source in the reviewer selection process at the Program Officer's discretion. Program Officers may obtain comments from assembled review panels or from site visits before recommending final action on proposals. Senior NSF staff further review recommendations for awards.

REVIEW CRITERIA

All NSF proposals are evaluated through use of two National Science Board approved merit review criteria. In some instances, however, NSF will employ additional criteria as required to highlight the specific objectives of certain programs and activities. For example, proposals for large facility projects also might be subject to special review criteria outlined in the program solicitation.

The two merit review criteria are listed below. The criteria include considerations that help define them. These considerations are suggestions, and not all will apply to any given proposal. While proposers must address both merit review criteria, Reviewers will be asked to address only those considerations that are relevant to the proposal being considered and for which he/she is qualified to make judgments.

What is the intellectual merit of the proposed activity?

- How important is the proposed activity to advancing knowledge and understanding within its own field or across different fields?
- How well qualified is the proposer (individual or team) to conduct the project? (If appropriate, the reviewer will comment on the quality of prior work.)
- To what extent does the proposed activity suggest and explore creative and original concepts?
- How well conceived and organized is the proposed activity?
- Is there sufficient access to resources?

What are the broader impacts of the proposed activity?

- How well does the activity advance discovery and understanding while promoting teaching, training, and learning?
- How well does the proposed activity broaden the participation of underrepresented groups (e.g., gender, ethnicity, disability, geographic, etc.)?
- To what extent will it enhance the infrastructure for research and education, such as facilities, instrumentation, networks, and partnerships?
- Will the results be disseminated broadly to enhance scientific and technological understanding?
- What may be the benefits of the proposed activity to society?

NSF staff will give careful consideration to the following in making funding decisions:

Integration of research and education
One of the principal strategies in support of NSF's goals is to foster integration of research and education through the programs, projects, and activities it supports at academic and

research institutions. These institutions provide abundant opportunities where individuals may concurrently assume responsibilities as researchers, educators, and students, and where all can engage in joint efforts that infuse education with the excitement of discovery and enrich research through the diversity of learning perspectives.

Integrating diversity into NSF programs, projects, and activities

Broadening opportunities and enabling the participation of all citizens, women and men, under-represented minorities, and persons with disabilities, are essential to the health and vitality of science and engineering. NSF is committed to this principle of diversity and deems it central to the programs, projects, and activities it considers and supports.

Administrative corrections to proposals

NSF recognizes that minor, non-content-related errors may occur in proposal development and that these errors may not be discovered until after the proposal submission to NSF. To enable organizations to correct such errors, FastLane provides a 60-minute "grace period," that begins immediately following proposal submission. This grace period does not extend the proposal deadline (e.g., if a proposal deadline is 5:00 pm, proposer's local time, the proposal must be submitted by 5:00 pm, and administrative corrections are allowed until 6:00 pm, proposer's local time). During this grace period, authorized sponsored project office personnel are authorized to make administrative corrections to proposal Cover Sheet and Budget data. These corrections do not include changes to identified PIs, co-PIs, or other senior project personnel. Access to the Administrative Corrections utility is via the Research Administration module on the FastLane Web site through use of the "Submit Proposals/Supplements/File Updates/Withdrawals" function.

Proposal file updates

It is the responsibility of the proposing organization to thoroughly review each proposal prior to submission. On occasion, however, a problem is identified with a portion of the proposal after the proposal has been electronically submitted to NSF.

The FastLane Proposal File Update module allows the organization to request the replacement of files associated with a previously submitted proposal. Proposal file update requests must be submitted by an individual who is authorized to submit proposals on behalf of the organization, and electronically signed by the Authorized Organizational Representative (AOR). Update requests must contain a justification that addresses:

1. why the file replacements are being requested

and

2. any changes between the original and proposed replacement files

A proposal file update request automatically will be accepted if submitted prior to the deadline/target date of the program announcement or solicitation, or anytime prior to review in the case of an unsolicited proposal. A request for a proposal file update after an established target or deadline date will require acceptance by the cognizant NSF Program Officer. Such requests only may be submitted in cases where a technical problem has been identified with the proposal (i.e., formatting or print problems). Therefore, **changes to the content of a previously submitted proposal after the established deadline or target date should not be requested.** When a request is accepted, the proposed files will immediately replace the existing files and become part of the official proposal.

PIs can access the proposal file update utility via the "Proposal Functions" section of FastLane. Authorized individuals in the organization's sponsored projects office (or equivalent) can initiate review proposal file update requests using the "Submit Proposals/Supplements/File Updates/Withdrawals" module via the FastLane "Research Administration Functions."

NSF will consider only one proposal file update request per proposal at a time. It is anticipated that it will be a rare occurrence for more than one file update request to be submitted for a proposal.

Revisions to proposals made during the review process

In the event of a significant development (e.g., research findings, changed circumstances, unavailability of PI or other senior personnel, etc.) that might materially affect the outcome of the review of a pending proposal, the proposer must contact the cognizant Program Officer to discuss the issue. **Submitting additional information must not be used as a means of circumventing page limitations or stated deadlines.**

Before recommending whether or not NSF should support a particular project, the NSF Program Officer may, subject to certain constraints outlined below, engage in discussions with the proposing PIs.

Negotiating budgets generally involves discussing a lower or higher amount of total support for the proposed project. The NSF Program Officer may suggest reducing or eliminating costs for specific budget items that are clearly unnecessary or unreasonable for the activities to be undertaken, especially when the review process supports such changes; however, this would generally not include faculty salaries, salary rates, fringe benefits, or tuition. Note: indirect cost rates are not subject to negotiation. The NSF Program Officer may discuss with PIs the "bottom line" award amount, i.e., the total NSF funding that will be recommended for a project. NSF Program Officers may not renegotiate cost sharing or other organizational commitments.

When such discussions result in a budget reduction of 10% or more from the amount originally proposed, a corresponding reduction should be made in the scope of the project. Proposers must use the FastLane Revised Proposal Budget module to submit this information. The components of a revised proposal budget generally consist of the following: the revised budget, and a Budget Impact Statement that describes the impact of the budget reduction on the scope of the project.

> **NOTE:** Revised Proposal Budgets must be electronically signed by the AOR. Paper copies of the revised budget should not be mailed to NSF.

Award recommendation

After scientific, technical, and programmatic review and consideration of appropriate factors, the NSF Program Officer recommends to the cognizant Division Director whether the proposal should be declined or recommended for award. Normally, final programmatic approval is at the division level. Because of the large volume of proposals, this review and consideration process may take up to six months. Large or particularly complex proposals may require additional review and processing time. For example, proposals for large facility projects also might require review in accordance with NSF's Guidelines for Planning and Managing the Major Research Equipment Account. If the program recommendation is for an award and final division or other programmatic approval is obtained, then the recommendation goes to the Division of Grants and Agreements for review of business, financial, and policy implications, and the processing and issuance of a grant or cooperative agreement. The Division of Grants and Agreements generally makes awards to academic institutions within 30 days after the program division makes its recommendation. Grants being made to organizations that have not received an NSF award within the preceding two years, or involving special situations (such as coordination with another Federal agency or a private funding source), cooperative agreements, and other unusual arrangements may require additional review and processing time.

Proposers are cautioned that only an appointed Grants Officer in the Division of Grants and Agreements may make commitments, obligations, or awards on behalf of NSF or authorize the expenditure of funds. No commitment on the part of NSF or the government should be inferred from technical or budgetary discussions with an NSF Program Officer. A PI or organization that makes financial or personnel commitments in the absence of a Grant or Cooperative Agreement signed by the NSF Grants Officer does so at its own risk.

Copies of reviews

When a decision has been made (whether an award or a declination), verbatim copies of reviews, excluding the names of the Reviewers, and summaries of review panel deliberations, if any, are provided to the PI. Proposers also may request and obtain any other releasable material in NSF's file on their proposal. Everything in the file except information that directly identifies either Reviewers or other pending or declined proposals is usually releasable to the proposer.

Examples illustrating activities likely to demonstrate broader impacts are available electronically on the NSF Web site at

http://www.nsf.gov/pubs/2004/nsf042/bicexamples.pdf

Detailed instructions on submitting proposal file updates are available on the FastLane Web site at

https://www.fastlane.nsf.gov/documents/pfu/pfu.jsp

APPENDIX V

SOME INFORMATION ABOUT APPLYING TO OTHER AGENCIES

AMERICAN ASSOCIATION FOR THE ADVANCEMENT OF SCIENCE (AAAS) CONGRESSIONAL FELLOWSHIPS PROGRAM

Congressional Fellows spend one year working as special legislative assistants on the staffs of members of Congress or congressional committees. The program includes an orientation on congressional and executive branch operations, and a year-long seminar program on issues involving science, technology, and public policy. The program provides a unique public policy learning experience, and demonstrates the value of science-government interaction and bringing technical backgrounds and external perspectives to the decision-making process in the Congress.

Prospective Fellows must

- demonstrate exceptional competence in some area of science or engineering
- have a good scientific and technical background
- be cognizant of and demonstrate sensitivity toward political and social issues
- have a strong interest—and some experience—in applying personal knowledge toward the solution of societal problems

AAAS invites Applications from individuals in any

- physical science
- biological science
- social science
- field of engineering
- relevant interdisciplinary field

Applicants must

- be a U.S. citizen
- have

  (1) a Ph.D. or an equivalent doctoral-level degree

  or

  (2) a master's degree in engineering and at least 3 years of post-degree professional experience

- **not** be Federal employees

AAAS will sponsor two Congressional Fellows for 2004–05. The fellowship stipend is $60,000 with allowances for health insurance and relocation.

Approximately 30 other national science and engineering societies sponsor Congressional Fellows. Applicants for these fellowships should apply directly to the appropriate professional society. Stipends, Application procedures, degree requirements, timetables, and deadlines vary. Fellows selected by these societies also will participate in the year-long program of activities administered by AAAS.

For information, contact:
Ms. Claudia J. Sturges, Director
AAAS Science and Technology Policy Fellowship Programs
Directorate for Science and Policy Programs
AAAS
1200 New York Ave. NW
Washington, DC 20005
Tel: 202-326-6700

Fax: 202-289-4950
E-mail: fellowships@aaas.org

http://www.fellowships.aaas.org/congressional/

AAAS also has other science and technology policy fellowship programs. If you are interested in the interaction of science, technology, and government in the United States and around the world, and would be willing to work in Washington, DC, to learn firsthand how the federal government operates and to help make decisions that result in national public policy, check out these programs at

http://www.fellowships.aaas.org/

NATIONAL TECHNICAL TRANSFER CENTER (NTTC)

A congressionally funded information center with the mission to put people in contact with researchers in a federal laboratory or facility. Most of the services are free.

In 2003, NTTC had over 700 laboratories/facilities in their database. There are also 6 regional Technical Transfer Centers in the United States. The regional centers deal with research in the private sector as well as with government laboratories and facilities.

For further information, contact:
National Technical Transfer Center (NTTC)
Wheeling Jesuit College
Wheeling, WV 26003
Tel: 1-800-678-6882
Fax: 304-243-2539

UNITED STATES ARMY RESEARCH OFFICE: LIFE SCIENCES RESEARCH PROGRAM

The core program **supports basic research** in the biological and neurosciences, exclusive of medical and social science research. Average core grant size is $100,000/year for 3 years. The program funds about 12 new core grants per year, with continuing support for about 24 grants. Funding is also available for minority institutions, small businesses, equipment, and others (see Web site).

For information, contact:
Dr. Elmar Schmeisser
Acting Associate Director
Life Sciences Division
Army Research Office (ARO)
P.O. Box 12211
Research Triangle Park, NC 27709-2211
Tel: 919-549-4318
E-mail: elmar.schmeisser@us.army.mil

http://www.aro.army.mil

STRATEGIC ENVIRONMENTAL RESEARCH AND DEVELOPMENT PROGRAM (SERDP)

SERDP funds environmental research and development via a competitive process. Both government and private sector parties may compete for SERDP funds. There are 2 announcements for each solicitation:

- a Broad Agency Announcement (BAA) for the private sector
- a Call For Proposals to the Federal sector

There are usually 2 solicitations annually.

The Core solicitation (usually released in mid-November) provides funding in various amounts for multi-year projects. **Pre-proposals** from the non-Federal sector are due in early January; Federal proposals are due in early March. Levels of possible support, detailed instructions for both Federal and non-Federal proposers, and additional information are available via links at

http://www.serdp.org/funding/funding.html

Foundations are private organizations that give grants to individuals and organizations for a broad range of projects. Some Foundations have very specific mandates; others have broader missions. For example, many family foundations are dedicated to specific fields or causes; others, such as corporate foundations, are a philanthropic arm of a parent corporation and provide money for a variety of causes.

The *Guide to U.S. Foundations for 2002* lists over 64,000 private foundations in the United States that provided grants totaling more than $30.5 million.

The *Foundation Directory* (2003 edition) divides foundations into 4 general types:

- Independent
- Company-Sponsored
- Operating
- Community

Independent Foundation: A fund or endowment designated by the Internal Revenue Service as a private foundation under the law, the primary function of which is the making of grants. The assets of most independent foundations are derived from the gift of an individual or family. Some function under the direction of family members and are known as "family foundations." Depending on their range of giving, independent foundations may also be known as "general purpose" or "special purpose" foundations.

Company-Sponsored Foundation: A private foundation under the tax law deriving its funds from a profit-making company or corporation but independently constituted, the purpose of which is to make grants, usually on a broad basis although not without regard for the business interests of the corporation. Company-sponsored foundations are legally distinct from contributions programs administered within the corporation directly from corporate funds. Direct corporate giving programs are not listed in *The Foundation Directory*, The Foundation Center's *National Directory of Corporate Giving*, Eighth Edition, published in 2002, includes complete corporate giving profiles on nearly 3,000 companies.

Operating Foundation: A fund or endowment designated under the tax law by the Internal Revenue Service as a private operating foundation, the primary purpose of which is to operate research, social welfare, or other programs determined by its governing body or charter. Most operating foundations award few or no grants to outside organizations, and therefore do not appear in *The Foundation Directory*.

Community Foundation: In its general charitable purposes, community foundation is much like a private foundation; its funds, however, are derived from many donors rather than a single source, as is usually the case with private foundations. Further, community foundations are usually classified under the tax law as public charities and are therefore subject to different rules and regulations.

The above information is summarized in Table V–1. The table is taken from Figure A (page viii) in *The Foundation Directory* (2004 edition).

SOME ADVICE FOR APPLYING FOR FOUNDATION GRANTS

It is useful to think of granting agencies as specialized venture capital companies. Although a venture capital company is generally looking for investments that are likely to bring large financial returns, such companies will "gamble" money on you only if the staff members think that you and your team have the background—and exhibit the capabilities—to accomplish what you set out to do.

Likewise, a granting agency will fund your project only if its staff members foresee that you will further the agency's cause—that is, in some substantive way help the agency meet its goal. Thus, you—the Applicant—must aim to **"sell" your idea** to the potential funding agency by convincing its staff members that your project will succeed and will fulfill the agency's mandate.

Foundations differ widely in "personality" and "style." Thus, in terms of the particulars, there are probably as many Application and Review procedures for private foundations as the number of such foundations that provide funding. However, the basic information that agencies need from Applicants is not so different for the different foundations, or from the large government agencies.

Almost every granting agency will want

- a description of your project (Long-Term Objectives and Specific Aims)
- information about what has already been done in the field (Background)
- to know what has already been done in the field by you (Preliminary Studies/Progress report)
- information about how you will do the project (Project Design and Methods)
- information about you (Biographical Sketch) and your Track Record
- information about your team, and what resources or help you have at your disposal (Resources and Environment)
- to know how much money you need (Budget) and why (Budget Justification)
- to know what other agencies have been interested in supporting you and/or your project (Other Support)

If you know how to write a good NIH Application and understand the correct way to approach, interpret, and meticulously respond to instructions, you should be able to write a good Application to any agency.

A few private foundations have "free-form" Applications, that is, Applications with no specified format. For such proposals it is useful to ask a relevant staff member at the organization what information is required. Also ask to see past successful proposals. If you

Table APPX V-1: Types of Foundations

Foundation Type	Description	Source of Funds	Decision-Making Activity	Grantmaking Requirements	Reporting
Independent Foundation	An independent grantmaking organization established to aid social, educational, religious, or other charitable activities.	Endowment generally derived from a single source such as an individual, a family, or a group of individuals. Contributions to endowment limited as to tax deductibility.	Decisions may be made by donor or members of the donor's family; by an independent board of directors or trustees; or by a bank or trust officer acting on the donor's behalf.	Broad discretionary giving allowed but may have specific guidelines and give only in a few specific fields. About 70% limit their giving to local area.	Annual information returns (990-PF) filed with IRS must be made available to public. A small percentage issue separately printed annual reports.
Company-Sponsored Foundation	Legally an independent grantmaking organization with close ties to the corporation providing funds.	Endowment and annual contributions from a profit-making corporation. May maintain small endowment and pay out most of contributions received annually in grants, or may maintain endowment to cover contributions in years when corporate profits are down.	Decisions made by board of directors often composed of corporate officials, but which may include individuals with no corporate affiliation. Decisions may also be made by local company officials.	Giving tends to be in fields related to corporate activities or in communities where corporation operates. Usually give more grants but in smaller dollar amounts than independent foundations.	Same as above.
Operating Foundation	An organization that uses its resources to conduct research or provide a direct service.	Endowment usually provided from a single source, but eligible for maximum deductible contributions from public.	Decisions generally made by independent board of directors.	Makes few, if any grants. Grants generally related directly to the foundation's program.	Same as above.
Community Foundation	A publicly sponsored organization that makes grants for social, educational, religious, or other charitable purposes in a specific community or region.	Contributions received from many donors. Usually eligible for maximum tax deductible contributions from public.	Decisions made by board of directors representing the diversity of the community.	Grants generally limited to charitable organizations in local community.	IRS 990 reutrn available to public. Many publish full guidelines or annual reports.

cannot get any guidance, simulate an NIH Application or follow the advice in some of the resources listed in the "Resources" Appendix posted online to accompany this book.

As is the case with Federal funding, the most important factor—and an absolutely essential component in seeking Foundation support—is **a good idea.** Ideally, the idea should be **unique—but not so "way out" that it is beyond the comprehension of the Reviewer(s).** The latter criterion is especially important with Foundation proposals. Although some of these organizations have review boards that include technical experts in your subject matter, others may use only a few Reviewers—or even only one Reviewer (sometimes an agency staff member) who may have an overall grasp of the subject but may not have an in-depth understanding of your project and field of research.

As is also the case with the NIH funding components, another important factor for success in getting funded is a **good match between your research idea and the mission or mandate of the funding agency.** Like other Grant Applications, those to Foundations take a lot of thought, planning, and hard work. Therefore, it pays to call a potential funding agency—before you begin writing a proposal—to find out whether the agency is really interested in your project and whether it provides funds sufficient to make it worthwhile for you to apply. Because subtle preferences in funding are often omitted from printed materials that an organization may provide, it is important to speak to the person in charge of the particular funding (giving) program, and try to **get accurate, detailed information about the organization's mandate and Application and Review procedures.**

Do your homework

Submitting an Application without previously contacting the Program Officer and discussing your project can lead to an enormous waste of your time. Finding the right foundation—one that is likely to be interested in your project—requires that you do some homework. Become acquainted with the various Foundation Center publications and Foundation indices and directories. Some of these listings are now available on computer databases, making it easier to search for those that may be a good match for your project.

Once you have determined which Foundations may be of interest to you—and interested in your work

- send for their annual reports
- ask to see a list of grants they have funded in recent years
- look at a roster of the agency board members and their professional backgrounds (the board members sometimes make the final funding decisions!)
- find out
  —who is the director of the grants program
  —how much funding is available for the period for which you are applying
  —what the Application process involves
  —what the eligibility requirements are
  —when Applications are due
  —how long the review process takes

Your institutional Office for Sponsored Research (OSR) may be able to help you.

For example, the Harvard University OSR

- maintains a library of literature about federal and private sponsorship of research
- subscribes to SPIN (Sponsored Programs Information Network, a computer database that provides information about Federal and non-Federal sponsors/ Funding Agencies)

- publishes a periodic newsletter that lists information about current funding opportunities, many of them excerpted from the Federal Register, Commerce Business Daily, etc. Listings are not limited to the sciences; they also cover arts and humanities.

Your institutional development office may also have information about Foundations. It is also important to **check with your OSR to determine whether it is cultivating a relationship with a foundation,** thereby—possibly—making it "off limits" to individual grant seekers from the same institution!

If you meet the two requirements outlined above—a good idea and a good match—submission of a well-thought-out, focused, clearly presented proposal that is meticulously responsive to the instructions provided by the agency should make you highly competitive for available funding.

If at all possible, it is useful to find and **study a successful proposal** to the foundation in question before you plan your own proposal.

Some Foundations require a **pre-proposal** or **letter of inquiry** prior to submission of a full-length proposal. In some cases the pre-proposals are reviewed and only a percentage of the Applicants are invited to submit a full proposal. Some Foundations have fairly lengthy and precise instructions for what they require in the pre-proposal or letter of inquiry. However, some Foundations provide no written instructions for proposal preparation. When this is the case, it is generally safe to provide the information required in an NIH or other major agency Application kit.

A number of agencies, once they determine that your project is of interest to them, will work with you to develop the written proposal. In any event, when instructions are provided, one of the **clues to success** is to

- read the instructions word for word
- make an extremely detailed outline of what the agency wants:
  —in what form
  —in what order
  —with what page limits

In my experience, people who simply read through the instructions and then write from the major headings in the instructions often overlook things and fail to provide some of the major items on which their proposals will be judged. That instructions sometimes have major topics buried in subtle places in the text may seem unlikely until you consider that the individuals who write the instructions are often not schooled in the art of writing instructions. Thus, the responsibility falls to the Applicant to decipher, understand, and respond to what the Reviewers need and want to know.

You should also be aware that, in contrast to public institutions, which readily disclose their Application Review Procedures, private Foundations are sometimes quite discreet about disclosing information about their review procedures. If you are unable to determine the level of professional sophistication of the potential Reviewer(s), it is best to assume that you are writing your proposal for an **intelligent and educated non-expert** who is familiar with the generalities of the programs funded by the agency but not conversant with the subtle intricacies of the field. You should be on target for the majority of foundation Reviewers if you

- write **clearly**
- submit a **complete** proposal
- include a **clear, succinct Abstract** that **parallels** the content of the proposal

- avoid professional jargon
- are careful to avoid a condescending tone

Letters of inquiry and pre-proposals

Some funding agencies require you to submit a letter of inquiry before they will send you the instructions for submission of a full proposal. Some of these agencies have very specific instructions about what is to be included in the letter of inquiry; if so, follow the instructions. If there are no specific instructions, consider the advice below.

- Write the letter from the point of view of the opportunity the agency has in supporting your project, not how their funding will fill your needs.

- Unless there are specific instructions that require you to write a longer letter, you should aim to summarize the essentials of your project in one page.

- Address the letter to the person responsible for funding.

- Address the mandate of the agency.

- Explain clearly and succinctly what you propose to do and what you hope to accomplish (or enclose a separate summary of the project).

- Discuss the suitability of your project for the agency's mandate.

- Discuss the amount of funding required.

- Include an up-to-date Resume.

- If appropriate, ask for an appointment with the relevant official.

  Subtle funding preferences of an agency, not made explicit in their brochures, can sometimes be clarified during verbal exchanges.

- Be persuasive but not overbearing.

Some agencies require a more formal pre-proposal. These pre-proposals are evaluated, and only a small number of the proposers may be invited to submit a full proposal. Making this "first cut" does not ensure success in getting funded in response to submission of the full proposal.

The review process at private foundations

- Specifics vary; the process may be more informal than at government agencies in some ways, but some aspects are very formalized.

- The review process is often not as codified as at government agencies and information about review procedures may not be readily available.

- The review committee is often ad hoc, and size varies from a single staff member to a group as large as an NIH Study Section. The review committee may become the advisory committee for the project.

- The Foundation may use outside consultants or Reviewers—often by mail.

- The Foundation may make a site visit.

- At some Foundations, Applicants may be asked to come to the Foundation to present their project.

- Because there may be considerable interaction between the Foundation staff and the grantee in the course of proposal preparation, the review process may be based much more on the project than on the written proposal.

- There may or may not be a rating of the project or proposal.
- If the review committee is composed largely of outside Reviewers, there may be a second level of review by an in-house staff committee.
- The Foundation board of directors (which may be composed entirely of business-people who may not be specialists in your field of interest) usually votes on the final recommendation of the review committee.

Some review criteria at private foundations

- Is there a good match between the proposed project and the mandate (mission) of the funding agency?
- Does the Applicant meet the guidelines and qualifications of the funding agency:
  —geography
  —tax status
  —etc.
- Has the Applicant conformed to all proposal submission guidelines of the funding agency:
  —submission deadline
  —page limits
  —appropriate print size
  —complete Application with all parts correctly filled out
  —appropriate appendices provided
  —assurances/certifications filed and attested to
  —neat presentation
- Is the project idea innovative and of high quality?
- Does the Applicant demonstrate insight into the problem?
- Does the Applicant present clear direction for solving the problem?
- Is there evidence of commitment to the project by the PI and the PI's institution as evidenced by:
  —track record
  —financial support (e.g., matching funds)
  —space and personnel commitment
- Is there evidence that the project will continue after funds provided by the funding agency in question run out?
- Is the project concept exportable?
  That is, is there a likelihood that the project results will be adaptable to other institutions and/or situations?
- Is the material presented accurate?
- Is there a discussion of **alternative approaches** for the project?
- Is there a reasonable approach to data analysis?
- Is the project presented clearly?
- Does the Applicant demonstrate attention to required details?
- Are there well-thought-out plans for periodic, ongoing evaluations of the project?
- Are there well-thought-out plans for dissemination of project results?

- Is the tone of the proposal positive and confident?
  - —Does it de-emphasize the PI's need and emphasize the PI's abilities and accomplishments?
  - —Is it enthusiastic but not arrogant?
  - —Is it optimistic but not unrealistic?

For more information about writing proposals to private Foundations, refer to references provided in the "Resources Appendix" such as

- *Tips for Applying to Private Foundations for Grant Money,* by Reif-Lehrer
- *Program Planning and Proposal Writing,* by Kiritz

INDEX

page numbers followed by t denote tables